美国针灸立法汇编

美国中西部地区针灸立法汇编

Collection of Acupuncture Laws in the Midwestern United States of America

（汉英对照）

总顾问

刘保延　沈远东

主　编

桑　珍　杨宇洋　宋欣阳　张博源

上海科学技术出版社

内 容 提 要

针灸于 19 世纪上半叶传入美国，在 20 世纪 70 年代"针灸热"的影响之下，开始在美国流行。针灸在美国流行的五十年间，经历了三次热潮，完成了法律本土化、教育本土化、职业本土化和医学属性本土化四个层次的本土化，广泛应用于变态反应性疾病、糖尿病、艾滋病、各种肿瘤、高血压、肥胖症、戒毒、戒酒、戒烟、化疗或手术后发生的恶心和呕吐等领域。美国 47 个州及华盛顿特区都在州议会法中专章规定了针灸师执业法律制度，广泛涉及针灸与东方医学的概念、针灸师的准入条件、教育培训、执业规范、行业组织管理和惩戒规则等内容。

本书为美国中西部十一州针灸立法汇编，包括艾奥瓦州、北达科他州、俄亥俄州、堪萨斯州、密苏里州、密歇根州、明尼苏达州、内布拉斯加州、威斯康星州、伊利诺伊州、印第安纳州十一州，从针灸人员的法律地位、准入与注册、日常管理机构、职业道德、惩戒报告等方面展开介绍。希望本书的出版能为中医药政策和法律的制定者、中医药政策和法制研究者以及高等院校、科研机构中医药学科的研习者们提供参考和借鉴。

图书在版编目（CIP）数据

美国中西部地区针灸立法汇编 = Collection of Acupuncture Laws in the Midwestern United States of America : 汉英对照 / 桑珍等主编. -- 上海 : 上海科学技术出版社，2025.2
（美国针灸立法汇编）
ISBN 978-7-5478-6563-7

Ⅰ．①美… Ⅱ．①桑… Ⅲ．①针灸学－立法－汇编－美国－汉、英 Ⅳ．①D937.122.16

中国国家版本馆CIP数据核字(2024)第051513号

美国中西部地区针灸立法汇编：Collection of Acupuncture Laws in the Midwestern United States of America（汉英对照）

总顾问 刘保延 沈远东

主 编 桑 珍 杨宇洋 宋欣阳 张博源

上海世纪出版(集团)有限公司
上海科学技术出版社 出版、发行
（上海市闵行区号景路 159 弄 A 座 9F-10F）
邮政编码 201101 www.sstp.cn
上海颛辉印刷厂有限公司印刷
开本 787×1092 1/16 印张 20.5
字数 400 千字
2025 年 2 月第 1 版 2025 年 2 月第 1 次印刷
ISBN 978-7-5478-6563-7/R·2976
定价：188.00 元

编委会名单

丛 书 前 言

　　针灸是我国历代劳动人民及医学家在长期与疾病作斗争中创造和发展起来的一种医学,具有悠久的历史。它是以中医理论为指导,运用针刺和艾灸防治疾病的一门临床学科。针灸具有适应证广、疗效明显、操作方便、经济安全等优点,数千年来深受广大劳动人民的欢迎,对中华民族的繁衍昌盛作出了巨大的贡献。

　　几千年来,针灸不仅对我国人民的保健事业作出重大贡献,而且很早就流传到国外,成为世界医学的重要组成部分,并产生积极而深远的影响。根据世界卫生组织统计,目前有113 个成员国认可使用针灸,其中 29 个成员国设立了相关法律法规,20 个成员国将针灸纳入医疗保险体系。针灸的神奇疗效引发全球持续的“针灸热”。针灸推拿等治疗手段成为奥运会运动员们缓解伤痛的新时尚。我国援外医疗队采用针灸、推拿、中药以及中西医结合方法治疗了不少疑难重症,挽救了许多垂危病人的生命,得到受援国政府和人民的充分肯定。不少国家先后对针灸进行了立法,成立了针灸学术团体、针灸教育机构和研究机构。

　　从 20 世纪 70 年代开始,世界卫生组织就积极地向全世界推广针灸,在多国设立针灸培训机构,支持创建世界针灸学会联合会,发布了针灸治疗的适宜病症、针灸经穴定位、从业人员培训指南等一系列国际标准,努力推进针灸的国际化与标准化进程。伴随着针灸的全球化应用,针灸针的国际贸易也逐年增长。2011 年 5 月,国际标准化组织/中医药技术委员会(ISO/TC 249)在第二次荷兰海牙年会上,决议成立专门的工作组承担针灸针的国际标准研制工作,由中国专家担任召集人的职位。《ISO 17218:2014 一次性使用无菌针灸针》于 2014年 2 月 3 日正式出版,成为首个在传统医药领域内由中国主导发布的 ISO 国际标准。截至目前,ISO/TC 249 已发布了 7 项针灸针的国际标准,为针灸的国际化推广应用作出了积极的贡献。

　　针灸于 19 世纪上半叶传入美国,在 20 世纪 70 年代“针灸热”的影响之下,开始在美国流行。针灸在美国流行的五十年间,经历了三次热潮,完成了法律本土化、教育本土化、职业本土化和医学属性本土化四个层次的本土化。起初,针灸在美国主要用于治疗疼痛症状,后来也广泛应用于变态反应性疾病、糖尿病、艾滋病、各种肿瘤、高血压、肥胖症、戒毒、戒酒、戒烟、化疗或手术后发生的恶心和呕吐、不孕症、性功能不全、神经衰弱、紧张综合征、网球肘、肌纤维组织炎、中风后遗症、骨性关节炎、美容、体外受精、血液病、哮喘等领域。针灸在美国的发展并没有昙花一现，而是入乡随俗，遍地开花。美国的医疗改革给低成本针灸提供了全新的发展契机。中医针灸疗法针对很多病症可以采取非手术的保守疗法，成本低廉，疗效显著。迄今为止，美国 50 个州除了南达科他州、亚拉巴马州、俄克拉何马州 3 个州没有专门的针灸立法之外，其余 47 个州及华盛顿特区都在州议会法中专章规定了针灸师执业法律制度，广泛涉及针灸与东方医学的概念、针灸师的准入条件、教育培训、执业规范、行业组织管理和惩戒规则等内容。

"美国针灸立法汇编"丛书编委会经过两年多的信息搜集，资料整理分析，将美国 47 个州针灸法律英文文本进行了收集、翻译、校对和法律评析，重点展示美国各州现行针灸法律制度的全貌。本丛书共 5 册，按照新英格兰地区、中西部地区、西部地区、南部地区、西南部地区划分。每一区域立法均从针灸人员的法律地位、准入与注册、日常管理机构、职业道德、惩戒报告等方面展开介绍。希望本丛书的出版能为中医药政策和法律的制定者、中医药政策和法制研究者以及高等院校、科研机构中医药学科的研习者们提供参考和借鉴。由于时间仓促、经验不足，可能存在不严谨之处，望广大读者朋友不吝指正。

编　者
2023 年 3 月

目　录

艾奥瓦州^①

艾奥瓦州针灸法

第 148E.1 条　定义

除文义另有所指外,下列定义适用于本章:

1. "针灸"系指从东方传统和现代医学观念中发展而来的一种保健形式,采用东方医学诊断、治疗及辅助疗法和诊断技术,旨在促进、维持、恢复健康和预防疾病。

2. "针灸师"系指从事针灸实践的人士。

3. "委员会"系指第 147 章中设立的医学委员会。

4. "针灸实践"系是指基于东方医学诊断的基础上,在人体的特定部位实施针刺和灸法为主的治疗方式。在针灸范围内的辅助治疗可能包括手动、机械、热、电、电磁治疗,以及基于传统东方医学概念推荐膳食指南和治疗运动。

第 148E.2 条　执业执照的获取——续期

1. 为了获得针灸执照,申请人应当向委员会提交以下所有证据:

a. 获得国家针灸师认证委员会颁发的有效证书。

b. 顺利完成三年高等教育培训课程或针灸学院课程,且课程经针灸及东方医学教育审核委员会的认证,或有资格得到认证,或达到了该委员会的相关标准。

c. 顺利完成国家针灸与东方医学认证委员会批准的洁针技术课程。

2. 尽管第 148E.1 条另有规定,在 2001 年 7 月 1 日当日或之前,如果该州居民顺利完成医学委员会批准的针灸学位课程,或者医学委员会批准的学徒或者指导计划,则医学委员会须向其颁发针灸师执照。

3. 根据本条所授予的执照须每两年续期一次。执照续期需要提供国家针灸师认证委员会的有效证明。

第 148E.3 条　本章范围

本章不适用于下列事项:

---

① 根据《艾奥瓦州法典》注释版第 4 卷第 3 编第 148E 章 "针灸" 译出。

1. 获得内科和外科、骨科医学和外科、脊椎治疗、足科或者牙科的执照，并且专职从事该专业活动的人。

2. 学生在执业针灸师的直接监督下从事针灸实践，作为委员会批准的学习课程的一部分。

第 148E.4 条　护理标准

根据本章获得执照的人应当遵守与获得从事内科和外科或者骨科医学和外科执照的人相同的护理标准。

第 148E.5 条　使用和处理针灸针

针灸师必须只使用预先消毒的一次性针灸针，并适当处理用过的针灸针。

第 148E.6 条　向患者出示证书和披露信息

针灸师应当在营业场所的显著位置出示根据第 148E.2 条颁发的执照。针灸师应当以书面形式向每一位初次接触的患者提供以下信息：

1. 针灸师的姓名、营业地址、工作电话。

2. 价目表。

3. 一份说明针灸师的教育、经验、学位、证书的清单，或者由专业针灸组织授予的针灸相关资格证明，获得学位或者资格证明所需的时间和经验。

4. 一份说明曾经被各个地方、州或者国家医疗卫生机构撤销医疗行业执照、证书或者注册情况的声明。

5. 一份针灸师遵守委员会通过的法规和规定的陈述，包括针灸师只使用预先消毒的一次性针灸针的声明。

6. 一份说明针灸实践受委员会管理的声明。

7. 一份说明针灸师执照并非授权某人在本州行医和实施手术，针灸师的服务不允许被视为行医执照者的诊断和治疗，也不允许被视为医疗意见或建议的声明。

第 148E.7 条　委员会职责

委员会应当采用履行其职责所必需的，与本章和第 147 章一致的法律规则。

第 148E.8 条　执照的撤销或吊销

除了第 147.55 条所述的撤销或吊销的理由外，当针灸师存在下列过错或者违法行为时，针灸执照将被撤销或吊销：

1. 未能按照第 148E.6 条的要求提供信息，或向患者提供虚假信息。

2. 将患者转诊给其他卫生保健专业人员并获取报酬。

3. 为转诊患者提供或给予报酬，不包括付费广告或营销服务。

4. 未能遵守本章、根据本章通过的规则或者第 147 章规定的规则。

5. 在执业范围内与患者进行或声称与患者发生性行为或生殖器接触的，无论患者是否同意发生性行为或生殖器接触。

6. 泄露患者的隐私信息。

第 148E.9 条　事故和健康保险的范围

本章不应解释为，需要根据本州已签发的或签发待交付的现有或者未来的合同或保险单,对针灸服务提供事故和健康保险,除合同或保单另有规定外。

第 148E.10 条　根据 2000 年法令(78 G.A.) 废除。

艾奥瓦州针灸行政法①

第 653‑17.1(148E) 条　目的

针灸执照的设立是为了确保从业者有资格为爱荷华居民提供安全和健康的治疗。《艾奥瓦州法典》第 147、148E 和 272C 章授权医学委员会制定执照考试要求;评估执照申请人的资格证明(147.2,148E.3) ;向合格的申请人授予执照(148E.2) ;制定继续教育要求(272C.2) ;调查指控执业针灸师违反针灸服务法规和规章的控诉和报告(147.55,148E.6) ;参与艾奥瓦州医生健康计划(272C.3) ;对违反州法律和委员会规则(147.55,148E.6) 的执业针灸师进行惩罚。

第 653‑17.2(148E) 条　章节范围

本章中的规则仅适用于根据《艾奥瓦州法典》第 148E 章获得执照的个人。根据《艾奥瓦州法典》第 148E.3 条,本章中的规则不适用于以下情况:

1. 由本州授予从事内外科、骨内外科、脊椎按摩、足科或者牙科的人,专门从事其专业领域的实践。

2. 学生在执业针灸师的直接监督下从事针灸实践,作为委员会批准的学习课程的一部分。

第 653‑17.3(148E) 条　定义

"针灸及东方医学教育审核委员会"或"ACAOM"系指美国的审核委员会,负责对针灸和东方医学培训计划和学院进行认证。ACAOM 监督美国所有专业的东方医学和针灸学位课程。ACAOM 前身为全国针灸和东方医学院校认证委员会。

"针灸"系指从传统和现代东方医学理念发展而来的一种卫生保健形式,它采用东方医学诊断和治疗,以及辅助疗法和诊断技术,以促进、维持和恢复健康,预防疾病。

"针灸针"系指一种实心器械,包括但不限于针灸针、皮针、皮内针、针灸钉、梅花针、三棱针、一次性采血针等。

"穴位"系指人体特定的解剖部位,作为针灸的治疗部位。

"申请人"系指根据《艾奥瓦州法典》第 148E.3 条未获授权从事针灸的人,向委员会申请执照。

"阿是穴"系指触诊时按压痛定位的穴位。阿是穴也被称为激痛点。

"委员会"系指在《艾奥瓦州法典》第 147 章中设立的医学委员会。

"执照委员会"系指医学委员会下设的执照委员会,负责监督针灸师执照的管理。

"部"系指艾奥瓦州公共卫生部。

---

① 　根据《艾奥瓦州行政法典》"行政机构"653 卷第 17 章"针灸师执照"译出。

"披露表"系指执业针灸师在初次接触时必须向患者提供的书面信息。

"一次性针灸针"系指根据《艾奥瓦州法典》第148E.5条在初次使用后丢弃的预消毒针灸针。

"执照"系指委员会根据《艾奥瓦州法典》第148E.2条颁发的执照。

"持证人"系指持有委员会根据《艾奥瓦州法典》第148E章颁发的针灸执照的人。

"国家针灸与东方医学认证委员会"或者"NCCAOM"系指通过专业认证来验证针灸和东方医学实践的入门级能力的美国委员会。

"针灸实践"系指在东方医学诊断基础上,在人体特定部位实施针刺或灸法为主的治疗方式。在针灸范围内的辅助治疗可能包括手法治疗、机械治疗、温针治疗、电针治疗、电磁治疗,以及基于传统东方医学概念推荐膳食指南和治疗性运动。

"服务费"系指委员会为在线提供服务而收取的费用,是对服务本身实际费用的补充。例如,在线续期执照的人将支付执照续期费和服务费。

第653-17.4(147,148E)条　获取执照的资格

17.4(1)资格条件。获得委员会颁发的针灸执照的人员,必须符合以下所有要求:

a. 满足第17.5条(147、148E)中指定的所有申请要求。

b. 持有现行有效的NCCAOM认证的文凭;或者在2004年6月1日之后,持有现行有效的NCCAOM针灸或者东方医学文凭。

c. 证明有足够的英语知识,以理解以及被患者、委员会和执照委员会成员理解。

(1)通过NCCAOM英语笔试和实践考试的申请人,可以视为具备足够的英语水平。

(2)通过NCCAOM除英语以外其他语言的笔试或者实践考试的申请人,应当通过由教育考试服务处管理的英语口语测试(TSE)或者托福考试(TOEFL)。TSE的及格分数至少为五十分。托福的及格分数系指在周五或者周六(以前称为特殊或者国际管理)进行的纸质托福考试中总分不低于五百五十分,在计算机管理的托福考试中最低总分不低于二百一十三分,或在互联网的托福考试中总分不低于七十九分。

d. 顺利完成经针灸及东方医学教育审核委员会认证或认证候选资格或符合标准的三年高等教育培训课程或者针灸学院课程。

e. 顺利完成NCCAOM批准的洁针技术课程。

f. 根据第653-9.3(3)款,申请人执照不会因为被取消资格行为而被委员会拒绝。

17.4(2)禁止豁免或变更。本章的规则不得根据第653卷第3章或任何其他法律规定予以豁免或变更。

第653-17.5(147,148E)条　申请要求

17.5(1)执照申请。要申请针灸执照,申请人应当:

a. 提交由委员会提供的完整的申请表格,包括所需的证书和文件、完整的指纹资料袋及证明申请人提供的所有资料真实性的宣誓声明。

b. 支付第653-8.2(2)款"a"项中规定的不可退还的初始申请费。

c. 支付第653-8.2(2)款"e"项中规定的用于由艾奥瓦州刑事调查局(DCI)和联邦调查局(FBI)进行的指纹资料评估和国家犯罪历史背景调查的费用。

17.5（2）申请表的内容。每位申请人应当在委员会提供的申请表上提交以下信息：

a. 申请人的法定全名、出生日期和地点、家庭地址、通信地址、主要营业地址，以及申请人或持证人经常用于与委员会通信的个人电子邮件。

b. 适用于身份鉴别的申请人照片。

c. 从申请人进入针灸和东方医学培训计划或者学院之日起至申请之日的所有时间段的年表。

d. 申请人在美国或者其他国家或准州的司法管辖区被授权从事针灸实践的证明，包括执照，注册证书或者证书编号以及颁发日期。

e. 充分披露申请人在美国、其他国家或者准州的司法管辖区参加与针灸实践相关的民事诉讼的情况。在审查过程中，如有需要，可以要求提供法律文件的副本。

f. 声明中披露和解释任何司法管辖区的医疗、针灸或者专业监管机构、教育机构、培训或研究项目或卫生机构中通过自愿协议或者正式行动的形式采取的任何非正式或非公开行动、发出的警告、开展的调查或者采取的纪律处分。

g. 声明中披露和解释在任何司法管辖区内提出的涉及申请人的轻罪或重罪的任何指控，无论为撤销定罪或抗辩是否存在未决的任何上诉或其他程序。

h. 由 NCCAOM 直接提交委员会的 NCCAOM 成绩报告核实表。

i. NCCAOM 证书，证明申请人目前持有有效的 NCCAOM 针灸或东方医学文凭。

j. 完成 NCCAOM 批准的洁针技术课程的证明。

k. 证明申请人身体和精神健康状况的充分披露和书面解释，包括可能影响申请人从事针灸服务和为患者提供安全健康治疗能力的功能障碍或损伤。

l. 申请人的临床针灸培训、工作经验及证明文件（如适用）的说明。

m. 由教育机构颁发的申请人针灸学位复印件。如果由于特殊情况无法提供针灸学位复印件，委员会可以接受其他可靠证据，证明申请人从特定教育机构获得了针灸学位。

n. 非英文文凭的完整翻译。一份由教育机构直接出具的官方英文成绩单，证明从针灸培训计划或者教育机构毕业是一个适当的替代方案。

o. 一份教育机构负责人的宣誓声明，证明申请人获得针灸学位的日期，并承认机构记录中存在关于申请人的贬损评论（如果有）。因特殊情况无法提供教育机构负责人宣誓声明的，委员会可以接受申请人获得特定教育机构针灸学位的其他可靠证据。

p. 一份申请人参加的针灸培训计划或者教育机构直接发送的正式成绩单，如果委员会要求，还需提供正式成绩单的英文译本。

q. 一份申请人英语语言能力的证明（当申请人未通过英文版的 NCCAOM 笔试和实践考试时）。

r. 如果委员会要求，申请人需要提供一份过去五年医院及临床工作人员经历及其他专业经验的证明。

s. 一份完整的指纹数据包，用于全国犯罪历史背景调查。指纹数据包的评估以及艾奥瓦州刑事调查局（DCI）和联邦调查局（FBI）的犯罪历史背景调查费用将由申请人承担。

17.5（3）披露表。2017 年 2 月 15 日撤销 IAB，2017 年 3 月 22 日生效。

17.5(4)申请周期。如果申请人在委员会首次要求提供更多信息的九十日内未提交所有材料,包括完整的指纹数据包,则该申请将被视为无效。委员会办公室应将申请状态变更通知申请人。

a. 如果要重新激活申请,申请人需要提交第653-8.2(2)款"b"项所述的不可退还的重新激活申请费,并且必须在委员会要求时更新申请材料。自通知申请人其申请未生效之日起,申请人重新申请的期限以三十日为限,除非执照委员会或委员会书面批准申请人延期。

b. 重新激活申请期限到期后,申请人必须重新提出申请,重新缴纳不可退还的初次申请费用,并提交所需的文件和证明材料。

17.5(5)申请人的责任。针灸执照申请人应对以下各项承担全部责任:

a. 支付第17.5(2)条所述监管机构、国家检测或认证机构、卫生机构和教育机构所收取的所有费用。

b. 在申请表上填写准确、最新和真实的信息,包括但不限于第17.5(2)条规定的与先前的专业经验、教育、培训、考试成绩、文凭、执照或注册以及受纪律处分情况有关的信息。

c. 提交非英语文件的英文译本,并附上翻译人员的宣誓书,证明该翻译是非英语原件的真实完整翻译版。且申请人应当承担翻译费用。

17.5(6)执照申请审核流程。下述程序应用于审核各项申请。如果申请人的主要服务对象为得不到充分医疗服务的人群,包括但不限于少数族裔、低收入人群或者居住在农村地区的人群,委员会办公室收到书面申请时,应优先处理其执照申请。

a. 自委员会办公室收到申请表和不可退还的初始申请费之日起,初始执照开放申请。

b. 在审核每项申请后,工作人员应当通知申请人如何解决审核人员发现的问题。工作人员或者委员会如有要求,申请人须提供补充信息。

c. 如果最终审查对申请人的执照资格没有提出问题或疑虑,工作人员可以行政颁发执照。工作人员可以在没有收到FBI关于申请人的报告的情况下颁发执照。

d. 如果最终审查发现问题或疑虑,且无法通过与申请人的持续沟通得到解决,则行政主管、执照主管和法律事务主管应确定此类问题或疑虑是否表明申请人当前的执照资格存在不确定性。

(1)目前没有问题的,由工作人员行政颁发执照。

(2)如有问题,应将申请提交执照委员会。

e. 工作人员应向执照委员会提交审查事项,包括但不限于:申请信息的伪造、犯罪记录、渎职、药物滥用、能力证明、身体或者精神疾病或者违纪历史。

f. 如果执照委员会能够在没有工作人员或者委员会成员异议的情况下消除问题或者疑虑,委员会可以指示工作人员行政颁发执照。

g. 如果执照委员会无法不引起工作人员或者执照委员会成员异议的情况下消除问题或者疑虑,应当建议委员会:

(1)要求调查。

(2)要求申请人出席面试。

(3)如果申请人在过去三年内未在美国任何司法管辖区积极执业,则要求申请人:

1. 顺利完成委员会或执照委员会认定的与安全、健康的针灸实践直接相关的继续教育或者再培训课程。

2. 顺利通过委员会批准的能力评估。

3. 顺利通过委员会批准的考试。

4. 顺利完成委员会批准的再执业计划或者监督计划。

（4）颁发执照。

（5）在某些条款和条件下，或在附加某些限制的情况下颁发执照。

（6）要求申请人撤回执照申请。

（7）拒绝颁发执照。

h. 委员会应当审议执照委员会的申请和建议，并且应当：

（1）要求进行调查。

（2）要求申请人出席面试。

（3）如果申请人在过去三年内未在美国任何司法管辖区积极执业，则要求申请人：

1. 顺利完成委员会或执照委员会认定的与安全、健康的针灸实践直接相关的继续教育或者再培训课程。

2. 顺利通过委员会批准的能力评估。

3. 顺利通过委员会批准的考试。

4. 顺利完成委员会批准的再执业计划或者监督计划。

（4）颁发执照。

（5）在某些条款和条件下，或在附加某些限制的情况下颁发执照。

（6）要求申请人撤回执照申请。

（7）拒绝颁发执照。委员会可以基于构成纪律处分的相关事由拒绝颁发执照。

17.5（7）拒绝颁发执照的理由。委员会根据执照委员会的建议，可以下列任何理由拒绝执照申请：

a. 未能满足《艾奥瓦州法典》第148E.2条或本章委员会规则对执照申请的要求。

b. 根据《艾奥瓦州法典》第147.4条规定，出现第147.55条和第148E.8或第653－17.12条（147,148E,272C）规定的撤销或吊销执照的理由。

17.5（8）初步拒绝通知。在拒绝向申请人颁发执照之前，委员会应当发出初步拒绝通知，该通知应按照申请人提供的地址通过邮件发送给申请人。初步拒绝通知是一份公开记录，应列举拒绝执照申请的事实和法律依据，将上诉程序通知申请人，并注明如不上诉，将最终决定拒绝颁发执照的日期。

17.5（9）上诉程序。收到初步拒绝通知的申请人可以就该通知提出上诉，并要求举行听证会，在初步拒绝通知邮寄之日起三十日内向执行主管提交听证请求。申请人当前地址应在听证请求中提供。该请求在委员会办公室收到之日起应视为已提交。如果收到带有美国邮政（USPS）邮戳的请求，委员会应将邮戳日期视为提交请求的日期。该请求应具体说明事实或法律错误，以及申请人希望进行证据听证，并且可以提供补充书面资料或者文件，以支持执照颁发。

17.5(10)听证会。如果申请人对初步拒绝通知提出上诉并要求举行听证会,听证应针对有争议案件,随后的程序应当根据第653 - 25.30(17A)条进行。

a. 拒绝颁发执照的听证会是向公众开放的有争议案件。

b. 如果专有信息或机密信息被提交为证据,任何一方均可以请求发布保护令。

c. 支持拒绝颁发执照的证据可由总检察长助理提出。

d. 尽管各方当事人均有责任确定所主张的事项,但申请人应对其执照资格承担最终说明责任。

e. 委员会在就拒绝颁发执照举行听证会后,可以批准或者拒绝执照的申请。委员会应说明其做出决定的理由,并可颁发执照、有限制颁发执照或者拒绝颁发执照。最终决定是一项公开记录。

f. 可以根据《艾奥瓦州法典》第17A.19条的规定对委员会拒绝颁发执照或者有限制颁发执照的最终决定进行司法审查,该条款适用于对任何机构在有争议案件中的最终决定进行司法审查。

17.5(11)最终决定。如果申请人未根据第17.5(9)条对初步拒绝通知提出上诉,初步拒绝通知将自动成为最终决定。最终拒绝执照申请是一项公共记录。

17.5(12)上诉失败。如果申请人根据第17.5(9)条对初步拒绝通知提出上诉,但申请人在初步拒绝通知发出之日起一年内未能上诉至最终决定,委员会可驳回上诉。只有在委员会通过普通邮件向申请人最后已知地址发送书面通知后,上诉才能被驳回。通知应当说明,如果申请人在从委员会办公室寄出信函之日起三十日内,未联系委员会安排上诉听证会,则上诉将被驳回,初步拒绝通知将成为最终决定。上诉驳回后,初步拒绝通知成为最终决定。根据本条最终拒绝执照申请是一项公共记录。

17.5(13)禁止豁免。本章的规则,不得因第653卷第3章或者任何其他法律规定予以豁免或者变更。

第653 - 17.6(147,148E)条 向患者展示执照和信息披露

17.6(1)执照展示。执业针灸师必须将委员会颁发的执照陈列在其主要营业场所的显著位置。

17.6(2)信息披露表的发放和保留。根据《艾奥瓦州法典》第148E.6条,获得执照的针灸师应当在与患者初次接触时发放一份信息披露表,并在治疗终止后至少五年内保留一份由患者签名并注明日期的副本。信息披露表应当包括以下内容:

a. 针灸师的姓名、营业地址、工作电话。

b. 价目表。

c. 由专业针灸机构颁发的针灸师的教育、经历、学位、证书或者与针灸相关的资格证明清单,以及获得学位或资格证明和经历所需的时间。

d. 被任何地方、州或国家卫生保健机构撤销的卫生保健职业的任何执照、证书或注册的声明。

e. 针灸师遵守委员会通过的法规和规章的声明,包括针灸师只使用预先消毒的一次性针灸针的声明。

f. 表明针灸实践由委员会监管的声明。

g. 表明针灸执照不授权个人在该州行医和外科手术的声明,针灸师的服务不得被视为有行医执照人员的诊断和治疗,也不得视为医疗意见或者建议。

第653-17.7(147,148E,272C)条 执照每两年续期一次

根据《艾奥瓦州法典》第148E.2条,执照将于偶数年的10月31日到期,并且可按第653-8.2(2)款中"c"项规定的费用续期。续期申请人应当提供NCCAOM证书,证明申请人持有现行有效的NCCAOM针灸或者东方医学文凭。

17.7(1)到期日期。针灸执照将于偶数年10月31日到期。

17.7(2)按比例收费。初始执照续期费用应当根据颁发日期按月按比例计算。

17.7(3)续期要求和超期续期的处罚。每个申请人应当在到期日前至少六十日收到续期通知。申请人有责任在执照到期之前续期执照。申请人未能收到通知并不免除其续期执照的责任。

a. 使用线上续期时,申请人必须在12月31日午夜之前完成线上续期,以确保执照不会失效。执照在1月1日凌晨十二时○一分变更为非执业和无效执照。

b. 工作人员在收到完整的续期申请后,应行政颁发执照,有效期至偶数年的10月31日。如果委员会收到有关续期申请的负面信息,委员会应颁发续期执照,但可以将负面信息提交进一步审议。

c. 每次续期均应在原始执照证书上展示。

d. 如果申请人未能在当前执照到期日前提交续期申请和续期费用,在宽限期内续期执照将被罚款五十美元,宽限期至1月1日,如不续期,执照将变更为非执业状态。

17.7(4)非执业执照。申请人未能在1月1日之前续期,则执照将变更为非执业状态。

a. 一旦执照变更为非执业状态,针灸师不得从事针灸实践。

b. 持有非执业状态的针灸执照,并不妨碍委员会采取《艾奥瓦州法典》第147.55条或者第148E.8条授权的纪律处分。

第653-17.8(147,272C)条 恢复执业执照

17.8(1)恢复要求。因未能续期而导致其执照失效的申请人可申请恢复执照。根据《艾奥瓦州法典》第147.11条,恢复执照的申请人应:

a. 根据委员会提供的表格提交完整的针灸执照恢复申请。申请书应当包括以下信息:

(1)申请人的法定全名、出生日期和地点、家庭地址、邮寄地址、主要营业地址以及申请人经常用于与委员会通信的个人电子邮件地址。

(2)每个授权或曾授权申请人从事针灸实践的司法管辖区,包括执照号码和颁发日期。

(3)充分披露申请人在美国、其他国家或准州的任何司法管辖区参加与针灸实践相关的民事诉讼。审查过程中可能会要求提供法律文件的副本。

(4)一份声明,披露和解释在各个司法管辖区的医疗、针灸或专业监管机构、教育机构、培训或研究计划或是卫生机构中通过自愿协议或者正式行动的形式发出的警告、开展的调查或者采取的纪律处分。

(5)申请人的身体和精神健康状况声明,包括充分披露和书面解释其任何功能障碍或

者损伤,可能影响其针灸实践能力以及为患者提供安全、健康的治疗。

（6）应根据委员会要求,核实申请人过去五年的医院和临床工作人员以及其他专业经历。

（7）从初始执照颁发日期算起所有时间段的年表。

（8）一份声明,披露和解释在任何司法管辖区内提出的涉及申请人的轻罪或重罪的任何指控,无论为撤销定罪或抗辩是否存在未决的任何上诉或其他程序。

b. 提交一份完整的指纹数据包,以便全国犯罪历史背景调查。第 653－8.2（2）款"e"项中规定的指纹数据包的评估以及艾奥瓦州刑事调查局(DCI)和联邦调查局(FBI)的犯罪历史背景调查费用将由申请人承担。

c. 支付四百美元的恢复费以及第 653－8.2（2）款"e"项中规定的费用,用于由艾奥瓦州刑事调查局(DCI)和联邦调查局(FBI)进行的指纹资料评估和国家犯罪历史背景调查。

d. 提供 NCCAOM 证书,证明申请人目前持有 NCCAOM 的针灸或者东方医学文凭的证明。

e. 满足自执照失效以来制定的任何新要求。

17.8（2）恢复限制。根据《艾奥瓦州法典》第 272C.3（2）条"d"项规定,委员会可要求过去三年在美国各个司法管辖区未积极从事针灸实践的申请人满足以下所有要求,任何恢复其非执业执照:

a. 顺利完成委员会或执照委员会认定的与安全、健康的针灸实践直接相关的继续教育或者再培训课程。

b. 通过委员会批准的能力评估。

c. 通过委员会批准的考试。

d. 通过委员会批准的再执业或者监督计划。

第 653－17.9（272C）条　继续教育要求

申请人应证明其目前持有有效的 NCCAOM 文凭。NCCAOM 要求每四年进行六十个学分的专业拓展活动。有效的 NCCAOM 认证满足《艾奥瓦州法典》第 272C.2 条中规定的继续教育要求。

第 653－17.10（147,148E,272C）条　一般规定

17.10（1）诊断和治疗方式。根据本章,持证人使用的诊断和治疗方式可能包括以下一项或者多项针灸服务:

a. 为以下目的而用针灸针刺激或者刺穿皮肤:

（1）在插入或者刺激区域的局部或者远端引起治疗性生理反应。

（2）缓解疼痛或者治疗神经肌肉骨骼系统。

（3）刺激阿是穴,以缓解疼痛和功能障碍。

（4）促进、维持和恢复健康并预防疾病。

（5）以耳针、手针、鼻针、面针、足针或者头针疗法刺激身体。

（6）使用或不使用草药、电流或加热的针灸针。

b. 使用东方医学诊断和治疗,包括:

（1）艾灸、拔罐、热法、磁石、刮痧、针灸贴、药膏、冷热敷、电磁波疗法、光色疗法、声音疗

法或者激光疗法。

（2）按摩、穴位按压、反射疗法、指压按摩、推拿按摩或者手法刺激,包括通过不刺穿皮肤的仪器或者机械装置进行刺激。

（3）草药和膳食补充剂,来源包括植物、矿物、动物和营养品等。

c. 根据经 NCCAOM 或者 ACAOM 批准的培训,持证人认为适宜临床应用的其他辅助服务或者程序。

17.10（2）针灸针的使用和处置。持证人只能使用预先消毒的一次性针灸针,并应当按照艾奥瓦州公共卫生部的要求对用过的针灸针进行处置。

17.10（3）治疗标准。持证人应遵守与获得执业内外科或整骨医学执照人员相同的治疗标准。根据《艾奥瓦州法典》第 272C.3 条,任何错误或者遗漏、不合理的技能缺陷,或者未能在针灸实践中保持合理的治疗标准,构成渎职行为,并且构成撤销或者吊销本州针灸执照的理由。

17.10（4）头衔。根据本标题获得执照的针灸师可使用"执业针灸师"或者"L.Ac"字样。根据《艾奥瓦州法典》第 147.74（18）条,在持证人姓名后表示专业地位。

17.10（5）联系方式的变更。持证人须在更改家庭地址、执业地点、家庭地址或电话号码,或者申请人或持证人经常与委员会通信的个人电子邮件地址后一个月内通知委员会。

17.10（6）责任委派。持证人须执行所有涉及刺入患者皮肤的针灸治疗。持证人可将其他方面的治疗委派给经持证人适当培训过的工作人员和患者。允许受过适当培训的工作人员和患者从患者身上取出针灸针。持证人负责为员工制定和维持书面培训标准。

17.10（7）更改法定全名。持证人应当在更改法定全名后一个月内告知委员会。需随附经过公证的结婚证副本或者经过公证的法庭文件副本。

17.10（8）已故。当委员会收到持证人的死亡证明副本或者其他关于持证人死亡的可靠信息时,应关闭持证人的档案并标记为"已故"。

第 653-17.11（147,148E,272C）条　一般纪律规定

委员会授权对任何违反有关针灸安全和健康服务的州法律和行政法规的持证人采取纪律处分。本规则不得根据 653-第 3 章或者任何其他法律规定予以豁免。

17.11（1）纪律处分方法。委员会可以实施下列任何纪律处分:

a. 撤销执照。

b. 吊销执照,直至委员会作出进一步指令。

c. 不予续期执照。

d. 永久或者暂时限制特定程序、方法、行为或者技术的实施。

e. 列入察看期。

f. 额外的补救教育或者培训。

g. 重考。

h. 在特定时间内由相关机构或委员会选定的从业者进行医疗或者身体评估,或者酒精或药物筛查。

i. 一千美元以下的民事处罚。

j. 必要时进行传讯和警告。

k. 法律允许的其他制裁。

17.11(2)委员会的自由裁量权。委员会在决定纪律处分的性质和严重程度时,可以考虑以下因素:

a. 违规行为的相对严重性,因为关系到保障艾奥瓦州公民接受高标准的专业治疗。

b. 特定违规行为的事实。

c. 任何减责情形或者其他抵消因素。

d. 先前违规或者投诉的数量。

e. 先前违规或者投诉的严重性。

f. 是否已采取补救措施。

g. 其他可能反映持证人能力、道德标准和专业行为的因素。

第 653 - 17.12(147,148E,272C)条　纪律处分理由

在确定执照持有人存在以下违法行为时,委员会可以采取第 17.11(1)条的纪律处分:

17.12(1)获取执照时存在欺诈行为,系指在申请针灸执照时故意歪曲事实或者使用欺骗手段,包括但不限于:

a. 在获得或者尝试获得执照时作出虚假或者误导性陈述。

b. 根据《艾奥瓦州法典》第 147 章和第 148E 章的规定,故意遗漏或者隐瞒委员会认为与安全健康的针灸实践相关的任何信息。

c. 谎报有关事实或者契约,以满足本章规定的申请或者资格要求。

d. 提交或者试图提交虚假、伪造或者涂改的文凭、证书、宣誓书,或者其他官方或者经认证的文件或译本,包括申请表,以证明申请人有资格在艾奥瓦州从事针灸实践。

17.12(2)不称职行为。不称职行为包括但不限于:

a. 在针灸师执业范围内严重缺乏履行专业义务的知识或者能力。

b. 持证人在相同或者类似情况下执业时,严重偏离其他针灸师通常拥有和应用的学习或者技能标准。

c. 针灸师在相同或者类似的情况下,未能在很大程度上行使普通针灸师通常会采取的谨慎程度。

d. 故意或反复偏离或未能遵守可接受的普遍针灸实践的最低标准。

17.12(3)针灸实践中的欺诈行为。针灸实践中的欺诈行为包括但不限于在针灸实践中以口头或者书面形式作出的任何误导性、欺骗性、虚假或者欺诈性陈述,违反针灸师的法律或公平义务、患者对针灸师的信任或信心,并被委员会视为违背良知,损害公共福利,并可能对他人造成伤害。无须提供实际伤害的证明。

17.12(4)不道德行为。由 NCCAOM 制定和批准的《道德准则》(2008 年)应被委员会作为本州针灸实践的指导原则。针灸实践中的不道德行为包括但不限于:

a. 未向患者提供《艾奥瓦州法典》第 148E.6 条要求的信息或者向患者提供虚假信息。

b. 接受将患者转诊给其他卫生保健专业人员的报酬。

c. 为转诊患者支付或提供报酬,不包括付费广告或营销服务。

d. 实施或者声称实施针灸执业范围内的治疗时,与患者发生性行为或者生殖器接触,无论患者是否同意该性行为或者生殖器接触。

e. 未经授权披露患者隐私。

f. 突破了针灸实践中可接受的职业行为界限。委员会认为该界限旨在确保针灸师为爱荷华人提供安全和健康的护理。

17.12(5)对公众有害的行为。针灸实践中对公众有害或不利的行为包括但不限于:

a. 在相同或者类似情况下,未能具备和运用一位理性、谨慎的针灸师应有的技能、学习和治疗水平。

b. 由于精神或者身体损伤、化学滥用或者化学依赖,无法以合理的技能安全从事针灸实践。

c. 开具、分配或者施用任何管制药物或者处方药。

d. 未经《艾奥瓦州法典》第148E章或者本章授权执行各种治疗或者康复程序。

17.12(6)习惯性使用麻醉剂或者吸毒成瘾。习惯性使用麻醉剂或者吸毒成瘾包括但不限于因持续过量使用酒精、毒品、麻醉品、化学品或者其他药物而无法以合理的技能和安全性从事针灸实践,或过量使用以上物质,以致损害其以合理的技能和安全性从事针灸实践的能力。

17.12(7)重罪判决。与针灸实践相关或者影响执业能力的重罪判决包括但不限于:

a. 根据美国、美国政府或者其他国家或者其政治分区的任何司法管辖区的法规,对与针灸服务直接相关或者与之相关的任何公共罪行的判决。

b. 根据美国、美国政府或者其他国家或者其政治分支机构的任何司法管辖区的法规,对影响针灸能力的公共罪行的任何判决被归为重罪,并且涉及道德败坏、文明、诚实、道德。

判决记录或认罪答辩或放弃答辩的副本,应作为重罪判决的确凿证据。

17.12(8)持证人谎报执业范围。持证人执业范围的谎报包括但不限于误导、欺骗、虚假陈述关于执业针灸师的能力、教育、培训、技能或者执行本章未授权服务的能力。

17.12(9)虚假宣传。虚假宣传是在提供给公众的信息中使用欺诈、欺骗或不可信的陈述。虚假宣传包括但不限于:

a. 未经证实的关于持证人的技能或能力、针灸的治疗效果或其中的特定技术或疗法。

b. 展示具有误导性或者可能会误导普通人的词汇、短语或者图片。

c. 声称拥有针灸行业不承认的非凡技能。

17.12(10)常规理由。出于以下原因,委员会也可以对针灸师采取纪律处分:

a. 未能遵守《艾奥瓦州法典》第148E章的规定或者《艾奥瓦州法典》第147章的适用条款,或未能遵守委员会根据《艾奥瓦州法典》第148E章通过的规则。

b. 在判决或和解之日起三十日内,未将医疗事故索赔和诉讼的不利判决或和解通知委员会。

c. 未能在针灸师最初得知该信息之日起三十日内,向委员会报告另一位获准在艾奥瓦州执业的针灸师的任何行为或者不作为,这些行为或者不作为将构成根据第17.12条(147,148E,272C)采取纪律处分的理由。

d. 未能遵守委员会发出的传票。

e. 未能遵守委员会给予针灸师的纪律处分。

f. 违反《艾奥瓦州法典》第 147 章或者第 148E 章中列出的撤销或吊销执照的任何理由。

第 653 - 17.13(272C)条 同行评审程序

规则第 653 - 24.3(272C)条应当适用于与执业针灸师相关事项的同行评审程序。

第 653 - 17.14(272C)条 报告职责和调查报告

653 - 第 22 章和第 24 章适用于执业针灸师的某些报告责任和涉及执业针灸师的渎职案件的调查。

第 653 - 17.15(272C)条 控诉、豁免和特许通信

653 - 24 章适用于与执业针灸师相关事项。

第 653 - 17.16(272C)条 调查文件的保密性

653 - 第 24.9(2)条应当适用于与执业针灸师相关的调查文件。

第 653 - 17.17 至 17.28 条 保留

第 653 - 17.29(17A,147,148E,272C)条 纪律处分程序

653 - 第 25 章适用于执业针灸师的纪律处分。

第 653 - 17.30(147,148E,272C)条 禁止豁免

本章中的费用,不得根据 653 - 第 3 章或者任何其他法律规定予以豁免。

北达科他州

北达科他州针灸法^①

第43-61-01条　定义

除文意另有所指外,下列定义适用于本章:

1. "针灸"系指一种东亚卫生保健体系,包括患者教育、植物医学、气功、太极等治疗手段,或者通过刺激体表或者体内的穴位,如传统经络穴位或者阿是穴来维持和恢复患者的健康,包括在使用或者不使用电刺激的情况下,插入预先消毒的、丝状的、一次性针灸针,或者使用手法或热技术。

2. "针灸师"系指依照本章获得针灸执照的人员。

3. "获批的针灸课程"系指由高等教育机构提供并经美国教育部认可的国家或者地区机构认证的经委员会批准的研究生教育课程,或者经委员会批准的另一同等课程,该课程须:

a. 获得认证,具有认可候选人资格,或者符合经委员会批准的针灸及东方医学认证委员会(ACAOM)机构的标准。

b. 通过调查确定该学院或者项目符合相当于 A 类认证机构建立的教育标准并符合委员会规则后,经委员会批准。

4. "委员会"系指根据第 43 卷第 57 章设立的州综合医疗委员会。

第43-61-02条　豁免

针灸师使用的一些疗法,如使用植物药、食物和诸如针灸和触摸等物理手段,并非专属于针灸师的疗法。本章不限制根据本州法律许可、认证或者注册的任何其他职业的执业范围。

第43-61-03条　执照的要求和称谓使用的限制

1. 自 2016 年 1 月 1 日起,未取得委员会核发的针灸执照,不得从事任何形式的针灸执业活动。

2. 针灸师可以使用"执业针灸师"的头衔和缩写"LAc"来表明其身份。自 2016 年 1 月

---

① 根据北达科他州法典注释版第 43 卷第 61 章"针灸师"译出。

1日起,未取得本章规定的针灸执照而使用这些术语或者首字母作为其身份证明的人员,即属无证从事针灸实践。

第43-61-04条 获得执照的资格条件

要获得在本州针灸执照,申请人应当向委员会提出申请。申请必须以委员会所采用的表格为准,并且必须按照委员会规定的方式提出。

第43-61-05条 执照的申请

1. 针灸执照申请人应当按照委员会提供的表格提出申请,证明申请人品行良好、符合本章和第43卷第57章规定的各项要求,包括:

a. 顺利完成获批的针灸课程。

b. 顺利完成国家针灸和东方医学认证委员会(NCCAOM)等委员会规定或者认可的考试。

c. 具备以委员会认可的方式从事针灸实践的身体、精神状态和专业能力。

d. 从未受到委员会、任何其他州执照管理委员会或者对委员会具有管辖权的法院针对根据本章和第43卷第57章规定构成纪律处分的任何行为做出的任何裁决。委员会可根据需要修改此限制。

2. 申请必须附有委员会确定的执照费和申请费,以及证明申请人具备所需资格的文件、宣誓书和证明文件。

第43-61-06条 首次申请及免除教育考试的条件

尽管有第43-61-05条第1款第a项和第b项规定的教育和考试要求,但是如果申请人在2015年1月1日至2015年12月31日期间是本州的真正居民,且在2016年1月1日之前曾在该国从事针灸实践,但是不符合教育或考试要求,或者两者都不符合,为了继续从事针灸实践,需要申请本章规定的执照,委员会在对申请人的教育和经历进行审查后,确定申请人有足够的教育和经验从事针灸实践的,可以向该申请人颁发执照或者受限执照。

第43-61-07条 向其他州持证人颁发执照并免予考试

1. 在符合执照要求的情形下,经许可机构认可的认证机构考核通过,并经委员会确认该考核在各方面均与本章规定的考试具有同等效力的,委员会可以向经认可的认证机构考试合格的申请人颁发针灸执照。

2. 委员会可以与其他州的执照机构签订互惠协议,规定互免进一步考试或者部分考试。

3. 依照本章规定免予考试的,申请人还应当符合其他执照条件。委员会可以通过制定规则,允许临时和特别执照在委员会会议间隔期间有效。

第43-61-08条 针灸实践

1. 根据第43-17-02条的规定,针灸师可以将针灸实践作为一种受限的医疗技术。针灸师不得实施下列行为:

a. 开具、调配、使用处方药。

b. 声称从事除针灸以外的任何需要执照的卫生保健专业或者治疗体系,除非持有该专业的单独执照。

2. 针灸师可以基于预防和治疗目的开具和使用下列治疗药物和方法:

a. 患者教育、植物药、气功、太极。

b. 刺激体表或体内的穴位,包括传统经络穴位和阿是穴,方法是在使用或不使用电刺激的情况下,插入预先消毒的、丝状的或者一次性的针灸针,或者使用手法或者热技术。

第43－61－09条 公共卫生职责

在公共卫生法、应报告的疾病和病症、传染病的控制和预防以及地方卫生委员会方面,针灸师与执业医师具有相同的职责,但是其权利和职责仅限于本章和第43卷第57章规定的与针灸师执业范围相一致的行为。

第43－61－10条 医院的就业情况

医院可以按照第43－17－42条规定的相同方式雇用针灸师。

北达科他州针灸行政法①

第112－04－01节 针灸实践许可

第112－04－01－01条 定义

《北达科他州世纪法典》第43－61章中的所有定义均适用于本规则,另有特别说明的除外。在本规则中,除文意或主题另有所指外:

1. "审核委员会"系指针灸及东方医学教育审核委员会(ACAOM)或其继受机构。继受机构必须是美国教育部认可的审核机构。

2. "认证委员会"系指美国针灸与东方医学认证委员会(NCCAOM)或其继受机构。

3. "遵循针灸和东方医学培训"系是指采用与获得认可的针灸学校的教育相一致的方法进行针灸和东方医学的实践,这被普遍认为是安全有效,并且符合针灸行业公认的实践标准。

4. "全国委员会考试"系指由认证委员会或者其继受机构设立的针灸专科或者东方医学专科认证考试。

5. "东方医学"系指一种医疗体系,它把体内能量的循环和平衡视为人体健康的根本。它通过专门的方法分析身体的能量以及针灸或者其他东方治疗方式,以强健身体,改善能量平衡,维持或者恢复健康,改善生理功能,减少疼痛。《北达科他州世纪法典》第43－61－01节对针灸的定义包括针灸师在其实践中所包含的东方医学的内容。

6. "处方药"系指《联邦食品、药物和化妆品法案》(21 U.S.C.353 等)第503(b)条定义的处方药。在其定义下,其标签必须注明"仅限处方产品"。

第112－04－01－02条 学校的批准

1. 委员会应当批准符合下列条件的针灸学校:

a. 已被认证或者已被认证委员会认证的申请者。

b. 提供至少为一千九百〇五个学时/一百〇五个学分的住宿研究生学位课程。

---

① 根据《北达科他州行政法典》注释版第112编第4章"针灸师执照"译出。

2. 符合第 1 款 b 项要求,并且毕业生经认证委员会批准参加国家委员会考试的国外学校则可考虑申请委员会批准。

3. 该委员会应当保留并在审查时提供一份最新获批的美国针灸学校名单。

第 112－04－01－03 条 执照申请

申请必须用委员会发布的正式表格提出。

1. 根据《北达科他州世纪法典》第 43－61－05 节的常规申请程序,在收到执照申请人以下所有材料时应对其申请予以考虑:

a. 一份签署并注明日期的正式申请表。

b. 由认证委员会直接寄给委员会的全国委员会考试的正式成绩单,证明其圆满通过全国委员会考试。

c. 由申请人毕业所在的获批的针灸学校直接寄给委员会的正式完整的成绩单,证明其毕业和完成临床培训的日期。

d. 申请费和初始执照费。

2. 根据《北达科他州世纪法典》第 43－61－06 节的豁免程序申请执照或者受限执照的申请人应当提交下列文件以供考虑:

a. 一份签署并注明日期的正式申请表。

b. 由认证委员会出具的正式成绩单,证明其为经过认证的学位证书持有者。

c. 研究生临床实践经验的文件,包括日期、临床联系信息和主管联系信息,以供核实。

d. 2015 年全年的北达科他州居民身份证明文件。

e. 2015 年北达科他州针灸实践的证明文件。

f. 申请费和授权费。

第 112－04－01－04 条 通过背书获得执照

以背书方式提出的执照申请,符合下列条件的,委员会应对其予以考虑:

1. 申请人毕业于获批的针灸学校并获得学位。

2. 申请人持有现行有效的执照,并在另一个州或者司法管辖区从事针灸实践,且信誉良好。委员会必须收到来自其他州或者司法管辖区官方的执照书面核实。

3. 其他州或者司法管辖区的考试要求与北达科他州基本相似。

4. 申请人已向委员会提交一份官方的执照背书申请,获批针灸学校的学位证书复印件,当前有效的执照复印件,以及所需的申请费。

第 112－04－01－05 条 照片

在向委员会提交申请前,申请人必须在申请书的空白处夹附申请人未装裱的护照照片。照片必须于申请日期起计一年内拍摄。

第 112－04－01－06 条 考试要求

1. 在全国委员会考试中成绩及格的执照申请人应当被视为符合《北达科他州世纪法典》第 43－61－05 节规定的考试要求。

2. 必须在毕业后四年内顺利完成执照考试要求。对于同时攻读另一个研究生学位的申请人,委员会可以给予例外,申请人提出可以验证的、合理的、有说服力的解释的,不受四年的时间限制。

3. 一个申请人最多具有五次机会参加国家委员会考试的单个部分。如果申请人在五次考试后未能通过国家委员会考试的单个部分,则申请人在一年后才有申请执照的资格,并必须作为新的申请人重新申请。

第 112－04－01－07 条　执照颁发

当委员会确定申请人已顺利毕业于获批学校,通过国家委员会考试,并是一个良好品德的人,委员会将向该申请人颁发针灸执照。

第 112－04－01－08 条　实践地点及执照展示

1. 如果执业针灸师更换主要执业地点,必须通知行政主管办公室针灸师执业地点的变化。由委员会颁发的现行证书或者证书副本必须随时展示在针灸师办公室的显著位置。如遗失或者毁坏,在收到符合要求的遗失或者毁坏的证明后,委员会可以发出一份证书副本。

2. 获得执照的针灸师在执业地点外提供临时服务时,必须携带一份执照钱包卡副本,并根据要求出示该卡。

第 112－04－01－09 条　执照续期

1. 每名获得委员会颁发执照的针灸师,必须于每一偶数年度的 12 月 31 日或者之前,缴纳续期费,并填写委员会提供的问卷,以续期执照。对于在偶数年 7 月 1 日之后获得初始执照的申请人,执照将在 12 月 31 日自动续期两年,无须支付额外的续期费。

2. 续期申请人必须在问卷上证明已经或者将于 12 月 31 日前符合继续教育要求。申请人必须保存完整的继续教育记录。委员会必须对持证人进行随机合规审核。未能完成继续教育将被认为是违反职业道德的行为。

3. 在奇数年的 1 月 1 日或者之后收到的执照更新申请属逾期续期,需要填写新的申请表格,缴纳续期费以及由委员会规定的逾期费。必须提供适当的继续教育学时数证明。在偶数年的 12 月 31 日之前没有续期的执照是失效执照。

第 112－04－01－10 条　失效执照

一旦执照失效,在新的执照颁发之前,持有失效执照的个人不得从事针灸实践或者使用州法律为获得委员会认证的个人保留的头衔。执照已经失效的个人,继续从事针灸实践或者使用受限头衔的,即违反州法律和本章的规定。这种违反法律和规定的行为,构成拒绝原持证人办理失效执照续期或者申请新执照的理由。

第 112－04－01－11 条　费用

委员会收取以下费用,且不可退还:

1. 申请。申请初始执照的费用是五十美元。

2. 初始执照。初始执照的费用是三百美元。执照周期为两年,每双数年份的 12 月 31 日到期。初始执照费应当在申请时根据两年周期内剩余的时间按季度按比例计算。

3. 临时执照。针灸师的临时执照费是一百美元。临时执照的费用将在收到初始许可申请时用于缴纳初始许可费。

4. 续期。执照在偶数年的 12 月 31 日续期。执业状态的续期费用为二百美元,非执业状态的续期费用为一百美元。

5. 状态的变更。将非执业状态变更为执业状态,费用应当按两年周期内剩余的时间按季度计算。

6. 逾期申请。每一个偶数年份,在 12 月 31 日前未收到续期申请的,将收取额外的逾期申请费。针灸师的逾期申请费为七十五美元。

7. 执照副本。针灸执照副本的费用为二十五美元。针灸师执照的钱包卡的副本费用为二十美元。

第112‑04‑02节 针灸师权限

第112‑04‑02‑01条 权利和特权

除法规另有限制外,执业针灸师应当遵循针灸和东方医学培训,具有北达科他州卫生保健从业人员的权利和特权。《北达科他州世纪法典》第43‑61‑01节的针灸实践包括一些东方医学方面的内容,例如:

1. 运用东方医学理论评估和诊断患者。

2. 运用东方医学理论制定患者治疗方案。

3. 作为患者治疗计划的一部分,开具处方和使用东方医学疗法。

第112‑04‑02‑02条 广告

执业针灸师具有以委员会根据第112‑01‑04‑02条通过的道德规范中规定的各种合法方式宣传他们的服务的特权,受法规限制或者禁止的除外。博士级别的执业针灸师可以根据已被认证的针灸博士学位,使用前缀"doctor"或者"Dr.",但是不可以宣传任何针灸头衔或者名称,根据《北达科他州世纪法典》第43‑61‑03节指定的除外。

第112‑04‑02‑03条 使用,开具以及分发的权限

针灸实践应基于东方医学原则,包括使用、开具、分发、指示或从事:

1. 食品,营养补充剂,草药和中草药专利疗法。

2. 健康咨询,营养疗法,草药疗法,东方按摩,功法,呼吸技巧。

3. 针灸穴位刺激,可采用针刺、耳穴、拔火罐、电疗、热疗、真皮摩擦、刮痧、触摸等方法。

第112‑04‑02‑04条 使用针刺;穴位刺激

1. 执业针灸师应当遵循针灸及东方医学培训使用针刺。用于针灸实践的只能是预先包装的、一次性使用的、无菌的针灸针。这些针头只能在单个治疗过程中用于单个患者,并且根据《联邦有害生物废料标准》进行处理。在插入针灸针之前,必须用酒精或者其他经批准的清洁针技术(CNT)消毒剂清洗穴位。

2. 执业针灸师必须有管理患者过敏等不良事件的计划。

第112‑04‑02‑05条 转诊要求

1. 面对具有潜在的严重障碍的患者,执业针灸师应当向执业医师要求咨询或者书面诊断。当患者出现以下症状或者体征时,必须转诊给执业医师:

a. 心脏疾病,包括高血压失控。

b. 急性严重腹痛。

c. 急性、未诊断的神经病变。

d. 在三个月内不明原因的体重减轻或者增加超过体重的 15%。

e. 疑似骨折或者脱位。

f. 疑似系统性感染。

g. 任何未确诊的严重出血性疾病。

h. 无既往病史的急性呼吸窘迫。

2. 在下列情况下,执业针灸师应当将患者转诊给执业医师:

a. 疑似气胸;或者

b. 针灸针断裂。

第 112‑04‑03 节　继续针灸教育

第 112‑04‑03‑01 条　继续教育要求

1. 在两年一次的执照周期内,所有持证人必须完成至少三十学时获批的继续教育学分。只有获得委员会认证的继续教育项目中的学时才被认可。实际上课时间每五十分钟可以获得一学时学分。

a. CPR 每两年需要重新认证一次,并且被授予四个继续教育单位。

b. 伦理或者安全课程每两年需要两个学分。

2. 如果持证人因疾病、服兵役、医疗或者宗教传教活动或者其他情有可原的情况而未能符合规定,则必须经过书面申请,准予延长时间或者其他豁免以完成第 1 款所规定的学时数。

第 112‑04‑03‑02 条　豁免

下列执业针灸师无须满足本章的继续教育要求:

1. 参加全日制针灸教育项目的针灸师(博士学位,住院医师和获得奖学金)。

2. 持有临时执照的针灸师,以及在获得委员会颁发的永久执照后首次未续期执照的针灸师。

3. 从执业针灸和东方医学领域退休的针灸师们。这一豁免只适用于已经完全退出针灸和东方医学实践的退休针灸师。任何寻求豁免以达到本款下所规定的继续针灸教育要求的针灸师必须向委员会提交一份宣誓书(在委员会的表格上),以证明其在下一个继续教育报告期内不会提供针灸服务。

第 112‑04‑03‑03 条　委员会的批准

1. 为了获得委员会批准,继续教育项目必须被认证委员会认证。

2. 持证人有责任利用项目来源核实适当的信用标识。所有持证人在参加任何特定的课程之前,必须核实其是否有资格获得继续教育学分和适当的指定学分。

第 112‑04‑03‑04 条　委员会审核

委员会应当每两年随机审核选定的针灸师,以检查其是否符合继续教育的要求。任何接受审核的针灸师都需要提供合规文件,包括继续教育提供者的名称、项目名称、完成的继续教育时间、入学日期以及出勤证明。任何针灸师如未能提供符合继续教育要求的证明,其执业资格将会撤销。为便于委员会的审核,每名针灸师都需要保存一份其参与所有继续教育活动的记录。向委员会报告包含教育活动在内的记录后,每名针灸师必须保存该记录至少两年。

第 112 - 04 - 03 - 05 条　非执业状态

在每个偶数年的 12 月 31 日或者之前，持证人可以选择将其执照续期为非执业状态。对于那些不执业、咨询，或者提供任何针灸行业服务的持证人，非执业状态的费用会降低。持有非执照执业持证人无须提供继续教育学时证明。任何非执业执照持证人在支付额外费用，并出示过去二十四个月内接受三十学时继续针灸教育的证明后，可以随时激活该执照。

俄 亥 俄 州

俄亥俄州针灸法[①]

第 4762.01 条　定义

下列定义适用于本章：

（A）"针灸"系指在使用或者不使用艾灸或者电刺激的情况下，在人体特定部位插入和取出专业针灸针的补充技术。

（B）"脊医"系指根据《法典修订版》第 4734 章获发脊医执照的人士。

（C）"一般非医疗营养信息"系指下列任何一项信息：

（1）良好的营养和食物准备原则。

（2）正常日常饮食中包含的食物。

（3）人体的必需营养物质及推荐量。

（4）含必需营养素的食物和补充品。

（5）营养物质对人体的作用以及营养不足和营养过剩对人体的影响。

（D）"草药疗法"系指使用食物、草药、维生素、矿物药、器官提取物和顺势疗法。

（E）"顺势疗法"系指一种非侵入性的天然替代医学系统，旨在通过使用以动物、植物或者矿物药为原料制备的小剂量高度稀释药物来刺激人体自愈的能力。

（F）"艾灸"系指使用草药热刺激一个或者多个穴位。

（G）"东方医学"系指在使用或者不使用草药疗法的情况下进行针灸的卫生保健形式。

（H）"医师"系指根据《法典修订版》的第 4731 章授权的人员，从事内外科、整骨医学或者足病学。

（I）"补充技术"系指使用一般非医疗营养信息、传统和现代东方疗法、热疗、艾灸、穴位按压和其他形式的中式按摩，以及有关改变生活方式的教育信息。

第 4762.01（1）条　本章对于东方医学医师的适用性

本条生效之日起，本章不再适用于东方医学医师。

---

① 根据《俄亥俄州法典》注释版第 47 卷第 4762 章"针灸师"译出。

第 4762.02 条　执照;豁免

（A）除本条（B）款、（C）款或者（D）款的规定外,任何人不得从事下列任何一项:

（1）从事东方医学实践,除非持有本州医学委员会根据本章颁发的东方医学医师有效执照。

（2）从事针灸实践,除非持有本州医学委员会颁发的针灸执照。

（B）本条（A）款不适用于医师。

（C）本条（A）款（1）项不适用于下列情况:

（1）作为东方医学培训计划的一部分,从事东方医学活动的人员,但是必须满足以下两个条件:

（a）培训计划由教育机构或者培训学校实施。教育机构应当持有根据《法典修订版》第 1713.02 条由高等教育校长颁发的有效授权证书;培训学校应当持有根据第 3332.05 条由州职业院校委员会颁发的有效注册证书。

（b）在持有根据本章颁发的东方医学执照的人员的监督下从事活动,但是未在《法典修订版》第 4762.10 条规定的监督期内实践。

（2）就针灸是东方医学的一个组成部分而言,持有根据本章颁发的针灸执照的人员或者根据《法典修订版》第 4734.283 条,持有州脊医委员会颁发的针灸执业证书的脊医。

（D）本条（A）款（2）项不适用于下列情况:

（1）作为针灸培训计划中从事针灸实践的人员,但是必须满足下列两个条件:

（a）培训计划由教育机构或者培训学校实施。教育机构应当持有根据《法典修订版》第 1713.02 条由高等教育校长颁发的有效授权证书;培训学校应当持有根据第 3332.05 条由州职业院校委员会颁发的有效注册证书。

（b）该人员在针灸师的监督下从事针灸实践,该针灸师持有根据本章颁发的针灸执照,并且未在《法典修订版》第 4762.10 条规定的监督期内从事针灸实践。

（2）持有根据本章颁发的东方医学执照的人员。

（3）根据《法典修订版》第 4734.283 条持有国家脊医委员会颁发的针灸执业证书的脊医。

第 4762.03 条　申请;资格;审查;费用

（A）个人申请东方医学或针灸执照,应当按照州医学委员会要求并提供的格式向其提出书面申请。

（B）为获得执照,申请者应当符合下列条件(如适用):

（1）申请人应当向委员会提交符合要求的证明,证明申请人至少已年满十八周岁。

（2）申请人如果想要取得东方医学执照,应当向委员会提交符合要求的证明并满足以下两个条件:

（a）申请人持有国家针灸与东方医学认证委员会认证的现行有效的东方医学或者针灸和中草药专科证书。

（b）申请人已在申请执照前的两年内顺利完成美国食品药品监督管理局药房管理和配方指南委员会批准的一门课程。

（3）申请人应当向委员会提交符合要求的证明,证明其持有国家针灸与东方医学认证委员会授予的有效的针灸学历证书。

（4）申请人须向委员会证明其熟练掌握英语口语,并须符合下列要求之一:

（a）通过《法典修订版》第4731.142条规定的考试。

（b）向委员会提交符合要求的证明,证明申请人必须证明其熟练掌握英语口语,作为从国家针灸与东方医学认证委员会获取东方医学、针灸和中草药学历证书或者针灸学历证明的学历证书。

（c）向委员会提交符合要求的证明,证明申请人在要求获取国家针灸与东方医学认证委员会指定的东方医学、针灸和中草药学历证明或者针灸学历证明时,已顺利地用英文顺利完成了国家针灸与东方医学认证委员会授予证书所需的考试。

（d）如申请人拟获得东方医学执照,应当向委员会提交符合要求的证据,证明其之前曾持有根据《法典修订版》第4762.04条颁发的针灸执照。

（5）申请人应当向委员会提交委员会要求的任何其他资料。

（6）申请人应当向委员会支付一百美元的费用,且该费用不予退还。

（C）委员会应当审查根据本条收到的所有申请。委员会在收到完整申请后六十日内,应当确定申请人是否符合颁发执照的条件。

第4762.03（1）条　犯罪记录检查

除本章规定的资格要求外,每名申请东方医学医师执照或者针灸执照的申请人都应当遵循《法典修订版》的第4776.01条至第4776.04条的规定。州医学委员会不得向申请人颁发执照,除非该委员会通过自由裁量决定刑事记录审查结果不会使申请人丧失《法典修订版》第4762.04条规定的颁发执照的资格条件。

第4762.04条　执照的登记和颁发

如果本州医学委员会根据《法典修订版》第4762.03条的规定确定申请人符合本州颁发东方医学执照或者针灸执照的要求,委员会秘书长应当酌情将申请人注册为东方医学医师或者针灸师,并向申请人颁发适当的执照。证书的有效期为两年,除被撤销或吊销外,有效期应当在颁发日期后两年届满,并可根据《法典修订版》的第4762.06条的规定延长两年。

第4762.05条　执照副本及费用

持有东方医学执照或者针灸执照的个人申请更换证书时,州医学委员会应当补发一份针灸执照副本,以替代缺失或者损坏的针灸执照,证书中应当显示姓名变化或者其他合法事由。执照副本的费用为三十五美元。

第4762.06条　执照续期

（A）东方医学执照或者针灸执照的续期,应当在证书有效期届满之日或者之前,向本州医学委员会申请续期。委员会应当在到期日之前至少一个月向证书持有人发送续期通知。

申请应当以规定的方式提交给委员会。每份申请应当附有每两年一百美元的续期费用。

自上次签署申请东方医学医师执照或针灸执照以来,申请人如有任何刑事罪行构成根据修订守则第4762.13条拒绝颁发执照的理由,且已认罪,或者已被裁定为有罪,或者已被认为符合干预而不是定罪的条件的，申请人必须进行上报。

（B）（1）为了有资格续期东方医学执照，申请人应当向委员会提供以下两项证明：

（a）作为东方医学申请人一直持有由国家针灸与东方医学认证委员会现行有效的东方医学或者针灸和中草药学历证书。

（b）申请人在其从该委员会获得东方医学学历证书或者针灸和中药学历证书之前的四年内，已顺利完成经国家针灸与东方医学认证委员会批准的一门为期六学时的草药和药物结合课程。

（2）为有资格续期针灸执照，申请人须向委员会证明，针灸师已取得国家针灸与东方医学认证委员会颁发的现行有效的针灸文凭。

（C）如申请人提交完整的续期申请，并有资格根据本条（B）款续期执照，委员会应向申请人颁发续期的执照。

（D）执照在到期日或者到期日期之前没有续期的，至到期日自动吊销。

如果根据本款吊销执照两年或者两年以内，委员会应在申请人提交续期申请、两年期续期费和适当的罚款后恢复执照。恢复执照的罚款为二十五美元。

如果根据本款的规定，执照已被吊销两年以上，可恢复执照。根据《法典修订版》第4762.061条，委员会可在申请人提交恢复申请、两年期续期费、适当罚款并遵守《法典修订版》第4776.01条至第4776.04条规定后恢复执照。委员会不得重新恢复执照，除非委员会酌情决定犯罪记录检查结果不会使申请人丧失根据《法典修订版》第4762.04条规定获得执照的资格。恢复执照的罚款是五十美元。

第4762.06（1）条　执照的恢复

（A）本条适用于下列两种情况：

（1）请求恢复根据本章颁发的、因任何原因处于吊销或者非执业状态两年以上执照的申请人。

（2）根据本章两年以上没有从事东方医学或者针灸实践的申请人，存在下列任一情形：

（a）积极执业人员。

（b）参加《法典修订版》第4762.02条规定的培训计划。

（B）在向受本条管辖的申请人颁发证书或者为其恢复良好信誉之前，本州医学委员会可规定包括下列任何一项或多项相关条款和条件：

（1）要求申请人通过口头或者书面考试，或者通过两者，以确定申请人目前是否适合恢复执业。

（2）要求申请人参加额外培训，并在完成培训后通过考试。

（3）要求对申请人的身体技能进行评估，以确定申请人的协调、精细动作技能和灵巧度是否符合最低护理标准。

（4）要求评估申请人在辨别和理解疾病和病症方面的技能。

（5）要求申请人进行全面的体格检查，其中可包括对身体能力的评估、对感觉能力的评估或者对是否存在神经疾病的筛查。

（6）限制申请人的执业范围或类型。

委员会应当考虑申请人在吊销或者非执业状态期间的道德状况和活动。委员会不得根据本条颁发或者恢复执照,申请人符合《法典修订版》第 4776.01 条至第 4776.04 条规定的除外。

第 4762.08 条　头衔的使用

(A) 根据本章持有东方医学医师执照者,可使用下列或者与此相当的头衔、首字母或者缩写,以表明其为东方医学医师:"东方医学医师""执业东方医学医师""L.O.M""NCCAOM 东方医学文凭持证人""Dipl.O.M""NCCAOM 国家委员会认证东方医学证书持证人""针灸师""执业针灸师""L.Ac 和 L.C.H""NCCAOM 针灸与中草药药证书持证人""NCCAOM Dipl.Ac 和 Dipl.C.H."或者"NCCAOM 国家委员会认证针灸与中草药证书持证人"。不得使用与其从事东方医学实践相关的头衔、首字母或者缩写,包括"医生"在内。

(B) 根据本章持有针灸执照的人,可使用下列或者与此相当的头衔、首字母或者缩写,以表明其为针灸师:"针灸师""执业针灸师""L.Ac""NCCAOM 针灸学历证书持证人",或者"NCCAOM Dipl.Ac.",或者"NCCAOM 国家委员会认证针灸师"。不得使用与其从事针灸实践相关的头衔、首字母或者缩写,包括"医生"头衔在内。

第 4762.09 条　执照展示及通知

根据本章的规定,持有东方医学医师执照或者针灸执照的人员,应当在其主要执业场所的显著位置展示下列各项:

(A) 针灸执照,作为授权其在本州从事针灸实践的证明。

(B) 一份载有东方医学和针灸实践由州医学委员会监管的说明,以及委员会办公室的地址以及电话号码。

第 4762.10 条　监督期及权力和职责的行使

下列条款适用于持有东方医学医师执照或者针灸执照的人员:

(A) 在收到初始执照后,东方医学医师或者针灸师的实践将受到监督期的约束。监督期应当从执照颁发之日起至一年后结束。在监督期内,如果本州医学委员会根据《法典修订版》第 4762.13 条对东方医学医师或针灸师进行纪律处分,则监督期应当重新计算,直至其在一年内未受到任何纪律处分。

(B) 在监督期内,除了适用本条(D)款和(E)款的要求外,下列两项均适用于东方医学医师或者针灸师的实践:

(1) 只有在患者收到医生的书面转诊或者处方,推荐其实施医师提供的东方医学或者针灸,或者脊医提供的针灸时,东方医学医师才可为患者进行东方医学或者针灸治疗。针灸师只有在患者收到医生或者脊医的书面转诊或者针灸处方时,才应当为患者进行针灸治疗。如果转诊或者处方中规定了相应的报告程序,东方医学医师或者针灸师应当向医生或者脊医报告患者的病情或者治疗进展,并遵守对东方医学医师或者针灸师治疗过程的条件或者限制。

(2) 东方医学医师或者针灸师应当在患者的转诊或者开方医师或者脊医的一般监督下进行东方医学或者针灸治疗,除非东方医学医师使用草药疗法患者,无须在脊医的一般监督下提供草药疗法。一般监督不要求东方医学医师或者针灸师和监督医生或者脊医在同一诊所实践。

（C）针灸师的监督期结束后,除了适用本条（D）款和（E）款的规定外,针灸师的实践也应当遵守下列两项规定:

（1）在治疗患者的特定病症之前,东方医学医师和针灸师应当确认患者是否曾在过去六个月内接受与其寻求针灸治疗的病症相关的由医师或者脊医在其执业范围内进行的诊断检查。可向患者索取一份其签署的表格确认其已接受诊断检查。

（2）若患者未提供本条（D）款（1）项规定的签字表格,或者针灸师确定患者未经过该条规定的诊断检查,针灸师应当向患者提供由医生或者脊医进行诊断检查的书面建议。

（D）从事东方医学或者针灸实践的持证人,应当适用下列内容:

（1）在治疗患者之前,针灸师应当告知针灸不能替代常规的医学诊断和治疗。

（2）初次会诊时,针灸师应当以书面形式提供其姓名、营业地址、营业电话、针灸的信息及使用的技术。

（3）针灸师治疗患者时,不得作出诊断。若患者病情无好转或者需要紧急治疗,针灸师应当及时咨询医生。

（4）持证人应当为每位接受治疗的患者保存记录。记录应当保密,并应当在治疗终止后保留至少三年。该记录应当包括在监督期内对患者进行治疗的书面转诊单或者处方,以及在监督期后对患者进行治疗的任何书面转诊单或者东方医学或者针灸处方。

（E）在个人的东方医学实践中对患者进行草药疗法,适用下列规定:

（1）东方医学医师为患者提供咨询和治疗指导。治疗说明应当包含下列所有内容:

（a）解释草药疗法的必要性。

（b）指导患者如何进行草药疗法。

（c）解释草药疗法的可能禁忌证,并在出现不良反应时提供护理。

（d）指导患者通知已提供草药疗法的其他医疗服务提供者,包括患者的药剂师。

（2）东方医学医师应当将下列各项记录在案:

（a）建议患者使用的草药疗法的种类、数量和强度。

（b）根据本条（E）款（1）项规定向患者提供咨询和治疗指导。

（c）患者在使用草药疗法时所反馈的任何不良反应。

（3）东方医学医师应当将本条（E）款（2）（C）项下患者的任何不良反应报告州医学委员会。

第 4762.11 条　督导医生或者脊医的权力和职责

在《法典修订版》第 4762.10 条所规定的针灸师监督期间内,下列规定均适用于监督针灸师的医生或者脊医:

（A）在开具针灸转诊或者处方前,医生应当对患者进行医学诊断检查或审查最近由另一位医生检查的结果,或者脊医应当对患者进行脊椎诊断检查或审查最近由另一位脊医检查的结果。

（B）医生或者脊医应当以书面形式提出转诊或者处方,并在转诊或者处方中指明下列各项:

（1）医生或者脊医对需要使用针灸治疗的疾病或者病症的诊断。

（2）针灸师必须向医师或者脊医报告患者的病情或者治疗进展。

（3）根据本条(C)款对针灸治疗过程施加的条件或者限制。

（C）医生应当根据公认的或者普遍的医疗保健标准对针灸师的治疗过程施加条件或者限制,或者脊医应当根据公认或者普遍的整脊护理标准对针灸师的治疗过程施加条件或者限制。

（D）医生或者脊医应当亲自与针灸师协商。若医生或者脊医在针灸治疗时无法到场,须通过某种电信方式与针灸师进行联系,以便提供帮助。通常情况下,医生或者脊医应距离进行针灸治疗的场所不超过 60 分钟的路程。

（E）脊医不应当监督东方医学医师使用草药疗法治疗患者的过程。

第 4762.12 条　督导医生或者脊医的补偿

对于根据《法典修订版》第 4121 章或者第 4123 章提出索赔的患者,针灸师的督导医生和脊医应当对其向东方医学医师或者针灸师转诊患者或者向患者开具东方医学或者针灸处方的行为进行补偿。除非医生具有对患者进行东方医学或者针灸治疗的知识,或者脊医具有对患者进行针灸治疗的知识,顺利完成由医学、骨科医学、足病医学或者整脊疗法的专修学院开设的相关学习课程,并且该学院应当是俄亥俄州劳工赔偿局所认可的学院或者由其认可机构所管理的学院。

第 4762.13 条　纪律处分

（A）若针灸执照申请人被州医学委员会证实采用欺诈行为申请或者取得执照,只要委员会有不少于六名成员的赞成票,即可撤销或者拒绝颁发其执照。

（B）在法律允许的范围内,只要委员会有不少于六名成员的赞成票,就可根据以下原因限制、撤销或者吊销针灸执照,拒绝向申请人颁发执照或者恢复执照,或者对持证人进行谴责或将其列入察看期:

（1）允许持证人的姓名或者证件被他人使用。

（2）未能遵守《法典修订版》第 4731 章的要求以及委员会通过的规章制度。

（3）违反或者企图违反、直接或者间接、协助或者教唆他人违反或者共谋违反第 4731 章的规定以及委员会通过的规章制度。

（4）在相同或者类似情形下,偏离或者未能达到同类从业者的最低护理标准,无论是否对患者造成实际损伤。

（5）由于精神疾病或者身体疾病,包括对认知、运动或者感知技能产生不利影响的身体退化,无法按照可接受和普遍的护理标准从事针灸实践。

（6）因习惯性或者滥用药物、酒精或者其他损害服务能力的物质而损害按照可接受和普遍的护理标准进行服务的能力。

（7）故意透露职业机密。

（8）为吸引患者或者为取得或者试图取得针灸执照,做出虚假性、欺诈性、欺骗性的或者误导性的陈述。

本条所述"虚假性、欺诈性、欺骗性的或者误导性的陈述"系指含有虚假事实的陈述,由于未披露重要事实而可能误导或者欺骗他人,有意或者可能造成对有利结果错误或者不合理的期望,或者意指含有在合理概率下会造成普通谨慎之人误解或者被欺骗的陈述或者暗示。

（9）为个人或者他人获得报酬或者其他利益之目的,谎称不治之症、损伤或者其他不可治愈的病症可永久治愈。

（10）在实践过程中通过欺诈性的虚假陈述获得或者试图获得金钱或者其他有价值的东西。

（11）存在对重罪的认罪、定罪或者对申请人虽判罪却获保释的司法判决。

（12）存在在本州构成重罪的行为,不论该行为在哪个司法管辖区实施。

（13）存在对在实践过程中所犯轻罪的认罪、定罪或者对申请人虽判罪却获保释的司法判决。

（14）存在对涉及道德败坏的轻罪的认罪、定罪或者对申请人虽判罪却获保释的司法判决。

（15）存在在本州开展执业过程中构成轻罪的行为,不论该行为在哪个司法管辖区实施。

（16）存在在本州涉及道德败坏构成轻罪的行为,不论该行为在哪个司法管辖区实施。

（17）存在对违反任何州或者联邦法律关于持有、散播、使用或者贩运任何毒品的监管的认罪、定罪或者对申请人虽判罪却获保释的司法判决。

（18）除不缴纳费用的原因外,负责规范另一个司法管辖区针灸实践的国家机构采取的下列行为：限制、撤销或者吊销执照；接受放弃执照；拒绝颁发执照；拒绝续期或者恢复执照；列入察看期；或者发出谴责或者其他斥责。

（19）违反委员会对东方医学执照和针灸执照的制度规范。

（20）未能使用根据《法典修订版》第4731.051条规定的通用血液和体液预防措施。

（21）未能配合委员会根据《法典修订版》第4762.14条进行的调查。包括未能遵守委员会发出的传票或者命令,或者未能如实回答委员会在证词或者书面质询中提出的问题,若有管辖权的法院已发出撤销传票或者允许个人隐瞒有关证词或者证据的命令,则不配合调查不构成根据本条规定受到纪律处分的理由。

（22）未能遵守国家针灸与东方医学认证委员会关于职业道德、对患者的承诺、对职业的承诺和对公众的承诺的标准。

（23）未能按照《法典修订版》第4762.22条的规定提供足够的职业责任保险。

（24）未能保持国家针灸与东方医学认证委员会授予的有效的东方医学学历证明、针灸和中草药学历证明或者针灸学历证明。包括被国家委员会撤销其称号,或者不符合国家委员会重新授予其称号的要求,或者没有通知委员会其未能保持相应的称号。

（C）委员会不得因申请人就某项罪行作出认罪答辩、司法裁定其有罪或者司法裁定其有资格介入而不将其定罪等原因,拒绝向申请人发出执照,根据修订后法典第9.79条的规定拒绝颁发执照的除外。

（D）委员会根据本条（A）款和（B）款采取的纪律处分应当根据《法典修订版》第119章的裁决进行,但是委员会可与针灸师或者申请人签订协议,共同解决违反本章或者其中任何规则的指控,以代替裁决。同意协议在经过不少于六名委员会成员的赞成票通过后,须包含委员会对协议所述事项的调查结果和命令。若委员会拒绝批准此项协议,则协议中所载的承认及调查结果将不具有法律效力。

(E)为本条(B)款(12)、(15)和(16)项规定之目的,委员会根据《法典修订版》第119章的裁决可判定申请人或者持证人犯下有关行为。若初审法院作出对持证人有利的最终判决且该判决是基于案情的裁决,则委员会不具有管辖权。若初审法院出于技术或者程序理由发出解雇令,则委员会具有管辖权。

(F)若基于申请人或者持证人已认罪、定罪或者对申请人虽判罪却获保释的司法判决的情形,在法院下令密封犯罪档案之前,委员会已发出了听证会通知或签订了同意协议,则根据本条规定,委员会先前发布的查看档案命令或者委员会采取行动的管辖权不受任何法院犯罪档案密封的影响。委员会无须密封、销毁、编辑或者以其他方式修改其档案记录,以反映法院对犯罪档案的密封。

(G)根据本款之目的,任何根据本章持有执照或者申请执照的个人在按照委员会书面指示进行的精神或者体格检查,均被视为同意进行检查,同时不得对构成对证词或者检查报告可采性的决定特权提出异议。

(1)在执行本条(B)款(5)项时,若有可能存在违规行为,委员会可强制任何根据本章持有证书或者申请证书的个人接受精神检查、体格检查。包括艾滋病毒检测,或者进行精神、体格双重检查。检查费用需由个人自行承担。未能接受精神或者体格检查或者同意委员会下令进行的艾滋病毒检测,即表示接受针对该个人的指控,除非是由于个人无法控制的情况,且最终命令可在未采取证词或者未提交证据的情况下做出。若委员会发现针灸师由于本条(B)款(5)项所述原因而无法从事针灸实践,委员会应当要求针灸师接受其批准或者指定的医生的护理、咨询或者治疗,作为获得初始、继续、恢复或者续期执照的条件。受本款影响的个人应给予机会向委员会证明其有能力按照可接受和普遍的护理标准恢复执业。

(2)为本条第(B)(6)款之目的,若委员会有理由相信任何根据本章持有执照或者申请执照的人遭受此类损害,委员会可强迫其进行精神或者体格检查或者精神、体格双重检查。检查费用需由个人自行承担。本条所要求的任何精神或者体格检查应当由有资格进行此类检查并由委员会选择的治疗提供者或者医生进行。

未能接受精神或者体检或者同意委员会下令进行的艾滋病毒检测,即表示接受针对该个人的指控,除非是由于个人无法控制的情况,且最终命令可在未采取证词或者未提交证据的情况下做出。若委员会确定个实践能力受损,应吊销其执照或者拒绝执照申请,并将接受治疗作为初始、继续、恢复或者续期执照的条件。

在有资格申请恢复根据本款吊销的证书之前,东方医学医师或者针灸师应当向委员会证明其有能力按照可接受和普遍的护理标准恢复执业。证明应包括下列内容:

(a)根据《法典修订版》第4731.25条获批的治疗提供者证明该人已顺利完成各种所需的住院治疗。

(b)继续完全遵守出院护理合同或者同意协议的证据。

(c)两份书面报告表明已对个人实践能力进行评估,且该个人有能力按照可接受的和普遍的护理标准实践。报告应当由委员会批准进行此类评估的个人或者提供者提供,并应当描述其确定的依据。

在提交此类证明及个人签署的书面同意协议之后，委员会可恢复根据本条吊销的执照。

当执业能力受损的针灸师恢复执业时，委员会应当要求继续对其进行监督。监督应包括监督恢复前签订的书面同意协议遵守情况，或者听证会后委员会命令中所做规定，以及在同意协议终止后，根据伪造所定惩罚，向委员会提交至少两年的年度书面进展报告，说明其是否一直保持清醒。

（H）对于秘书长和监督成员确认同时出现以下情形，可以建议委员会在不进行事先听证的情况下吊销其执照：

（1）存在明确且具有说服力的证据表明东方医学医师或者这针灸师违反了本条(B)款规定。

（2）该人持续实践对公众健康构成直接严重的威胁。

书面指控应当准备妥当，以供委员会审议。委员会在对指控进行审议后，经不少于六名成员（不包括秘书长和监督成员）的肯定投票，可直接吊销证书，而无须事先听证。电话会议可用于审查指控，并对吊销执照进行即时表决。

委员会应当根据《法典修订版》第119.07条，以挂号邮件的形式发出或者亲自发出书面吊销令。在根据《法典修订版》第119.12条提出的任何上诉的未决期间，法院不得中止该命令。若针灸师请求委员会举行裁决性听证，除委员会和持证人另有协定外，听证日期应当在针灸师请求听证之日起十五日内，但是不得早于七日，委员会和持证人均同意的除外。

在委员会根据本条和《法典修订版》第119条发布的最终裁决令生效前，根据本条施加的吊销执行仍然有效，上诉被推翻的除外。委员会应当自听证会结束之日起六十日内发布最终裁决令。六十日内未作出裁定的，撤销吊销令，但是不影响其后的终审裁定。

（I）若委员会根据本条(B)款(11)和(13)项或者(14)项采取行动，且对有罪的司法调查结果、认罪，或者对申请人虽判罪却获保释的司法判决在上诉中被推翻，在用尽刑事上诉途径之后，持证人还可向委员会提交重新审理该命令的呈请书以及适当的法院文件。委员会在收到呈请书及有关法院文件后应当恢复执照。执照恢复后，委员会可根据《法典修订版》第119章进行裁决，以确定个人是否已实施该行为。听证通知应当根据《法典修订版》第119章发出。若委员会根据本条裁决认定该个人已实施该行为，或者未要求举行听证会，则可下令执行本条(B)款所规定的制裁措施。

（J）东方医学医师或者针灸师的执照及其执业活动，自其自认有罪，或者被法官或者陪审团认为有罪，或者在本州或者其他州需要基于司法裁决是否有资格采取干预或者治疗代替定罪之日起自动中止。这些犯罪行为包括：严重谋杀、谋杀、故意杀人罪、重罪攻击、绑架、强奸、性殴打、强制性交、加重纵火罪、加重抢劫罪或者加重盗窃罪。吊销执照后继续执业的，视为无证执业。

委员会应当根据《法典修订版》第119.07条，以挂号邮件的形式发出或者亲自发出书面吊销令。如果根据本部门吊销执照的个人未能及时要求根据《法典修订版》第119章作出裁决，委员会应当作出永久吊销执照的最终命令。

（K）根据《法典修订版》第119章的要求，委员会应当发出听证会通知，且受通知的个人未根据《法典修订版》第 119.07 条及时要求举行听证的情形下,委员会无须举行听证,但是可通过不少于六名成员的赞成票通过包含委员会调查结果的终审裁定。在终审裁定中,委员会采用本条(A)款或者(B)款所列任何制裁。

(L)委员会根据本条(B)款吊销执照的,均应当随附一份书面声明,说明恢复执照的条件。委员会应当根据《法典修订版》第 119 章的规定制定恢复执照的条件。恢复根据本条(B)款吊销的执照,需要不少于六名委员会成员的赞成票。

(M)当委员会拒绝向申请人颁发执照、吊销个人执照、拒绝续期执照或者拒绝恢复执照时,可指明其行为是永久性的。此后,被采取永久行动的个人无权获得针灸执照,委员会不得接受恢复执照或者颁发新执照的申请。

(N)尽管《法典修订版》另有规定,下列规定也应当适用:

(1)放弃根据本章颁发的东方医学医师执照、针灸师的执照均无效,委员会接受的除外。恢复放弃的执照需要至少六名委员会成员的赞成票。

(2)未经委员会批准,根据本章提出的执照申请不得撤回。

(3)如果未能按照《法典修订版》第 4762.06 条的规定续期执照,不得撤销或者限制委员会根据本条对该人士采取纪律处分的管辖权。

第 4762.13(1)条　因拖欠儿童抚养费而吊销执照

在收到《法典修订版》第 3123.43 条规定的通知后,州医学委员会应当遵守《法典修订版》第 3123.41 条至第 3123.50 条、第 3123.63 条通过的有关东方医学医师和针灸执照的规则。

第 4762.13(2)条　精神疾病或者不称职;吊销执照

若州医疗委员会有理由相信根据本章被授予针灸执照的人员患有精神疾病或者精神上的能力丧失,则可向该人合法居住县的遗嘱认证法院提出申请。以《法典修订版》第 5122.11 条规定的格式提交一份宣誓书,并由委员会秘书长或者委员会秘书长办公室成员签署,签署宣誓书后,应当按照《法典修订版》第 5122 章的规定进行相同的程序。总检察长可在根据本条提起的各个诉讼中代表委员会。

若获得执照的人被遗嘱认证法庭判定患有精神疾病或者精神上无能力,则其执照自动吊销,直至该人向州医疗委员会提交经遗嘱认证法庭认证的关于其已恢复实践能力的裁决副本,或者已向委员会提交证明书,证明其已按照《法典修订版》第 5122.38 条规定的方式和形式恢复能力。遗嘱检验法院的法官应当将精神疾病或者精神无能力的判决立即通知州医学委员会,并在法庭记录的页边空白处记载吊销证书的情况。

第 4762.13(3)条　民事处罚

(A)(1)如果东方医学医师或者针灸师违反本章或者根据本章通过的规则,本州医学委员会可根据《法典修订版》第 119 章作出的裁决和不少于六名成员的赞成票,对其予以民事处罚。民事处罚的数额由委员会根据本条(A)款(2)项通过的规定确定。除了根据《法典修订版》第 4762.13 条规定的其他行动外,也可对其予以民事处罚。

(2)委员会应当通过并可修订关于根据本条应当判处的民事处罚数额的准则。准则的通过或者修正需要至少六名委员会成员的批准。

准则规定,任何民事处罚金额不得超过两万美元。

（B）委员会应当根据《法典修订版》第 4731.24 条的规定,交存根据本条规定缴纳的民事罚款的款项。因违反《法典修订版》第 4762.13 条（B）款（6）项而受民事处罚的款项,只应当用于该委员会的调查、执行和遵守情况监测。

第 4762.14 条　违法行为调查

（A）州医疗委员会应当对违反本章或者本章通过的规则的证据进行调查。任何人如有任何信息表明某人违反本章的各项规定或者本章通过的规则,均可以书面形式向委员会报告。在没有不诚实的情况下,在根据《法典修订版》第 119 章进行的裁决中向委员会报告这类信息或者作证的人,对因举报或者提供证据而造成的民事损害,不承担民事责任。委员会收到的每项违规控诉或者指控均应当分配案件编号并进行记录。

（B）对违反本章或者根据本章通过的规则的指控所进行的调查,应当由委员会根据《法典修订版》第 4731.02 条选出的监督委员,并由秘书长按照《法典修订版》第 4762.15 条的规定监督。委员会主席可指定其他委员会成员代替监督成员进行监督调查。监督案件调查的委员会成员不得参与案件的进一步裁决。

（C）在调查可能违反本章或者根据本章通过的规则时,委员会可管理誓词,下令取证,发出传票,强制证人出庭,出示书籍、账目、文献、记录、文件和证词,但是未经咨询总检察长办公室、委员会秘书长及监察委员的批准,不得发出有关病历信息的传票。在发出病历信息的传票之前,秘书长和监督成员应当确定是否有理由相信提出的申诉违反本章或者其所采用的规则,且所寻求的记录与指控及调查的材料有关。传票仅适用于涵盖涉嫌违规行为的合理时间段的记录。

如果当事人未能遵守委员会发出的任何传票,在向被传唤人发出合理通知后,委员会可根据民事诉讼规则,要求发出命令,强制要求出示人或者记录。

由委员会发出的传票可由治安官、副治安官或者委员会指定的委员会员工送达。送达委员会发出的传票,可将传票副本送交该人,或者将传票内容读给该人,或者将传票副本留在该人通常居住处。当被送达人士为针灸师时,传票可通过挂号信、限制递送、要求回执等方式送达,传票在递送日期或者拒绝接受递送日期即视为送达。

副治安官应当收取与治安官相同的送达传票费用。每位服从传票出席委员会的证人,均应当收到《法典修订版》第 119.094 条规定的费用和交通补贴。

（D）为《法典修订版》第 2305.252 条之目的,所有听证会和委员会调查均应当视为民事诉讼。

（E）委员会根据调查所收到的信息须保密,禁止在任何民事诉讼中予以披露。

委员会应当以保护向委员会提出投诉的患者和个人隐私的方式进行所有调查和程序。委员会不得公布患者或者投诉人的姓名或者任何其他识别信息,得到适当同意的除外。

委员会可与执法机构、其他许可委员会和其他正在起诉、裁决或者调查涉嫌违反法规或者行政规则的政府机构共享根据调查所收到的任何信息,包括患者病历和病历信息。收到信息的机构或者委员会应当遵守与州医疗委员会必须遵守的相同的保密要求,尽管其与《法典修订版》条例存在冲突或者与其他机构或者委员会根据该要求在处理其他信息的程序上存在冲突。在司法程序中,信息只能根据证据规则被采纳为证据,但是法院应要求采取适当措施,确保委员会掌握的患者或者投诉人的姓名或者其他身份识别信息的保密性。为确保保密性,法院可采取的措施包括密封记录或者从记录中删除特定信息。

(F)州医疗委员会应当为委员会聘用的调查员制定要求并提供适当的初步培训和继续教育,以履行本章规定的职责。培训和继续教育可包括俄亥俄州治安官员培训委员会根据《法典修订版》第109.79条规定的条件开办或者批准的课程。

(G)委员会应当每季度编制一份报告,说明前三个月所有案件的处理情况。就委员会完成其活动的每一案件,本报告应当载有下列资料:

(1)被投诉或者涉嫌违法的案件编号。

(2)被投诉的人持有的执照类别(若有)。

(3)对投诉书所载指控的说明。

(4)案件的处理。

报告应当说明尚未处理的案件数量,并应当以保护每个案件中所涉及的每个人员身份的方式编写。该报告是为《法典修订版》第149.43条而作的公共记录。

第4762.15条　针灸师或者东方医学医师的定罪将由检察官通知本州医学委员会

(A)如本条所适用,"检察官"的含义与《法典修订版》第2935.01条中的含义相同。

(B)根据本章取得有效执照的东方医学医师或者针灸师,因违反《法典修订版》第2907章、第2925章或者第3719章,或者存在任何与该人执业相关联的市政法人的实质性类似条例,自认有罪、司法裁决有罪或者司法裁决干预代替定罪的资格,案件的检察官应当根据州医疗委员会规定和提供的形式,及时将定罪通知委员会。在收到该信息后的三十日内,委员会应当根据《法典修订版》第119章启动诉讼,以确定是否根据《法典修订版》第4762.13条吊销或者撤销其执照。

(C)检察官在根据本章由州医学委员会规定和提供的形式颁发有效执照的各个案件中,应将下列情况通知委员会:

(1)对重罪的认罪、定罪或者干预代替定罪的司法判决,或者初审法院根据技术或者程序理由对重罪指控发出驳回诉讼的裁定。

(2)对在执业过程中所犯轻罪的认罪、定罪或者干预代替定罪的司法判决,或者若指控的行为是在实践过程中发生的,则初审法院根据技术或者程序理由对轻罪指控发出驳回诉讼的裁定。

(3)对涉及道德败坏的轻罪的认罪、定罪或者干预代替定罪的司法判决,或者初审法院根据技术或者程序理由对涉及道德败坏的轻罪指控发出驳回诉讼的裁定。

报告应当载明持证人的姓名、住所、犯罪的性质,以及经法院认证的记载该行为的证明文件。

第4762.16条　卫生保健机构记录处分、向本州医学委员会或者监督组织报告及医疗事故诉讼

(A)由任何医疗机构,包括医院、由健康保险公司运营的医疗机构、门诊手术中心或者类似机构,对任何持有执照的东方医学医师、针灸师实施的各种纪律处分后的六十日内,该机构的首席行政官或者执行官应当向州医疗委员会报告个人姓名、机构采取的行动以及导致采取行动的基本事实的摘要。根据要求，机构应向委员会提供病历的认证副本，以作为机构采取行动的依据。向委员会提供摘要之前，审查案件的同行评审委员会或者机构的管理委员会应当批准该摘要。

向委员会提交报告或者决定不提交报告、委员会的调查或者纪律处分，并不妨碍医疗机构对针灸师予以纪律处分。

在没有欺诈或者不诚实的情况下，任何向委员会提供病历的个人或者实体，均不对因提供记录而对任何人造成损害承担责任。

（B）（1）除本条（B）款（2）项另有规定外，东方医学医师或者针灸师、东方医学医师专业协会或者针灸师协会、医师，认为有违反本章规定、经《法典修订版》第4731章或者委员会规则的情况发生的，应当向委员会报告其所依据的资料。

（2）东方医学医师或者针灸师、专业协会或者东方医学医师或针灸师协会、医师或者专业协会或者医师协会，认为有违反《法典修订版》第4762.13（B）（6）条规定的情况发生的，应当根据经修订的《法典修订版》第4731.251条制定的方案的监测机构报告有关的信息资料。如果向委员会提交了此类报告，则还应当将其提交给监测组织，除非委员会知道作为报告对象的个人不符合《法典修订版》第4731.252条的方案资格要求。

（C）任何主要由因违反职业道德、专业能力不足或者渎职而被吊销或者撤销个人成员资格的东方医学医师、针灸师组成的专业协会或者社团，在最终决定宣布后的六十日内，按委员会规定和提供的形式向其报告，包括个人姓名、专业组织采取的行动，以及导致采取行动的基本事实的摘要。

向委员会提交报告或者决定不提交报告、委员会的调查或者纪律处分，并不妨碍专业组织对针灸师予以纪律处分。

（D）承保东方医学医师、针灸持证人或者其他机构提供职业责任保险的保险人，应当在最终处置任何超过二万五千美元损害赔偿的书面请求后三十日内通知委员会。通知应当包含下列信息：

（1）提交通知的人的姓名和地址。

（2）作为索赔主体的被保险人的姓名和地址。

（3）提出书面索赔的人的姓名。

（4）最终处置日期。

（5）适用最终处置索赔的法院。

（E）委员会可调查因本条的报告引发其关注的、可能违反本章或者根据本章通过的规则的行为。除非委员会违法行为可能涉及多次医疗事故。在本条中，多次医疗事故是指在过去五年有三次或者三次以上的医疗事故索赔，每一次都导致对索赔人有利的超过二万五千美元的判决或者和解，且每一次都涉及针灸师的过失行为。

（F）委员会根据本条收到的摘要、报告和记录均应当保密，且不得在任何涉及本条要求的报告对象如东方医学医师、针灸师、监督医师或者医疗机构的任何联邦或者州民事诉讼中作为证据使用。委员会只可将所取得的资料作为调查的依据，作为对针灸师或者监督医师进行纪律处分听证的证据，或者在随后对委员会的行动或者命令进行的各个审判或者上诉中使用。

委员会仅可将根据本条收到的摘要和报告披露给本州内外的医疗机构委员会,医疗机构委员会负责为针灸师或者监督医师颁发证书或者重新颁发证书,或者审查其在特定机构内执业的特权。委员会应当说明信息是否得到核实。委员会传递的信息应当遵守与委员会保存时相同的保密规定。

(G)除个人根据本条(B)款提交的报告外,委员会应当将根据本条收到的任何报告或者摘要副本送交针灸师。针灸师有权就信息的正确性或者相关性向委员会提交一份声明。该声明应当始终与有争议的记录部分一起提交。

(H)向委员会报告、向经《法典修订版》第 4731.251 条所述的监督组织报告,或者将存在创伤的东方医学医师或者针灸师,转诊给经委员会根据经修订的《法典修订版》第 4731.25 条批准的治疗提供者的个人或者机构,不应当因报告、转诊或者提供信息而受到民事损害起诉。

(I)在没有欺诈或者不诚实的情况下,由东方医学医师或者针灸师组成的专业协会或者协会赞助的委员会,向有药物滥用问题的东方医学医师或者针灸师、该委员会或者计划的代表或者代理人、第 4731 条所述监测组织的代表或者代理人提供同行协助。经《法典修订版》第 251 条规定,本州医学委员会成员对于因将东方医学医师或者针灸师转诊至《法典修订版》第 4731.25 条批准的治疗提供者接受检查或者治疗而受到损害,不承担任何责任。

第 4762.17 条　法律执行

州医疗委员会秘书长负责执行有关东方医学或者针灸实践的法律。若秘书长知道或者被告知有违反本章或者根据本章通过的规则的行为,应当调查此事,并在合理根据出现时向犯罪者提出控诉和起诉。当秘书长提出要求时,本县的检察官负责并进行起诉。

第 4762.18 条　禁令救济

(A)根据本条(E)款,总检察长、犯罪发生地或者违法者居住县的检察官,州医疗委员会或者任何人知晓某人未持有针灸执照、但是直接或者共谋从事东方医学或者针灸实践,可按照《法典修订版》禁令规则的规定,以州的名义支持诉讼,通过向有管辖权的法院申请禁令,禁止任何人直接从事或者共谋从事针灸非法实践。

(B)在根据本条(A)款规定申请禁令之前,州医疗委员会秘书长应当收到充分的信息,证明该人直接或者共谋从事非法针灸实践,通过挂号邮件通知该人已受指控。该人应当在三十日内答复秘书长,证明其已获得适当的许可从事所述活动,或者未违反本章的规定。若在秘书长发出通知后三十日内仍未得到答复,秘书长应当要求总检察长、犯罪发生地或者罪犯居住地的检察官或者州医疗委员会按照本条的授权进行调查。

(C)在向法院提交经核实的申诉书后,法院应当就申诉书举行听证会,并应当给予本诉讼程序与根据《法典修订版》第 119 章提出的所有诉讼程序同等优先权,不论该程序在法院审案日程表上处于何种位置。

(D)本条授权的禁令程序应当作为对本章规定的所有处罚和其他补救措施的补充,而非替代。

(E)本条(A)款所规定的禁令程序,不得对《法典修订版》第 4762.02 条(B)款所述人士或者持有根据《法典修订版》第 4734.283 条颁发的有效针灸证书的脊医实施。

第 4762.19 条　规则

州医疗委员会可采用任何必要规则来管理东方医学和针灸实践、东方医学医师或者针灸师和监督医师之间的监督关系，或者管理东方医学医师的草药疗法，以及本章制度的实施。上述规则的采用，应当与《法典修订版》第 119 章的规定一致。

第 4762.20 条　费用

州医疗委员会经监督管理委员会批准，可设置超过本章规定数额的费用，但是不得超过规定数额的百分之五十以上。

委员会收到的所有费用、罚款和其他款项，均应当按照《法典修订版》第 4731.24 条的规定存放。

第 4762.21 条　州医学委员会豁免

在没有欺诈或者不诚实的情况下，州医疗委员会、现任或者前任委员会成员、委员会代理人、被委员会正式任命担任委员会代表的人员或者委员会员工，无须对根据本章执行与公务相关的法令、过失、诉讼、行为或者决定而对任何人承担赔偿责任。若任何此类人员要求州为任何与该人执行与公务相关的法令、过失、诉讼、行为或者决定所引起的任何索赔或者诉讼进行辩护，并且若该请求是在合理时间之前以书面形式提出的，且该人在请求或者诉讼的抗辩中诚实合作，则由州承担答辩费用，并支付由此产生的判决、协商、和解费用。州在任何时候都不得支付惩罚性或者惩戒性损害赔偿请求或者判决中的任何部分。

第 4762.22 条　职业责任保险

持有根据本章颁发的执照的东方医学医师或者针灸师，应当办理承保金额不低于五十万美元的职业责任保险。

第 4762.23 条　遵守第 RC4776.20 条

本州医学委员会应当遵守《法典修订版》第 4776.20 条。

第 4762.99 条　处罚

（A）首次违反《法典修订版》第 4762.02 条的罪行，属一级轻罪；其后续的每一次罪行均属四级重罪。

（B）首次违反《法典修订版》第 4762.16 条（A）款、（B）款、（C）款或者（D）款的，属于轻微轻罪；在后续的每一次罪行中，属四级轻罪。但对后续的每一次罪行，不判处监禁，而是单处一千美元以下的罚款。

俄亥俄州针灸行政法[①]

第 4734－10－01 条　获得针灸执业证书

（A）每位获委员会颁发针灸执业证书的脊医，需持有俄亥俄州现行有效的整脊执照。

---

① 根据《俄亥俄州行政法典》注释版第 4734 卷第 10 章"针灸服务认证"译出。

（B）在任何情况下,当脊医在俄亥俄州的整脊执照被吊销、撤销、置于非执业状态或者没收时,其持有的委员会颁发的针灸执业证书也将同样被吊销、撤销、置于非执业状态或者在没有进一步措施下被没收。

（C）在任何情况下,未持有现行有效脊医执照的,不能持有在俄亥俄州从事针灸实践的有效执业证书。

第 4734－10－02 条　针灸课程批准

（A）每个获得委员会批准的针灸教育提供机构的目标,是培养脊医提供针灸服务的专业能力。

（B）请求委员会批准的针灸服务教育提供机构,需要提交委员会所需的申请。申请应包括:

（1）该计划符合《法典修订版》第4734.211条所述要求的证明。

（2）该课程的大纲。

（3）受到教育提供机构的认可,包括认证的课程。

（4）课程能够培养合格的针灸实践提供机构的证明。

（5）每位讲师的个人简历,包括讲师在请求批准的教育提供机构的教师身份。

（6）该课程被国家脊医审查委员会认可,允许学生参加针灸考试的证明。

（7）委员会认为适当的其他信息。

（C）委员会可审查申请文件和证明文件或指派一个部门审查此类材料。

（D）获委员会批准的针灸教育机构,可以接受脊医先前取得的针灸教育学时数,并计入规定的三百学时针灸教育之中。教育机构应当确保任何转移学时都是适当并合理的,以满足修订后的《教育法典》第4734.211条中所述的三百学时课程要求。经委员会批准的针灸教育机构应将所有转入课程反映在脊医的最终成绩单上。

（E）教育机构应当确保学习的适当性并在学习过程中设有监控程序。

（F）根据本条规定,如果课程不符合规定,委员会可以随时撤销对针灸课程的批准。如果委员会认为,有证据表明被批准的针灸教育机构不符合本规则,委员会将向该教育机构发出警告函,随函说明委员会的批准可能被撤销,以及委员会采取行动的原因。委员会将在拟采取行动前三十日发出警告函。若教育机构提供证据,委员会可以恢复对其的批准状态。

第 4734－10－03 条　针灸执业证书的申请

（A）每位针灸执业证书申请人,应当按照委员会规定的方式提出申请并提交不可退还的一百美元申请费。申请和申请费的有效期为自申请之日起为期一年。申请人应当提交符合要求的证明,证明其符合根据《法典修订版》第4734.282条规定,获得俄亥俄州针灸执业证书的条件。所有需要的资格证明必须由发证机构直接发出。

（B）如果申请人无法满足《法典修订版》第4734.282条的要求,或者其实施的行为表明其不具备从事针灸实践所需的品格和能力,包括《法典修订版》第4734.31条规定的任何可能导致纪律处分的行为,委员会可以拒绝其申请。申请人有责任向委员会提供明确和令人信服的证据,证明其符合领取针灸执业证书的条件。

（C）任何遭到委员会提议拒绝颁发针灸执业证书的申请人,有权就该提议举行听证会。

第 4734－10－04 条　针灸执业证书续期条件——废止

第 4734－10－05 条　针灸转诊——废止

第 4734－10－06 条　非执业状态的针灸执业证书;针灸执业证书的恢复

（A）非执业状态的持证人,可以按照委员会规定的方式申请恢复其证书,并应当完成申请且提供申请所需的所有信息。除非脊医执照现行有效,否则不得恢复针灸执业证书。

（1）如果委员会在继续教育期间的第二年第一日之前收到恢复申请,申请人应当提交不可退还的一百美元费用,并提供在申请日期前的二十四个月内获得《行政法典》第 4734－7－01 条规定的十二学时针灸继续教育的证明。

（2）如果委员会在继续教育期间第二年的第一日之后收到申请,申请人应当提交不可退还的五十美元费用,并提供在申请日期前的二十四个月内获得《行政法典》第 4734－7－01 条规定的六学时针灸继续教育的证据。

（B）委员会将考虑申请人处于非执业状态期间的时长、道德品质和行为,以及适用《法典修订版》第 4734.286 条(B)款的恢复条款。

（C）如果申请人不符合《法典修订版》第 4734.286 条的要求,或者其行为不具备从事针灸实践所需的品格和能力,包括任何《法典修订版》第 4734.31 条规定的可能导致纪律处分的行为,委员会可以拒绝恢复其执业证书的申请。申请人有责任向委员会提供明确和令人信服的证据,证明其符合恢复执业证书的条件。

堪 萨 斯 州

堪萨斯州针灸法[①]

第 65－7601 条　法令的引用

堪萨斯州法第 65－7601 条至第 65－7624 条及其修正案,应称为并引用为《针灸实践法》。

第 65－7602 条　定义

下列定义适用于《针灸实践法》:

(a)"针灸及东方医学教育审核委员会"系指美国教育部认可的针灸和东方医学教育计划国家认证机构。为《针灸实践法》之目的,术语 ACAOM 还应包括被委员会视为与 ACAOM 等同的实体。

(b)"本法"系指《针灸实践法》。

(c)"针灸"系指将针灸针插入人体穿刺皮肤和相关治疗方式,通过控制和调节体内能量的流动和平衡,并刺激身体恢复其正常功能和健康状况,来评价、评估、预防、治疗或者调节任何生理异常或者疼痛。

(d)"委员会"系指州治疗艺术委员会。

(e)"咨询委员会"系指由堪萨斯州法第 65－7813 条及其修正案所设立的针灸咨询委员会。

(f)"执业针灸师"系指根据《针灸实践法》获得针灸执照的人员。

(g)"国家针灸与东方医学认证委员会"(NCCAOM)系指通过管理专业认证考试来验证入门级的针灸和东方医学执业能力的国家组织。就《针灸实践法》而言,NCCAOM 还应当包括被委员会视为与 NCCAOM 等同的实体。

(h)"医师"系指在堪萨斯州获得行医、外科或者整骨治疗执照的人。

(i)"针灸实践"包括但不限于:

(1)有时被称为"干针""激痛点疗法""肌内注射疗法""耳穴戒毒疗法"及类似术语的技术。

---

① 根据《堪萨斯州议会法》注释版第 65 章第 76 节"针灸服务法案"译出。

（2）机械、热力、压力、吸力、摩擦、电、磁、光、声、振动、人工和电磁处理。

（3）使用、应用或者推荐进行治疗性功法、呼吸技术、冥想和饮食营养咨询等。

（4）根据针灸师的培训水平和 NCCAOM 或者同等级别的认证，使用和推荐草药产品和营养补充剂。

（j）"针灸实践"不包括：

（1）开处方、配药或者给予根据《堪萨斯州法》第 65－4101 条及其修正案所规定的受管制物质或者各种处方药。

（2）医学和外科手术，包括产科和激光或者电离辐射的使用。

（3）整骨医学和外科或者整骨疗法。

（4）脊椎按摩。

（5）牙科治疗。

（6）足科治疗。

第 65－7603 条　针灸执照作为执业必要条件、针灸师身份及处罚措施

（a）自 2017 年 7 月 1 日起，除本法另有规定外，任何人未持有根据本法颁发的现行有效针灸执照的，不得从事针灸实践。

（b）（1）任何人在未持有本法规定的现行执照时，都不得以口头或者书面形式明示或者暗示自己持有执照。

（2）只有根据本法获得执照的，才有权使用"执业针灸师"或者指定的"L.Ac"头衔。

（3）本条的各项规定均不得解释为禁止执业针灸师列出或者连同其名称一起使用任何字母、单词、缩写或其他标志来表示其获得的任何教育学位、证书或者资格证书。

（4）违反本条规定的，构成 B 类轻罪。

第 65－7604 条　针灸针使用要求

在针灸实践中使用的针灸针应当是一次性、无菌且预先包装的。这些针头只能用于单个患者的单次治疗。

第 65－7605 条　无须持有针灸执照的人士

（a）依照本法规定，下列人员可以免除持有针灸执照的要求：

（1）任何在本州有执照从事内科和外科、骨科、牙科或者足科治疗的人，执业脊椎按摩师或执业自然疗法医师，并且该人将其活动或者执业限制在其卫生专业许可法授权的执业范围内，且不向公众表明该人根据本法获得了执照。

（2）任何未声称自己是执业针灸师的草药师或者草药零售商。

（3）美国各武装部队、联邦设施和其他军事服务机构在本州执行公务时的卫生保健提供者。

（4）任何被指定为针灸、东方医学或者草药学的学生、学员或者客座教师，并在经咨询委员会核准的项目中根据本法获得许可的针灸师的监督下参加课程学习或者培训的。这包括继续教育课程和任何被 NCCAOM 或者同等级别认证的针灸或者草药课程。

（5）任何在紧急情况或者救灾中提供援助的人。

（6）任何从事自我护理的人士或者提供免费护理的家庭成员，只要该等人士或者家庭

成员不宣称或者对公表示自己是针灸师。

（7）任何提供按摩的人，只要不从事针灸实践或者宣称其为执业针灸师。

（8）任何根据本法取得执照的从业者委托在其监督下提供专业服务的人。

（9）随国（境）外或国家队临时来本州参加训练、比赛，负责随行治疗的针灸、中草药医师。

（10）任何持有理疗师执照进行干针、激痛点治疗或者《理疗服务法案法》特别授权的服务的人。

（b）本条款自 2017 年 7 月 1 日起生效。

第 65－7606 条　通过考试获得针灸执照的先决条件

申请针灸执照，应当填写委员会提供的表格递交申请，并应当使委员会相信该申请人：

（a）年满 21 周岁。

（b）已顺利完成中学教育或者同等学力。

（c）已顺利完成经认证的针灸学校的针灸课程学习，该学校的教育标准实质上与 ACAOM 或者 NCCAOM 为针灸学院制定的最低教育标准基本等同。

（d）已顺利通过委员会核准的执照考试。

（e）具有一定的英语沟通能力。

（f）已支付根据堪萨斯州法第 65－7611 条及其修正案规定的所有执照所需费用。

第 65－7607 条　凭背书办理针灸执照的先决条件

（a）委员会可以不经审查，向在其他州、准州、哥伦比亚特区或者其他国家从事针灸实践的人员颁发执照，该类人员须经该州、地准州、哥伦比亚特区或者其他国家的适当许可机构认证，证明申请人已正式取得执照，申请人的执照从未被限制、吊销或撤销。持证人从未受谴责或者受到其他惩罚措施，而就该授权机构的记录而言，申请人有权获得该授权机构的背书。申请人还须提交符合委员会要求的证明：

（1）申请人最后执业所在的州、准州、哥伦比亚特区或者国家的执业标准至少与堪萨斯州的执业标准等同。

（2）申请人的原始执照须建立在至少与本州考试具有同等质量的基础上，获得该原始执照所需的及格分数与本州要求的及格分数相当。

（3）申请人的原始执照和所有已核准的执照的日期，以及获得任何执照的日期和地点。

（4）申请人自获发该等执照或者许可后一直积极从事执业活动。委员会可以通过制定定性和定量的执业活动的规则和条例，使之符合积极执业的条件。

（5）申请人具有一定英语沟通能力。

（6）申请人已支付堪萨斯州法第 65－7611 条及其修订案所规定的执照所需的所有费用。

（b）通过背书申请执照的申请人不应当获得许可，除非根据委员会的决定，该申请人的个人资格在本质上等同于堪萨斯州《针灸实践法》下的执照要求。

第 65－7608 条　执照要求的豁免

对于在 2018 年 1 月 1 日或者之前提交申请的申请人，以及在 2017 年 7 月 1 日或者之前提交申请的申请人，委员会将免除教育和考试要求：

（a）已满二十一周岁。

（b）已成功完成中学教育或者其同等学力。

（c）（1）（A）已经完成至少一千三百五十个学时的学习,不包括针灸领域网课学习。

（B）2017 年 7 月 1 日之前五年中的三年参加至少一千五百名患者的针灸实践问诊,具有诊所合作伙伴,诊所主管或者其他委员会批准的个人出具的两份宣誓书,这些人应了解针灸申请人的执业年限和就诊患者数量。委员会可以通过规则和条例,进一步核实申请人的针灸实践情况。

（2）顺利通过委员会核准的针灸考试。

（d）具有一定英语沟通能力。

（e）已支付堪萨斯州法第 65－7611 条及其修订案所规定的所有执照费用。

第 65－7609 条　执照续期日期、维持执照的要求、续期及失效的通知、注销执照、恢复执照和执照的分类

（a）执照于每年 3 月 31 日失效,除非按照委员会规定的方式进行续期。执照续期少于十二个月的情况下,委员会可以按堪萨斯州法第 65－7611 条及其修正案规定的费用比例进行调整。续期申请须填写委员会提供的表格,并须附上规定的费用,费用须在执照续期日期之前缴付。

（b）关于执业执照。委员会有权发放执业执照,只要持证人以委员会提供的表格提出书面申请,并缴纳堪萨斯州法第 65－7611 条及其修订案规定的费用。委员会应当要求每名在职持证人提交证据,证明其顺利完成了委员会所要求的继续教育课程。继续教育的要求应当由委员会通过的规则和条例规定。

（c）在执照续期前,委员会应当要求持证人向委员会提交符合委员会要求的证据,证明持证人持有一份职业责任保险。委员会应当根据规则和条例确定此种职业责任保险的最低承保范围。

（d）委员会应在持证人执照续期日期至少三十日前,以邮件方式通知持证人续期日期,并寄往持证人最后登记的邮寄地址。如果持证人在续期日期前未提交申请并支付续期费,应当通知持证人在续期日期前提交申请并支付费用,如未续期,执照将在续期日期后三十日内认定失效。根据相关规章制度,续期申请和需要缴纳的续期费以及在三十日的期限内不超过五百美元额外的逾期费;如果在三十日的期限内没有收到该两项费用,执照将被依法认定失效,无须进一步诉讼。

（e）任何未能续期而失效的执照,可以在失效后两年内,经委员会推荐、支付到期的续期费用,并证明已符合委员会规定的继续教育要求后恢复其效力。在申请恢复效力前的两年内,没有积极从事针灸实践或者没有参加正式教育课程的人,可能需要完成委员会认为必要的额外测试、培训或者教育,以确认持证人目前具有合理的技能和安全服务的能力。

（f）关于豁免执照。委员会有权向各个持证人颁发豁免执照,只要持证人以委员会提供的表格提出书面申请,并将堪萨斯州法第 65－7611 条规定及其修订案规定的费用及其修订款汇回。委员会可以颁发豁免执照给在堪萨斯州不定期从事针灸实践,也不向公众表明其从事该项实践的人士。豁免执照持证人有权享有与针灸相关的所有特权。豁免执照可以根据本条的规定进行续期。除本款另有规定外,豁免执照应符合《针灸实践法》的所有规定。

豁免执照持证人可以被要求提交本条要求的完成继续教育项目的证据。豁免执照持证人的继续教育,应当由委员会通过的规则和条例规定。豁免执照持证人可以向委员会提交书面申请,申请定期从事针灸实践的执业执照。应当按照要求填写委员会提供的表格,并附上根据堪萨斯州法第 65－7611 条及其修订案规定的执照费用。对于持有豁免执照不到两年的持证人,委员会应采取相应规章制度,为其建立适当的继续教育制度,以便获得在堪萨斯州定期从事针灸实践的执照。对于豁免执照持有超过两年但没有积极从事针灸实践的持证人,委员会认为有必要可以要求其完成执照持证人额外测试、培训或教育以确认持证人目前有能力以合理的技能和安全的技术从事针灸实践。本款的任何内容均不得解释为禁止豁免执照持证人作为以下机构的受薪雇员:(1)堪萨斯州法第 65－241 条及其修正案规定的地方卫生部门。(2)堪萨斯州法第 75－6102 条及其修正案定义的贫困保健诊所。

(g)关于非执业执照。委员会有权颁发非执业执照,只要持证人以委员会提供的表格提出书面申请,并将堪萨斯州法第 65－7611 条及其修订案规定的费用及其修订款汇回。委员会可以颁发非执业执照,给在堪萨斯州不定期从事针灸实践,也不向公众表明其从事针灸实践的人士。非执业执照的持证人不得在该州从事针灸实践。非执业执照可根据本条规定进行续期。除本款另有规定外,非执业执照应符合《针灸实践法案》的所有规定。非执业执照持证人不应当被要求提交第(b)款要求的继续教育项目完成的证据。每个非执业执照持证人可以向委员会提交书面申请,且应当按照要求填写委员会提供的表格,并附上根据堪萨斯州法第 65－7611 条及其修订案规定的执照费用。对于非执业执照持有两年以内的持证人,委员会将通过规章制度,为其建立适当的继续教育要求,以获得在堪萨斯州提供针灸实践的执照。对于持有非执业执照两年以上的人员,委员会认为必要时,可以要求其完成持证人额外测试、培训或者教育以确认持证人目前有能力以合理的技能和安全的技术提供针灸实践。

(h)本条款自 2017 年 7 月 1 日起生效。

第 65－7610 条　被撤销执照的恢复、要求和程序

被吊销执照者,自撤销执照之日起满三年,可以申请恢复执照。申请应当以委员会提供的表格递交,并须附上委员会根据堪萨斯州法第 65－7611 条及其修正案所规定的费用。申请人有责任提供清晰和令人信服的证据,表明其已充分恢复工作状态,以证明恢复执照的正当性。如果委员会决定不予恢复,该人在被拒绝之日起的三年内没有资格再次申请恢复。申请恢复执照的所有程序都应当按照《堪萨斯行政程序法》进行,并应当按照《堪萨斯司法审查法》进行复审。委员会可以根据内部提议,保持撤销执照命令的有效性。

第 65－7611 条　费用由州医疗技术委员会收取

根据委员会制定的规则和条例,委员会应当预先向针灸师收取不可退还的费用,但费用不得超过:

首次申请执照	700 美元
执业执照的年度续期——纸质版	300 美元
执业执照的年度续期——线上版	250 美元

续　表

非执业执照的年度续期——纸质版	200 美元
非执业执照的年度续期——线上版	150 美元
豁免执照年度续期——纸质版	200 美元
豁免执照年度续期——线上版	150 美元
后期续期	100 美元
非执业执照到执业执照的转换	300 美元
豁免执照到执业执照的转换	300 美元
申请恢复被撤销的执照	1 000 美元
执照核证副本	25 美元
执照书面证明	25 美元

第 65 - 7612 条　惩罚费用

委员会应当根据堪萨斯州法第 75 - 4215 条及其修正案的规定,将委员会收到的或者用于委员会的所有费用、收费或者罚款汇给州财务主管。财务主管收到汇款后,应当将全部款项存入州财务库。其中 10% 计入普通基金,其余部分计入医疗费用基金。医疗费用基金的所有支出均应符合《拨款法案》并在账务主管的授权下进行,并根据委员会主席或者主席指定的一名或者多名人士核准的凭证发出报告。

第 65 - 7613 条　针灸咨询委员会成员的任命和任期、会议及报销细则

(a)设立针灸咨询委员会,以协助州医疗技术委员会执行本法。咨询委员会应当由五名成员组成,均为堪萨斯州的公民和居民,任命如下:

(1)咨询委员会须委任一名获发执照从事内科及外科或者整骨治疗的医生为成员。由咨询委员会委任的成员须按委员会的意愿任职。咨询委员会负责人应当委任三名在委任前至少有三年针灸经验,并在本州积极从事针灸实践或者针灸教学的针灸师。其中,应当至少有两名成员从堪萨斯州东方医学协会提交的四名提名者名单中选出。负责人还须从公共部门委任一名并非直接或间接提供保健服务的成员。由咨询委员会负责人任命的成员,应尽可能来自不同区域。

(2)咨询委员会负责人任命的咨询委员会成员任期为四年,直至任命继任者为止。咨询委员会出现空缺职位时,任命机构应当任命一名具有相同资格的人填补空缺,直至任期届满。

(b)咨询委员会应当每年至少召开一次会议,时间由其自行决定,并在主席要求或者咨询委员会成员过半数要求时举行其他必要的会议。

(c)咨询委员会的过半数成员构成法定人数。除非经出席并参加表决的成员有过半数的赞成票,否则咨询委员会不得采取任何行动。

(d)出席咨询委员会会议或者委员会的小组委员会的成员,应当由医疗费用基金支付

堪萨斯州法第 75－3223(e)条及其修正案规定。

第 65－7614 条　咨询委员会的职责

针灸咨询委员会应当就以下事项向州医疗技术委员会提出建议：

(a)考试,执照和其他费用。

(b)为实施本法规定而拟制定的规章制度。

(c)维持执业执照所需的每年继续教育学时数。

(d)针灸领域的变化和新要求。

(e)委员会指派的其他职责。

第 65－7615 条　规章制度

委员会应当颁布必要的规章制度,以管理或者补充本法案的规定。

第 65－7616 条　对持证人的纪律处分、处分理由、程序及调查记录的保密性

(a)持证人的执照可能会被撤销、吊销、限制或者列入察看期。持证人可能会被公开谴责。持证人申请执照、恢复执照的要求可能因存在下列情形而被拒绝:

(1)持证人作出了委员会通过的规则和条例所界定的违反职业道德的行为。

(2)持证人在申请或者取得原始执照、续期执照或者恢复执照时存在欺诈或者谎报的行为。

(3)持证人作出了委员会通过的规则及规例所界定的不称职行为。

(4)持证人被判犯有重罪。

(5)持证人违反《针灸实践法》的任何规定。

(6)持证人违反委员会任何合法的命令或者规章制度。

(7)持证人已被认定患有精神疾病、残疾、因精神失常不予定罪,或者因持证人患有精神疾病或者缺陷而不予定罪,或者没有能力接受有管辖权法院的审判。

(8)持证人未向委员会报告,由于根据本条可构成纪律处分的理由,其他州或者司法管辖区、同行评审机构、卫生保健机构、专业协会或者组织、政府机构、执法机构或者法院对持证人采取的任何不利行动。

(9)持证人由于可能遭受纪律处分的行为和举动,放弃在另一个州或者司法管辖区的针灸执照或者授权,或者已同意限制其在医疗机构的特权,或者放弃其在专业协会或者社团的成员资格。

(10)持证人并未向委员会报告,由于可能遭受纪律处分的行为和举动,其放弃了在另一个州或者司法管辖区的针灸执照,或者放弃在专业协会或者社团的成员资格。

(11)持证人因医疗事故或者类似的行为,遭受不利的判决、裁决或者和解,涉案的相关行为可构成纪律处分的理由。

(12)持证人没有向委员会报告各个因医疗事故责任而受到的不利判决、裁决或者和解事宜,相关的涉案行为可构成纪律处分的理由。

(13)由于身体或者精神疾病,或者使用酒精、毒品或者管制药物,持证人无法以合理的技能和安全的方式对患者提供针灸服务。当合理怀疑存在隐患时,委员会可以根据《堪萨斯州法》第65－2842条及其修正案采取行动。所有与隐患有关的信息、报告、调查结果和其他记录均应保密,不得被委员会程序之外的任何人或者单位发现或者披露。关于保密的条款

将于 2022 年 7 月 1 日到期,除非立法机构在 2022 年 7 月 1 日之前根据《堪萨斯州法》第 45 - 229 条及其修正案审查并重新制定该条款。

(b)委员会裁定违反《针灸实践法案》后,可以采取拒绝申请、拒绝续期、吊销、限制、列入察看期、撤销执照或者其他处罚。根据本法进行的所有行政诉讼应当按照《堪萨斯行政程序法》进行,并应当按照《堪萨斯司法审查法》进行复审。

(c)本条自 2017 年 7 月 1 日起生效。

第 65 - 7617 条　管辖权执行程序、相关规定及紧急裁决令

(a)委员会拥有诉讼管辖权,可以对根据《针灸实践法案》执业的任何持证人实施纪律处分。采取此类行动应当符合《堪萨斯行政程序法》。

(b)在正式指控提出前后,委员会及持证人可以订立一项对双方具有约束力的规定,委员会可以根据该等规定提出其事实调查结果及执行令,而无须就有关个案提出任何正式指控或者举行听证。基于某一规定的执行令可以命令对同意订立该规定的持证人采取任何纪律处分。

(c)如果委员会确定有理由相信需要对持证人实施纪律处分,并且持证人的继续行为将对公共健康和安全构成紧迫的危险,则委员会可以根据《堪萨斯行政程序法》下的紧急裁决令规定吊销或者暂时限制其执照。

(d)本法规定的任何机构行为的司法审查和民事执行应当符合《堪萨斯司法审查法》。

第 65 - 7618 条　非纪律处分决议及程序

委员会或者委员会小组可以执行与堪萨斯州法第 65 - 2838(a)条及其修正案规定的执业针灸师有关的非纪律处分决议。

第 65 - 7619 条　行政罚款

除《针灸实践法案》规定的其他罚款外,州医疗技术委员会在进行通知和听证后,可以对违反《针灸实践法案》的持证人进行民事罚款,第一次罚款不超过两千美元,第二次罚款不超过五千美元,第三次和任何后续罚款不超过一万美元。按照《堪萨斯州法》第 7575 - 4218 条及其修正案的规定,所有根据本条评估和收取的罚款均应当汇给州财务主管。财务主管收到每笔汇款后,应当将全部款项存入州财务库,计入普通基金。根据本条收取的罚款应当按照《美国法典》第 11 章第 523 条规定被视为行政罚款。

第 65 - 7620 条　申诉及有关报告、记录或者信息的保密及例外情况

(a)委员会收到、获取或者维护的与申诉有关的任何诉求或者报告、记录或者其他信息均应当保密,委员会或其员工不得以识别或者能够识别信息主体或者来源人员的方式披露,但以下可能披露的情形除外:

(1)在委员会根据法律规定进行的任何程序中披露,或在对进入程序的委员会命令的上诉中披露,或者向程序或上诉的任何当事方或该方的律师披露。

(2)向作为信息主体的人员披露,或者在信息主体提出要求时向任何个人或者单位披露,但委员会可能要求以防止识别信息主体或任何其他来源人员的方式披露。

(3)向对信息主体具有司法管辖权的州或者联邦许可、监管或者执法机构披露,或者向对根据本法构成诉讼理由的类似行为有管辖权的机构披露。

(b)除非法律另有授权,否则委员会根据本条授权披露的任何机密申诉或者报告,记录或者其他信息不得由接收机构重新披露。

（c）这一关于保密的条款将于 2022 年 7 月 1 日到期,除非立法机关在 2022 年 7 月 1 日之前根据堪萨斯州法第 45－229 条及其修正案审查并重新制定该条款。

第 65－7621 条　举报涉嫌渎职事件、民事豁免权及何时豁免

（a）善意地向州医疗技术委员会报告信息的人,不得因为此类举报而遭受民事损害赔偿诉讼。即使报告者与委员会授权、注册或者认证的人员的相关纪律处分、能力、品性、专业资格或者渎职行为等存在关联。

（b）由获得针灸执照的人员及其各个委员会的个人成员组成的州、地区或者地方协会,向州医疗技术委员会或者其各个委员会或者代理人,基于善意调查或者传达了有关持证人、注册人或者证书持有人的与涉嫌渎职事件有关的信息,或者资格、能力或者品性,或者纪律处分诉讼的有关信息,将免于因此遭受民事诉讼。前提是此类调查和信息传递是基于善意的,并且不把任何缺乏依据的情形作为事实加以描述。

第 65－7622 条　针灸师及患者的特权

（a）根据《堪萨斯州法》第 60－427 条及其修正案,执业针灸师和患者之间的保密关系和通信与医生和患者之间的保密关系和通信是建立在相同的基础上的。

（b）本条款自 2017 年 7 月 1 日起生效。

第 65－7623 条　对违法行为的禁令

（a）任何人违反各项条款时,委员会可以以州的名义向具有司法管辖权的法院提起诉讼,要求对这种违反行为下达禁令,而不考虑是否已经或者可能向委员会提起诉讼,或者是否已经或者可能提起刑事诉讼。

（b）本条款自 2017 年 7 月 1 日起生效。

第 65－7624 条　法案的可分割性

如果《针灸实践法案》规定的适用被认定为无效,并不应当影响《针灸实践法案》其他规定在不适用无效规定的情况下生效。因此,《针灸实践法案》的各项规定是可分割的。

堪萨斯州针灸行政法[①]

第 100－76－1 条　费用

（a）委员会应当收取以下费用：

（1）执照申请费	165 美元
（2）执业执照的年度续期费：	
（A）线下续期	150 美元

① 根据《堪萨斯州行政法规机构》第 100 卷第 76 章"针灸师"译出。

续　表

（B）线上续期	125 美元
（3）非执业执照的年度续期费：	
（A）线下续期	125 美元
（B）线上续期	100 美元
（4）豁免执照的年度续期费：	
（A）线下续期	125 美元
（B）线上续期	100 美元
（5）非执业执照转换为执业执照	75 美元
（6）豁免执照转换为执业执照	75 美元
（7）逾期续期费：	
（A）线下续期	50 美元
（B）线上续期	25 美元
（8）恢复作废执照申请费	165 美元
（9）恢复被撤销执照申请费	500 美元
（10）执照的认证副本费	20 美元
（11）执照的书面证明费	20 美元

（b）如果在第一个年度续期执照之前,执业针灸师的初始执照期限为六个月或不足六个月,首次年度续期费用应按比例收取,满月或不足月的每月为十美元整。

第 100 - 76 - 2 条　颁发执照的考试

通过考试申请执照的申请人须提供以下或者委员会确定的具有同等效力的文件:

（a）顺利完成国家针灸与东方医学认证委员会（NCCAOM）或者委员会确定的申请人完成考试时与 NCCAOM 标准等同的单位提供的认证考试的文件。认证考试应当包括以下内容:

（1）东方医学基础。

（2）穴位取穴针灸。

（3）生物医学,于 2005 年以前完成 NCCAOM 认证或者同等学力的申请人不需要进行生物医学部分的考试。

（b）由针灸与东方医学学院委员会（CCAOM）或者 NCCAOM 颁发的洁针技术证书（CNT）副本。

第 100 - 76 - 3 条　放弃参加考试和接受教育的资格

（a）根据《堪萨斯州针灸法案》（2017）第 65 - 7608 条及其修正案,对于在 2018 年 1 月 1

日或者之前提交申请并提供以下文件材料的申请人,委员会应当放弃关于教育及考试的某些先决条件:

(1)证明申请人在针灸领域已经完成了不少于一千三百五十个学时的课程学习、获批的学徒计划或者辅导课程,或者以上课程的组合(不包括在线学习)。学时证明可以通过完成以课程为基础的项目、获批的学徒计划、辅导课程,或者以上课程的组合,以满足 NCCAOM 的标准或者任何由委员会确定的与 NCCAOM 具有同等效力的单位所要求的标准。为证明已顺利完成要求,申请人应当提交以下材料:

(A)(1)证明学徒的导师在其从事针灸实践的州获得了针灸执照,或者是拥有执照的针灸专科医生。

(2)由指导学徒计划或者辅导课程的导师保存的笔记、记录或者其他文件的副本,提供学徒计划使用的教育材料的文件,并记录学时数和涵盖的科目。

(B)学校正式成绩单。

(2)从 CCAOM、NCCAOM 或者委员会确定的与以上两者具有同等效力的单位获得的当前洁针技术(CNT)证书的证明文件。

(3)证明申请人从事针灸实践,在过去五年中有三年完成至少一千五百次诊疗。申请人须提供下列任何一项文件供委员会复核:

(A)至少两名曾与申请人一起从事针灸实践人员的宣誓书,包括营业机构合伙人、诊所主管和委员会核准的其他人员。

(B)过去三年内取得的继续教育证书副本。

(C)申请人的患者预约簿副本。

(D)申请人的患者病历副本。

(b)申请人须提供委员会要求的任何额外文件。

第 100‐76‐4 条　豁免执照及从事专业活动的说明

(a)申请豁免执照的,应当在申请中指明该人在获得豁免执照后将从事的与针灸实践相关的所有专业活动。

(b)持有豁免执照的个人从事的专业活动应当限于以下情况:

(1)履行同行评审、实用评审、专家意见等行政职能。

(2)无偿提供直接的患者护理服务或者无偿提供监督、指导、咨询。本款不得禁止豁免执照持有人领取生活津贴或者提供这些服务而产生的实际和必要的开支。

(c)持有豁免执照的人,在执照续期时,应当在续期申请上指明该人在续期期间将从事的与针灸实践相关的所有专业活动。

(d)要求在豁免执照的申请或续期申请中对专业活动进行修改的,应当在三十日内将修改情况告知委员会。修改申请应当以委员会提供的表格提交。

(e)持有豁免执照不到两年的针灸师,要求获得执业执照,应当按照本法第 100‐76‐6 条中的规定,提交证明文件,证明其在前一年已完成至少十五个面授学时的继续教育。

(f)违反第(a)款、第(c)款或者第(d)款中规定的行为,均应当构成堪萨斯州针灸法案(2017)第 65‐7616 条及其修正案规定的违反职业道德行为的初步证据。

第100-76-5条 职业责任保险及申请执业执照

(a) 申请执业执照的人应当连同申请一起向委员会提交证明文件,证明该人已获得堪萨斯州针灸法案(2017)第65-7609条及其修正案要求的职业责任保险,其中对于每项索赔,该保险的责任限额至少为二十万美元,保险期间的所有索赔的年度赔偿总额总计至少为六十万美元。

(b) 执业针灸师应当向委员会提交年度执照续期申请,证明针灸师持续保持且目前持有第(a)款规定的职业责任保险。

(c) 执业针灸师在提交变更为执业执照的申请时,应当连同申请一起向委员会提交针灸师目前持有第(a)款规定的职业责任保险的证明文件。

第100-76-6条 继续教育

(a) 除(b)款规定的情形外,执业针灸师应当在偶数年的每次续期日期前的二十四个月内,完成最少三十个面授学时的获批的继续教育。

(b) 执业针灸师在续期日期前不足十二个月即须接受继续教育时,无须在第一个续期期间提交第(A)款所规定的完成继续教育的证明。执业针灸师在执照续期日期前持有执照一年以上但不超过两年的,应当在持有执照期间完成至少十五个面授学时的获批的继续教育。

(c) 执业针灸师应当保存完成所有继续教育活动的证明文件,有效期为活动完成日期起计的五年内。委员会可以要求申请人提供完成第(a)款及第(b)款所规定的继续教育活动的证明。

(d) 执业针灸师如因有实证的健康状况、自然灾害、配偶或者直系亲属死亡,或者任何其他类似情况而不能符合第(a)款或者第(b)款的规定,委员会可以根据针灸师的要求,给予最长六个月的延期。每项要求应当包括完成所规定的继续教育活动的计划。

(e) 面授学时应当包括五十分钟获批的继续教育活动。面授学时的计算不包括用餐和休息。

(f) 所有继续教育活动应当与针灸实践有关,并属于下列任何一项:

(1) 临床技能。

(2) 临床技术。

(3) 为患者、家庭、卫生专业人员、卫生专业学生或者社区提供服务时的教育原则。

(4) 卫生保健和卫生保健提供系统。

(5) 问题处理、批判性思维、医疗记录保存和道德规范。

(6) 政策。

(7) 生物医学课程。

(8) 研究。

(g) 继续教育活动应当包括下列内容:

(1) 提供的产品。"产品"系指 NCCAOM 批准的、NCCAOM 附属机构批准的或者与NCCAOM 标准基本同等的单位批准的任何产品,或者委员会批准的其他产品,但不受本条中(g)(9)(A)项规定的限制。

（2）讲座。"讲座"系指在听众面前进行的以教学为目的的现场演讲。

（3）专家组。"专家组"系指由多位专业人士就某一特定主题提出多项意见，但不视为最终解决方案。

（4）研讨会。"研讨会"系指为深入研究、工作或者讨论某一特定感兴趣领域而设计的一系列会议。

（5）培训会。"培训会"系指在某一特定感兴趣领域的有指导性的高级研究或者讨论。

（6）专题讨论会。"专题讨论会"系指为从不同观点讨论某一特定主题而组织的一次以上的会议，由不同的发言者参加。

（7）在职培训。"在职培训"系指员工在受雇期间所接受的，仅与提高在患者的评估、检查或者治疗中所需的针灸技能有关的教育讲座。

（8）行政培训。"行政培训"系指提高针灸师在质量保证、风险管理、报销、法律要求或者索赔程序等方面知识的介绍。

（9）自我指导。"自我指导"系指下列任何一种：

（A）阅读专业文献。每个继续教育周期最多奖励四个面授学时。执业针灸师应当保存继续教育活动期间阅读的所有专业文献的日志。

（B）完成 NCCAOM 或者 NCCAOM 附属机构或者由委员会确定的与 NCCAOM 标准基本同等的单位批准的函授、音频、视频或者互联网课程，或者由委员会批准的任何其他继续教育课程，并由提供该课程的个人或者组织提供完成的书面证明。

（10）继续教育活动展示。"继续教育活动展示"系指符合本款要求的继续教育活动的准备及展示。每展示一个学时，将授予三个面授学时。

（h）在四十八个月内重复进行的继续教育活动，不得计入继续教育面授学时。

第 100‐76‐7 条　违反职业道德的行为及定义

堪萨斯州针灸法案（2017）第 65‐7616 条及其修正案和委员会规定中使用的术语，应当具有本法中所规定的含义：

（a）"违反职业道德的行为"系指以下任一行为：

（1）利用欺诈、虚假广告招揽患者，或者自称为执业针灸师代理人进行牟利的。

（2）向患者声称明显无法治愈的疾病、病症或者损伤可以永久治愈的。

（3）未经患者或者其法定代理人同意，协助护理或治疗患者的。

（4）在信笺或者广告中使用任何字母、词汇或者术语作为词缀，或者以其他方式表明该人有资格从事该委员会或者其他州执照委员会或者机构规定的职业，但该人未获取执照的。

（5）故意泄露隐私的。

（6）以夸大的方式宣传专业优势或者提供专业服务的。

（7）发布保证提供专业服务或者提供无痛专业服务的广告的。

（8）从事与针灸实践有关的可能欺骗、诈骗或者危害公众利益的行为。

（9）对针灸师在治疗疾病或者其他身体或精神病症方面的技能或者其所规定的治疗或者疗法的效果或者价值作出虚假或者误导性陈述。

（10）与患者或者负责有关患者的医疗决策的人发生任何性虐待行为、不当行为或者其他利用诊疗关系进行的不当性接触。

（11）在与针灸实践有关的任何文件中使用任何虚假的、欺诈性的或者欺骗性的陈述，包括故意伪造或者欺诈性地更改患者记录。

（12）通过欺诈、欺骗或者虚假陈述获得任何费用。

（13）不按照患者本人或者其法定代理人的要求将患者的病历转交给其他针灸师的。

（14）进行不必要的化验、检查或者无正当目的提供服务。

（15）对提供的服务收取过高费用。

（16）多次未能达到合理谨慎的针灸从业者认为在类似条件和情况下可接受的治疗水平。

（17）未能保存准确记载每位患者病史、有关发现、检查结果和化验结果的书面病历。

（18）将专业责任委派给某人，且针灸师知悉或者有理由知悉该人在培训、经验或者执照方面不具备履行职业责任的资格。

（19）未能适当地监督、指导或者委托构成针灸实践的行为，而这些行为是根据执业针灸师的指导、监督、命令、转诊、委托或者实践协议进行的专业服务。

（20）在申请、取得初始执照、续期执照、恢复执照过程中欺诈或者谎报的。

（21）故意或者多次违反法令、任何实施条例或者卫生和环境部长发布的关于针灸实践的任何条例。

（22）非法从事受委员会规管而针灸师未获发相应执照的职业。

（23）未报告或者披露根据《堪萨斯州针灸法案》（2017）第65－7621条及其修正案要求报告或者披露的内容。

（24）未向委员会及其调查人员、代表提供委员会依法要求提供的资料。

（25）因可能构成根据委员会规则或者本章规定采取纪律处分的理由而招致同行评审委员会、政府机构或者部门或者专业协会或学会的任何制裁或者纪律处分的。

（26）未按照《堪萨斯州针灸法案》（2017）第65－7609条及其修正案和本规则第100－76－5条的要求维持职业责任保险。

（27）在理赔表、单据、报表上故意作出误导、欺骗、不真实或者欺诈性陈述。

（28）开出一张虚假支票，或者停止使用借记卡或者信用卡支付委员会合法应得的费用或者款项。

（29）因故意或者过失丢弃病历。

（30）违反患者信任，利用诊疗关系谋取私利的。

（31）妨碍委员会调查的，包括从事下列一项或者多项行为：

（A）伪造或者隐瞒重大事实。

（B）故意作出或者使他人作出任何虚假或者误导性的声明或者书面陈述的。

（C）作出任何其他可能欺骗或者欺诈委员会的行为。

（b）"广告"系指为直接或者间接诱导或者可能诱导专业服务的购买而以任何方式或者方法传播的所有陈述。

（c）"虚假广告"系指在实质性方面具有虚假、误导性或者欺骗性的任何广告。判断广告是否具有误导性，应当考虑以下因素：

（1）以陈述、文字、设计、装置或者声音或者其任何组合作出建议或者描述。

（2）广告在陈述中未能揭示重要程度的事实。

第 100‑76‑8 条　不称职行为的定义

《堪萨斯州针灸法案》（2017）第 65‑7616 条及其修正案和委员会规定中使用的术语"不称职行为"指以下任一情况：

（a）存在一项或者多项不遵守适用的护理标准的情况，经委员会确定，构成重大过失。

（b）存在多次不遵守适用的护理标准的情况，经委员会确定，构成一般疏忽。

（c）执业模式或者有其他事实表明其不能从事针灸实践。

第 100‑76‑9 条　患者病历的完整性

（a）每名执业针灸师应当为其提供专业服务的每名患者保存内容充分的记录。

（b）每一份患者记录应当符合以下要求：

（1）清晰。

（2）仅包含类似针灸师可以理解或者应当理解的术语和缩写。

（3）有充分的患者身份证明。

（4）注明提供各项专业服务的日期。

（5）包含与患者病情相关的所有临床相关信息。

（6）记录已获得、实施或者要求进行的检查、生命体征和检验及其结果。

（7）写明患者最初寻求针灸实践的原因和最初诊断。

（8）说明已进行或者建议进行的治疗。

（9）在治疗期间记录患者的病情。

（10）包含从其他卫生保健提供者处收到的所有患者病历，如果这些病历构成针灸师作出治疗决定的依据。

（c）除非整个患者病历是由针灸师自行书写，否则每项记录均须由记录人加以核实。

（d）每一份患者病历应当包含任何拟作为最终记录的文字，一旦这些信息转换为最终记录后，即不应当要求保留草稿、笔记、其他文字或者记录。最终记录应当准确反映向患者提供的护理和服务。

（e）为法案和本规则之目的，如果满足以下两个条件，患者的电子病历应当被视为书面病历：

（1）电子病历内的每一项均经针灸师核证。

（2）电子病历中的条目经核证后不得更改。

第 100‑76‑10 条　公开的记录

（a）执业针灸师在收到患者签署的授权书后，应当向患者、患者指定的另一针灸师或者患者的法定代理人提供一份患者记录的副本，除非法律允许扣留记录或者法律禁止提供记录。

（b）执业针灸师可以向个人或者单位收取检索或者复制患者记录的合理费用。针灸师不得以提前支付这些费用为条件向另一名针灸师提供患者记录。

（c）根据《堪萨斯州针灸法案》（2017）第 65‑7616 条及其修正案，违反该项规定的行为均构成违反职业道德的初步证据。

第 100 - 76 - 11 条　免费提供

为患者提供免费检查、服务或者程序的执业针灸师只能执行指定的检查、服务或者程序。在进行任何额外检查、服务或者程序之前，执业针灸师应当解释检查、服务或者程序的性质和目的，并尽可能向患者明确披露额外检查、服务或者程序的费用。

第 100 - 76 - 12 条　与患者的商业交易及违反职业道德的行为

（a）非健康相关商品或者服务。执业针灸师在经常从事针灸实践的地点向患者出售非健康相关产品或者服务的，除非本款另有准许，否则构成违反职业道德的行为。执业针灸师出售非健康相关产品或者服务的，如同时符合下列所有条件，不构成违反职业道德的行为：

（1）销售是为了公益组织的利益。

（2）销售没有直接或者间接给针灸师带来经济收益。

（3）没有患者受到不当影响而购买。

（b）商业机会。在符合下列所有条件的情况下，执业针灸师构成违反职业道德的行为：

（1）针灸师招募或者招揽患者参与涉及销售产品或者服务的商业机会，或者招募或招揽其他人参与商业机会。

（2）销售产品或者服务直接或者间接给针灸师带来经济收益。

（3）针灸师在患者出现在其经常从事针灸实践的地点时，随时招募或者招揽患者。

密 苏 里 州

密苏里州针灸法[①]

第 324.475 条　定义

第 324.475 条至第 324.499 条的术语含义如下:

(1)"针灸"系指通过刺穿皮肤将针头插入人体的治疗方法,以及通过控制和调节体内能量的流动和平衡来评估、评价、预防、治疗或者减缓各种生理或者疼痛的相关方式,以使身体恢复正常的功能和健康状态。

(2)"针灸师"系指根据第 324.475 条至第 324.499 条获得执照,实施本条第(1)款规定的从事针灸实践的人。

(3)"耳穴戒毒技师"系指专门接受耳穴戒毒疗法培训,并且只从事耳穴戒毒疗法的人。耳穴戒毒技师应当在获得执照的针灸师的监督下执业。此种治疗应当在医院、诊所或者治疗机构内进行,这些机构应提供包括综合药物滥用服务咨询并具有所有必要和适用的执照和证书。

(4)"耳穴戒毒疗法"系指一种有限制性的程序,将针灸针插入因吸毒、酗酒或同时吸毒和酗酒而接受治疗者的外耳特定穴位。

(5)"委员会"系指根据第 331 章规定的脊医考试委员会。

(6)"咨询委员会"系指密苏里针灸咨询委员会。

(7)"部门"系指商业保险部。

(8)"主管"系指专业注册主管。

(9)"处"系指专业注册处。

(10)"执照"系指由委员会为从事针灸实践的人员颁发的授权文件。

第 324.478 条　密苏里州针灸师咨询委员会成立以及其职责、成员和任期

1. 在专业注册处内部创建一个"密苏里州针灸师咨询委员会"。该咨询委员会由五名成员组成,所有成员均为美国公民和密苏里州已登记选民。咨询委员会成员由专业注册处

---

① 根据《密苏里州法律汇编》注释版第 22 卷第 324 编"针灸"专章译出。

主管任命,任期四年,本条第 2 款另有规定的除外。其中的三名成员必须是针灸师,且应当始终持有该州的针灸执照,符合第 324.475 条至第 324.499 条的许可要求的第一咨询委员会成员除外。其中一名成员应当是密苏里州脊医考试委员会的现任成员,其余成员均为公众成员。所有成员均须从专业注册处主管提交的名单中选出。在位的密苏里州针灸协会会长应当在委员会成员(公众成员除外)任期届满前至少九十日,或者在委员会出现空缺后尽快向专业注册处主管提供一份由五名资质合格并且愿意填补空缺的针灸师名单,并列出要求和建议,以供选择。密苏里州针灸协会应当在其送文函中说明协会选择候选人的方式。

2. 针灸咨询委员会最初任命的五名委员,其中三名委员任期分别为一年、两年和三年;另外两名委员的任期为四年。

3. 咨询委员会的公众成员不得是且从未是受第 324.475 条至第 324.499 条监管的专业人士或者此类人员的配偶;不得且从未与该专业服务或与其直接相关的活动或组织存在重大性经济利益关系。

4. 咨询委员会的任何成员存在如渎职、不称职、不道德或者不诚实的行为,专业注册处主管可将其免职。咨询委员会成员去世、辞职、取消资格或者被免职时,主管应当委任一名继任者。继任者只能在任期未届满时填补。

5. 针灸师咨询委员会应当:

（1）审查所有执照的申请。

（2）就有关针灸师的执照事宜,向委员会提出建议。

（3）审查所有的投诉和/或者调查中有可能违反第 324.475 条至第 324.499 条或者法规的行为,向委员会提供建议,以便委员会针对投诉采取进一步行动,包括建议向检察官或者巡回检察官起诉违反第 324.475 条至第 324.499 条的行为。

（4）在执行公务时,应当遵守委员会行政惯例程序的规定。

（5）在需要和委员会提出要求时,协助委员会根据第（3）款的建议而展开的任何调查或者纪律处分程序。

第 324.481 条　委员会的职责、制定规则的权力以及创立、使用针灸师基金

1. 委员会将根据咨询委员会的建议,向符合针灸师资格、申请针灸执照并支付针灸执照所需所有费用的申请人颁发执照。

2. 委员会应当:

（1）保存关于第 324.475 条至第 324.499 条的所有委员会和咨询委员会会议记录以及该州所有获得针灸执照的针灸师记录。

（2）每年准备一份本州所有获得针灸执照的针灸师姓名和地址的名册,并应当向任何支付复制件费用的人提供该名册的副本。

（3）确定名册费用的数额足以支付出版和分发名册的实际费用。

（4）加盖公章。

（5）确定根据第 324.475 条至第 324.499 条向所有申领针灸执照的人士提供的表格。

（6）确定根据第 324.475 条至第 324.499 条颁发的针灸执照的样式。

（7）通知执照持有人政策、规则或者规章的变化。

（8）根据咨询委员会的建议,依规设置执行第 324.475 条至第 324.499 条规定的所需的费用。

3. 经咨询委员会批准,委员会可以:

（1）发出传票,强制证人在诉讼中作证或者出示证据,拒绝颁发、吊销或撤销针灸执照。

（2）根据第 536 章颁布规则执行第 324.475 条至第 324.499 条的规定,包括但不限于下列规定:

（a）针灸的实施标准。

（b）针灸服务的道德行为标准。

（c）继续专业教育标准。

（d）耳穴戒毒技师的培训和实践标准,包括具体列举可能使用的特定穴位。

4. 根据第 536.010 条中的定义,为管理和执行第 324.475 条至第 324.499 条而颁布的各项规则或者部分规则,只有在机构完全符合第 536 章的所有要求时,包括但不限于第 536.028 条(如果适用的话),才会自 1998 年 8 月 28 日起生效。如果第 536.028 条的规定适用,则本节的规定是不可以分割的,如果根据第 536.028 条授予大会的任何审查、推迟生效日期、否决和废除一项规则或者规则的一部分的权力被认为是违反宪法或者无效的,则所谓的规则制定权力的授予以及规则制定命令中如此提议和包含的各项规则将无效。但是本条不得影响在 1998 年 8 月 28 日以前通过及公布的规则的效力。

5. 委员会根据第 324.240 条至第 324.275 条的规定收到的所有资金均应由主管收取并将资金转交税务局存入国库,记入特此设立的"针灸师基金"。

6. 尽管第 33.080 条的规定与此相反,在两年期结束时,该基金的数额超过上一财政年度针灸师基金拨款数额的三倍之前,不得将该基金中的资金转入一般收入的贷方。超过前一财政年度针灸师基金中的拨款的适当倍数后,此数额不再有效。

第 324.484 条　获得针灸豁免执照的人士

1. 第 324.475 至 324.499 条不得解释为适用于根据第 334.010 条至第 334.265 条获发执照的医生或者根据第 331 章获发执照的脊椎按摩医生。此类医生无论其是否持有经络疗法现行证书,只要其使用的头衔是"执业针灸师",都将适用第 324.475 条至第 324.499 条的规定。

2. 任何耳穴戒毒技师均不需要获得针灸执业执照,只要其在持证针灸师的监督下,根据第 324.475 条至第 324.499 条颁布的规定,仅实施第 324.47 条规定的耳穴戒毒疗法。耳穴戒毒技师不得在耳穴或者身体的各个其他穴位插入针灸针,也不得使用"执业针灸师"的头衔。

第 324.487 条　获得针灸执照的条件

1. 除下列人士外,任何人在本州从事针灸实践均属违法行为:

（1）持有委员会根据第 324.475 条至第 324.499 条颁发的有效执照。

（2）从事委员会批准的咨询委员会授权的监督学习课程,并清楚表明学员身份的头衔,且在获得执照的针灸师的监督下进行。

2. 申请人在本州内从事针灸实践,需要具备的条件包括:

（1）年满二十一周岁,具有被国家针灸与东方医学认证委员会认证的针灸文凭。

（2）以咨询委员会规定的形式向咨询委员会提出申请。

（3）支付适当的费用。

3. 委员会应当向每一位符合本条第 2 款规定的个人颁发执照,以证明持证人在本州合法从事针灸实践。持证人在进行针灸实践时,应当始终持有根据第 324.475 条至第 324.499条颁发的执照。

第 324.490 条　到期执照

1. 根据第 324.475 条至第 324.499 条颁发的执照每两年续期一次。续期申请应当连同适当的续期费用一并提交本部门。

2. 在有效期届满日或者届满日前未续期的针灸执照无效。可以根据第 324.493 条的规定恢复执照。

第 324.493 条　恢复执照的程序

任何未能在该针灸执照到期日或者到期日前续期的针灸师,可以按以下方式恢复该执照:

（1）如果申请人在最后一份执照期满后两年内向咨询委员会提出续期申请,则应当支付适当逾期费并按规则提供咨询委员会要求的所有文件。

（2）如果申请人在最后一份执照期满两年后向咨询委员会提交续期申请,则需要支付适当逾期费,并按照第 324.487 条第 2 款第(1)项和第(2)项的规定重新申请。

第 324.496 条　委员会的权力、投诉程序及责任限制

1. 根据咨询委员会的建议,委员会可以拒绝根据第 324.475 条至第 324.499 条的规定颁发、续期或者恢复任何执照,理由可以是本条第 2 款所述情形的一种或者多种。委员会须书面告知申请人拒绝的理由,并告知其有权根据第 621 章的规定向行政听证委员会投诉。

2. 根据咨询委员会的建议,委员会可以根据第 621 章的规定,基于以下理由的一项或者多项,针对未能续期或者放弃执照的人向行政听证委员会提出申诉:

（1）该人由于违反第 324.012 条规定的职责,根据州、美国或者其他国家的法律规定,在刑事诉讼中被最终裁决、认定有罪,或者认罪或不抗辩,无论其是否判刑。

（2）为取得第 324.475 条至第 324.499 条规定的执照,或者为获得参加第 324.475 至324.499 条规定的考试资格,使用欺诈、欺骗、谎报或者贿赂的手段。

（3）通过欺诈、欺骗或者谎报获得或者试图获得酬劳、费用、学费或者其他报酬。

（4）在履行第 324.475 条至第 324.499 条所规定的专业职能或者职责时,存在不称职、行为失当、重大疏忽、欺诈、失实陈述或者不诚实的情形。

（5）违反或者协助他人违反第 324.475 条至第 324.499 条的规定,或者根据前述规定所采用的规则或者制度。

（6）冒充或者允许他人使用学校、认证单位颁发的证书、毕业证书。

（7）对其他州、地区、联邦机构或者国家根据第 324.475 条至第 324.499 条规定授予的执照持有人或者其他从事该职业的权利的惩戒,理由是该州授权撤销或者暂停。

（8）最终被有管辖权的法院裁定为精神失常或者不称职的。

（9）基于实质性的错误事实颁发执照的。

（10）对公众或者主要受众使用虚假、误导、欺骗性的广告或者招揽方式。

（11）使用第 195 章所界定的管制药物或者酒精类饮品，达到了足以损害从事第 324.475 条至第 324.499 条规定执照持有人的执业能力的。

3. 任何个人、组织、协会或者公司出于善意且无过失地，根据第 324.475 条至第 324.499 条的规定向商业和保险部、委员会或者咨询委员会报告或者提供资料，不得因此被提起民事损害赔偿诉讼。

4. 依照本条第 2 款提出申诉后，程序应当依照第 621 章的规定进行。在行政听证委员会发现本条第 2 款所述的情节成立的情况下，委员会可以根据咨询委员会的建议，采取商业和保险部认为适宜的下列纪律处分：谴责、列入察看期、吊销或者撤销其执照。

第 324.499 条　违规、罚款及起诉的权利

1. 任何人违反第 324.475 条至第 324.499 条的规定，即属 B 类轻罪。

2. 因违反第 324.475 条至第 324.499 条规定提供服务而收取的所有费用或者其他补偿，应予以退还。

3. 为执行第 324.475 条至第 324.499 条的规定，委员会可以代表咨询委员会在该州的各个法院以自己的名义提起诉讼。委员会可以调查咨询委员会所提述的任何涉嫌违反第 324.475 条至第 324.499 条的行为，并可以依据第 324.475 条至第 324.499 条的规定就本条规定的罚款提起诉讼。

4. 根据委员会的申请，州司法部长可以代表委员会要求有管辖权的法院发出禁制令、限制令或者其他适当的命令，禁止相关当事人的下列行为：

（1）提出从事或者从事任何需要注册证书、授权、许可或者执照的业务活动，但是需要证明该种活动是在没有注册证书、授权、许可或者执照的情况下进行或者提议的。

（2）从事根据第 324.475 条至第 324.499 条颁发的注册证书或者主管机关、许可证或者执照授权的各种业务，前提是证明持有人具有严重损害该州任何居民或者被许可人的客户或者患者的健康、安全或者福利的重大可能性。

5. 根据本节提起的诉讼可以是对第 324.475 条至第 324.499 条所规定的各种处罚的补充或者代替，并且可以与其他旨在强制执行第 324.475 条至第 324.499 条的规定同时提起诉讼。

密苏里州针灸行政法[①]

第一节　总　　则

第 20 CSR 2015－1.010 条　申诉的管理及处置

目的：本条规定了接收、处理和处置控告和申诉请求的程序。

（1）所有申诉应当以书面形式提交给密苏里州针灸咨询委员会，密苏里州杰斐逊市密苏里州大道 3605 号，邮政信箱 1335 号，邮编 65102，并确定申诉人的姓名和地址。口头交流

---

① 根据《密苏里州行政法规》第 20 卷"部门"第 2015 章"针灸师咨询理事会"译出。

或者电话联络将不会被视为证据或者作为申诉处理依据。申诉人应当提交一份书面声明。针灸师咨询委员会的成员不得在担任该职务期间向咨询委员会提出申诉,除非该成员不参与咨询委员会对申诉后续事项的进一步审议或者活动。任何部门工作人员或者咨询委员会,均可以与任何公众成员相同的方式根据本条提出申诉。

(2)在收到适当形式的控诉后,州脊医考试委员会(以下简称委员会)或者咨询委员会可以调查被申诉的持证人、申请人、注册人或者未经许可的个人或者实体的行为。根据本条收到的每项控诉均须以书面形式予以承认,并将申诉的最终处理情况告知申诉人。

(3)咨询委员会将保留根据本条收到的每一项申诉。申诉文件将包含如下每位申诉人的记录:姓名和地址;申诉的主题;咨询委员会收到每份申诉的日期;申诉的简要陈述,包括因所称行为或者做法而受伤或者受害的人的姓名;以及申诉的最终处理结果。

第 20 CSR 2015 - 1.020 条　针灸师的执业证书,姓名和地址的更改

目的:本条规定了执业针灸师使用的头衔以及持证人信息维护要求。

(1)执业针灸师应当使用缩写 L.AC.,或者在执业者姓名后使用 Licensed Acupuncturist 作为执照头衔,确保该执照使用了合法的称谓。

(2)姓名或者地址已变更的持证人应当在变更后三十日内更新变更信息:

(A)名称变更需要提供授权名称变更的文件副本,普通邮件至密苏里州杰斐逊市邮政信箱 1335,传真 573/751/0735 或者电子邮件通知咨询委员会。

(B)销毁含有先前名称的执照。

(3)执业针灸师只能使用在第 20 CSR 2015 - 4.020 条中规定的合法教育机构获得的与针灸相关的教育证书。

第 20 CSR 2015 - 1.030 条　费用

目的:本条规定了针灸师咨询委员会的各种费用和收费。

(1)所有费用应当通过银行本票、个人支票、汇票或者本部门获批的其他方式支付,并支付给针灸咨询委员会。

(2)执照颁发后,一旦被收回、吊销或者撤销,不退还任何费用。

(3)费用规定如下:

(A)针灸师申请费为二百美元。

(B)针灸师两年一次的续期费一百美元。

(C)指纹识别费将由密苏里州高速公路巡警确定。

(D)支票账户资金不足管理费,二十五美元。

(E)逾期续期费五十美元。

(4)费用可以由咨询委员会自行决定退还给申请人或者持证人,申请人或者持证人可以向咨询委员会提交书面请求,解释应退还费用的原因。

第二节　颁发针灸执照的条件

第 20 CSR 2015 - 2.010 条　申请执照

目的:本条涉及针灸师申请执照应当符合的条件。

（1）执照申请应当根据针灸师咨询委员会提供的表格提出。申请可以通过书面请求向密苏里州 65102 －杰斐逊市 672 号信箱咨询委员会提出，或者致电（573）751 －1655 的咨询委员会办公室或者通过电子邮件 acupunct@ mail.state.mo.us 联系咨询委员会。

（2）申请书应当用黑色印刷，署上签名、经公证后，并附上咨询委员会要求的所有文件和 20 CSR 2015 －1.030（3）（A）中规定的申请费。文件包括且不限于以下内容：

（A）录入两组指纹。指纹背景检查的所有费用应当由申请人直接支付给密苏里州高速公路巡警或者其批准的供应商。

（B）证明申请人须年满二十一岁，由以下一种方式证明。

1. 美国州或者司法管辖区签发的驾照或者身份证（ID），身份证包括照片和出生日期。

2. 联邦、州或者地方政府机构或者实体签发的身份证，身份证包括照片和出生日期。

3. 美国的州、县、市当局或者司法管辖区签发的印有公章的出生证明的核证复印件。

4. 美国公民身份证，包括出生日期。

5. 作为美国居民公民使用的身份证，包括出生日期。

（3）根据国家针灸与东方医学认证委员会（NCCAOM）认证的执照申请人，应当视为 NCCAOM 确认的执业针灸专科医生。申请人负责授权 NCCAOM 的验证事宜，并通知咨询委员会。

（A）在美国以外的学校学习或者接受培训的执照申请人，如果获得 NCCAOM 的针灸证书，可以被认为符合这些规则。

（4）在美国其他州或者司法管辖区颁发的执照、认证或者注册证书基础上申请执照，申请人应当遵守本条第（1）款和第（2）款的规定，并提交以下文件：

（A）针灸师直接向咨询委员会办公室提供的、美国监管机构的州或者管辖机构有关执照、认证或者注册文件的验证文件，应当包括：

1. 申请人的执照状态。

2. 执照原颁发日期和执照是否失效情况。

3. 执照的有效期。

4. 有关任何申诉、调查或者纪律处分的信息。

第 20 CSR 2015 －2.020 条　执照续期、恢复和继续教育

目的：本条概述了执照的续期和恢复的要求，以及保持执照有效所需的继续教育。

（1）执照应当在到期日或者之前，提交填妥的续期申请表格，提交续期费用。持证人未收到通知和续期执照的申请，并不能免除持证人基于本州针灸法第 324.487 条的义务。

（2）有效期到期日后收到执照的续期表格和费用的，执照不再生效，持证人在缺乏有效执照的情形下继续执业的，应视为违反了本州针灸法第 324.475 条至第 324.499 条的规定，并应接受处罚。

（3）在执照到期之前，作为执照续期的条件，执业针灸师应当在两年的执照期内完成三十个学时的继续教育。继续教育应当与针灸实践有关，并包括普遍的预防措施、感染控制和心肺复苏（CPR）认证。在获得执照的第一年内不受此限。

（4）在执照到期的两年内，当事人可以申请恢复执照。应当按照第 20 CSR 2015 －2.010

条的标准提交申请,交付所需的费用,其中包括根据第 20 CSR 2015－2.020(3)条的标准完成继续教育的证明文件。

（5）违反本条的任何规定,均应作为根据本州针灸法第 324.496 条给予纪律处分的理由。

第三节　实践标准,道德规范,专业行为

第 20 CSR 2015－3.010 条　实践标准

目的：本条规定执业针灸师的实践标准。

（1）强烈鼓励执业针灸师投保职业责任保险。

（2）每个针灸师应当：

（A）根据本州针灸法第 324.475 条中定义的教育和培训范围内从事针灸实践。

（B）在所有有关针灸实践和广告的文件上披露针灸师的法定名称。

（C）在提供与针灸有关的免费服务或者折扣时,报价应当清楚、显著地说明,相关服务是否可能产生额外费用及其范围。

（D）在执业地点张贴执照或者向患者提供执照文件。患者系指接受本州针灸法 324.475(1)中定义的针灸治疗的任何个人。

（E）在提供最初的针灸服务之前,以书面形式记录患者的评估信息。书面的患者评估信息应当包括但不限于以下内容：

1. 本次就诊的目的。

2. 疼痛的存在和位置以及持续的情况。

3. 过敏情况和目前使用的药物及用药目的。

4. 患者是否由卫生保健或者精神保健专业人员照护。

5. 手术史。

6. 签署的治疗同意书及签署日期。

7. 告知患者有关的费用和预计费用。

（F）在每次会见中更新患者病历。更新的病历信息应当包括但不限于以下内容：

1. 患者评估的变化或补充信息。

2. 提供针灸服务的日期和类型。

3. 针灸师的签名,以及提供针灸服务的耳穴戒毒技师或针灸学员的姓名(如适用)。

（G）提供有关预期疗程的当前信息。

（H）保障病历的维护、保存和处理,未经授权者不得查阅。

（I）提供服务时,告知患者保密的例外情形。

（3）针灸师不得将针灸职责委托给没有资格或者没有针灸执照的人。

（4）为本规则之目的,针灸师应当在服务日期后保存患者病历至少五年,若其他适用法律或者法规要求的时间超过五年,则保存期限应不低于此期限。

（5）如果执业针灸师终止在密苏里州的执业,持证人应当在停止执业前至少三十日书面通知患者。患者或者患者选择的其他执业针灸师可以获得患者病历。如果持证人存在无

法遵守此规定的正当理由,则咨询委员会可以放弃三十日的要求。

(6)如果要由针灸学员或者耳穴戒毒技师提供服务,应当事先告知患者。

(7)在执业针灸师的指导下,针灸师、耳穴戒毒技师和针灸学员应当遵循全国针灸基金会发布的洁针技术(CNT)标准,并遵循普遍的预防措施。

(A)为了本规则之目的,"普遍预防措施"是由疾病控制中心(CDC)定义的一种感染控制方法。根据普遍预防措施的概念,所有人类血液和某些体液都被视为已知具有人类免疫缺陷病毒(HIV)、乙型肝炎病毒(HBV)和其他血源性病原体的传染性。

(8)所有一次性针头应当根据美国劳工部、职业安全与健康管理局(OSHA)的规定,在使用后立即处理,并放置在生物有害回收容器中。

(9)当使用可重复使用的针头时,应当采用基本的双重灭菌程序方案。全国针灸基金会出版的《洁针技术手册》概述了该方案的具体程序。

(10)每个患者就诊后,所有不穿透皮肤、直接接触针头或者由橡胶或者塑料制成的设备都应当使用抗菌产品。

第 20 CSR 2015-3.020 条　道德规范

目的:本条为申请人和针灸师确立了道德规范。

(1)所有申请人和持证人应当:

(A)在针灸专业中表现出诚信、支持客观性和培养信任感的行为。

(B)诚实、正直地开展与针灸有关的业务和活动。

(C)尊重和保护患者/客户的法律和个人权利,包括获得知情同意、拒绝治疗的权利,并避免危及患者的健康、安全或者福利。

(D)拒绝参与违法、不道德的行为,或者拒绝隐瞒他人的违法、不道德、不称职行为。

(E)在进行研究时,应当遵守联邦、州和地方的法律或者法规,以及与人类受试者研究相关的伦理程序的适用标准。

(F)遵守所有有关针灸实践的州和联邦法律和法规。

(G)不允许因追求经济利益或者其他个人利益而妨碍正确的专业判断和技能的运用。

(H)在法律允许的范围内,向咨询委员会报告所有已知的或者怀疑的违反有关针灸实践的法律法规的行为。

(2)针灸师不得:

(A)鼓励不必要或者不合理的针灸服务。

(B)对患者、耳穴戒毒技师或者学员实施任何口头或者身体虐待行为。

(C)剥削患者、耳穴戒毒技师或者学员,以获得经济利益。本条所称的"剥削"系指针灸师、患者、技术人员或者学员之间存在的,可能对患者、技术人员或者学员造成伤害的任何关系。

(D)接受旨在影响转诊、决定或者治疗的礼物或好处,主要是为了个人利益。

(E)在与患者建立持续的职业关系期间或者在该职业关系终止后六个月内,与患者、学员或者耳穴戒毒技师发生性行为。

第四节　耳穴戒毒技师和针灸学员的监督

第 20 CSR 2015－4.010 条　对耳穴戒毒技术人员的监督

目的：本条概述了对监督耳穴戒毒技师的要求。

（1）耳穴戒毒技师（以下简称技师）只能在耳郭内插入和摘除针灸针。技师插入针的点仅限于国家针灸戒毒协会（NADA）或者咨询委员会批准的其他国家实体所描述和定位的神门、肺、肝、肾和交感神经点。

（2）对技师进行监督时，执业针灸师每月应当与技师进行至少四小时的监督会议，当技师提供第 20 CSR 2015－4.010(1)条中定义的服务时，可以通过电话或者对讲机在现场提供督导。

（A）每月至少两小时面对面的监督，每次监督会议不少于连续五十分钟，包括观察技师耳郭插针的过程。

（B）每月其余的两小时监督会议可以是面对面的或者通过电子通信，包括电话联系、互联网，如电子邮件、录像带，或者通过互联网同时进行的视觉和口头互动。

（3）执业针灸师在确定其能够安全有效监督的技师数量时，必须做出专业判断，以确保其始终提供高质量的服务。

（4）技师的职责必须由执业针灸师确定和监督，不得超过被监督的耳穴戒毒技师的培训水平、知识、技能和能力。针灸师可以只把非评估性的、非评估导向的、非任务选择性的或者非推荐的特定任务委托给技师。

（5）对技师进行监督时，执业针灸师只负责监督耳穴戒毒程序。当提及技师的操作程序时，应当只使用"auricular detoxification"（耳穴戒毒）或者"auricular detox"（耳穴戒毒）的术语。

（6）技师应当履行的职责或者职能不包括且不限于：

（A）对针灸服务的转诊或处方的解释。

（B）评估程序。

（C）制定、计划、调整或者修改针灸疗程。

（D）在任何患者直接护理中需要判断或者决策时代表针灸师。

（E）独立或者在缺乏执业针灸师监督的情形下实施针灸。

第 20 CSR 2015－4.020 条　对针灸学员的监督

目的：本条概述了对针灸学员的监督要求。

（1）针灸学员应当在执业针灸师的直接监督下，对公众提供针灸治疗。本条所称的直接监督系指对学生全程的控制、指导、教学和管理。

（2）为获得学员资格，个人应当报名参加咨询委员会授权的学习课程，且不得就学员提供的针灸治疗收取报酬。

（3）由针灸及东方医学教育审核委员会（ACAOM）认证的针灸项目被认为是合法针灸培训计划。

（4）未经 ACAOM 认证的课程，应当包括至少三个学年的课程，至少一百〇五个学期学分或者一千九百〇五学时的学习。课程应当包括以下内容：

（A）四十七个学期学分七百〇五学时的相关东方医学理论、针灸诊疗技术及相关研究。

（B）二十二学期学分，六百六十学时。

（C）生物医学临床科学的三十学期学分，四百五十个学时。

（D）六个学期的咨询、沟通、道德和实践管理学分达九十学时。

（5）针灸学员的职责应当由执业针灸师监督，并且不得超过被监督人的培训水平、专业知识、专业技能和能力。在针灸服务机构中，执业针灸师对针灸学员的行为或者行动负责。

密歇根州

密歇根州针灸法[①]

第 333.16501 条　定义

（1）下列定义适用于本法：

（a）"指压"系指将压力施加在身体的各个穴位上的一种物理疗法。

（b）"针灸"系指针刺穿人体皮肤的过程和操作。针灸包括但不限于激光针灸、电针、刺痛疗法、干针和肌肉刺激疗法。

（c）"针灸师"系指根据本法获得针灸执照从事针灸实践的个人。

（d）"拔罐"系指将一个特殊设计的杯子放置在身体上以产生吸力的医疗手法。

（e）"刮痧"系指在身体的润滑区域上使用光滑的工具反复、定时、单向按压的动作。

（f）"食疗咨询"系指根据东亚医学理论，向患者提供健康食物选择和健康饮食习惯建议的过程。

（g）"干针"系指使用毫针穿透皮肤或者皮下组织，仅针对肌筋膜激痛点和肌肉和结缔组织，以此来影响身体结构和功能的变化，并且评估和管理神经肌肉骨骼疼痛和运动损伤的一种康复过程。干针不包括刺激耳穴或者其他穴位。

（h）"东亚医疗技术"包括但不限于：针灸、推拿治疗、艾灸、热疗、食疗咨询、复健运动、穴位按压、拔罐、刮痧、顺势疗法、生活方式指导和中药治疗。

（i）"热疗"系指利用热进行治疗，例如利用热缓解疼痛和进行保健。

（j）"草药"系指内服或外用植物或者植物提取物、矿物或者动物药，但不是第 17708 条定义的处方药。

（k）"顺势疗法"系指使用来自植物、矿物和动物的高度稀释的天然药物的疗法。

（l）"生活方式指导"系指根据东亚医学理论，就健康的生活方式选择和习惯向患者提供建议的过程。

（m）"推拿治疗"系指对身体施加精确控制的、指向明确的手法力量的疗法，不包括对

[①]　根据《密歇根州法律汇编》注释版第 333 卷第 15 编第 165 章"针灸"译出。

脊柱施加的高速、低幅度的推力。

（n）"艾灸"系指一种在皮肤表面或者附近焚烧干燥的植物艾蒿的治疗形式。

（o）"针灸实践"，系指利用传统和当代东亚医学理论对患者进行评估和诊断，制定治疗患者的计划，以及通过东亚医学技术治疗患者的行为，第（2）款另有规定的除外。

（p）"脊椎按摩实践"系指第 16401 条所定义的术语。

（q）"推拿疗法实践"系指第 17951 条所定义的术语。

（r）"执业"系指第 17001 条所定义的术语。

（s）"骨科医学和外科疗法"系指 17501 条中定义的术语。

（t）"理疗实践"系指 17801 条中定义的术语。

（u）"注册针灸师"系指在根据第 16525 条颁布的规则生效日期之前根据本章注册或者以其他方式获得授权的个人。

（v）系统针灸教育包括针灸科学与理论基础、经穴定位、针刺技术、诊疗方法、患者管理等内容的教育课程。

（w）"复健运动"系指一系列有助于恢复和建立身体力量、耐力、灵活性、平衡和稳定性的身体活动。

（2）为本章之目的，针灸实践不包括内科、正骨疗法及外科手术、物理疗法、职业疗法、足科医学和足科手术、护理、牙科、推拿疗法或者脊椎按摩疗法实践。

（3）除本章的定义外，《密歇根州法律汇编》注释版第 333 卷第 1101 条以下内容包含了适用于法典所有条款的一般定义和解释原则，第 161 章包含了适用于本章的定义。

第 333.16511 条　词汇、头衔和字母的使用

（1）除本章另有规定外，自第 16525 条颁布的关于许可等规则的生效日期起，除非根据本章授权使用本章规定的词汇，其他个人不得使用"针灸师""认证针灸师""注册针灸师""执业针灸师""L.Ac"等词汇、称谓或头衔。然而，在根据第 16525 条颁布的关于执照的规则生效之日起不超过三十六个月的时间内，注册针灸师可以在没有获得本章规定的执照的情况下继续使用"针灸师""注册针灸师"或"认证针灸师"的头衔并从事针灸实践。

（2）除本章另有规定外，自第 16525 条颁布的执照规则生效之日起，除非根据本章授权使用本章规定的词汇，其他个人不得使用"针灸师""认证针灸师""注册针灸师""执业针灸师"等词汇、头衔，或者表明该人是针灸师的类似词汇或者缩写。

（3）自第 16525 条颁布的执照规则生效之日起，本章不适用于下列任何一项：

（a）根据第 170 章或者第 175 章获得执照的医生。

（b）由国家针灸戒毒协会认证的个人。

第 333.16513 条　执照要求及适用性

（1）自第 16525 条颁布的执照规则的生效之日起，个人不得从事针灸实践，除非其具有根据本章颁发的执照或者本条的其他授权。

（2）除根据第 16171 条获得豁免外，自第 16525 条颁布的执照规则生效之日起，本章不适用于下列任何一项：

（a）除第（e）款另有规定外，根据任何其他章或法案取得执照、注册或者获得其他授权

的个人，如果从事的活动属于针灸执业范围，且该个人没有使用第 16511 条保护的词汇、头衔或者字母，则该个人从事的活动属于针灸执业范围。

（b）根据第 170 章或者第 175 章规定，如果该医生已完成总计不少于三百个学时的系统针灸教育，包括不少于一百个学时的针灸现场讲座、示范和受监督的临床培训，则该医生具备获得执照的资格。

（c）满足下列要求的个人：

（i）满足由国家针灸戒毒协会或者委员会确定为继受机构的组织认证颁发的针灸戒毒专家培训证书所需要求。

（ii）只使用由国家针灸戒毒协会或者委员会确定为继受机构的组织制定的有关预防药物滥用和听觉治疗方案。

（iii）当使用第（ii）项所述的方案时，应当在一名针灸师，或者根据第 170 章或者第 175 章的规定获得执照的医生的监督下进行。

（iv）没有使用第 16511 条保护的词汇、头衔或者字母。

（d）当个人从事穴位按压、拔罐、刮痧、食疗咨询、热疗、草药、顺势疗法、生活方式指导、推拿疗法、复健运动等具有既定标准和道德规范的职业时，若这些服务未被指定为或者暗示为针灸实践，则其不得使用受第 16511 条所保护的头衔、词汇或者字母。

（e）由根据任何其他章规定取得执照、注册或以其他方式授权的个人在其执业范围之内从事干针疗法。

第 333.16515 条　颁发针灸执照和受限执照及资格

（1）除第（2）款和第（3）款另有规定外，监管部门应向满足第 16174 条要求以及第 16525 条规定的执照要求的申请人颁发执照。

（2）在第 16525 条规定的有关执照的规则生效日期后三十六个月届满日或者之前，监管部门应当向符合第 16174 条和第 1 条以及符合以下要求的申请人颁发执照：

（a）申请人为注册针灸师。

（b）根据第 16525 条颁布的执照规则的规定，申请人应当具有与针灸实践相适应的教育、培训和经验。在确定申请人是否符合本款项下的执照要求时，监管部门在与委员会协商后，应颁布相关规定，确定提交给委员会的患者记录、账单记录、教育记录、培训记录或其他申请人教育、培训和经历证明的考量标准。申请人应当确保提交给本款项下监管部门的各个文件中患者身份的保密性。

（3）在根据第 16525 条颁布的有关执照的规则生效之日后三十六个月届满或者之前，监管部门应当向符合第 16174 条要求的申请人颁发受限执照，并且该申请人在申请时应当满足以下所有要求：

（a）自加入本条的修正法案生效之日起，申请人至少在根据第 170 章或者第 175 章获得执照的医生的监督下从事针灸实践两年。申请人应当在受限执照申请表上注明从事针灸实践的医生姓名。

（b）申请人持有从事其他卫生保健职业的执照。

（4）根据第（3）款获得受限执照的个人须遵守下列所有规定：

（a）受限执照持证人只可以在受限执照申请书所指明姓名的医生的严格监督下从事针灸实践，如申请书所指明的医生不再愿意或者不能监督该持证人，该持证人应当立即通知监管部门。

（b）受限执照持证人不得就针灸执业范围内的服务向保险人收取费用。在本款中，"保险人"系指1956年《保险法》第106条、1956年颁布的第218页中定义的术语。

第333.16517条　针灸执照或受限执照的续期、颁布的规则及继续教育需求

（1）尽管有第161条的规定，监管部门在与委员会协商后，应当颁布相关规定，要求申请执照续期执照的持证人向监管部门提供符合要求的证据，证明在申请续期前的执照周期内，持证人参加了与针灸实践相关的继续教育课程或计划，该课程或计划是由委员会批准的，旨在对持证人进行进一步教育。如果监管部门确定该个人符合国家针灸戒毒协会和东方医学认证委员会的继续教育标准或者委员会确定的同等标准，则该个人视为符合本款规定的继续教育要求。

（2）根据第16204条的规定，在与委员会协商后，监管部门应颁布相关规定，要求续期执照的申请人完成适当学时的疼痛和症状控制课程，作为第（1）款所要求的教育课程或计划的一部分。

（3）除了本条的继续教育要求外，监管部门还应要求申请续期根据第16515（3）条取得受限执照的申请人在申请续期执照时同时持有从事另一卫生专业的执照，以此作为续期受限执照的条件。

第333.16521条　针灸委员会的创建以及委员会成员

（1）密歇根州针灸委员会在监管部门成立，由以下十三名有投票权的成员组成，每位成员都应满足第161章的要求：

（a）七名针灸师，或者是在第16525条颁布的规则生效之日起的三十六个月内获得执照的七名注册针灸师。根据本条任命的成员必须符合第16135条规定的要求。

（b）根据第170章或者175章取得执照的三名医生中至少有一名符合第16513（2）（b）条的要求。

（c）三名公众成员。

（2）除获委任以填补空缺的成员外，本部设立的委员会成员的任期至第16122条规定的届满年度的6月30日届满。

第333.16525条　颁布的规则及执照标准

（1）在至2021年3月4日的期限内，监管部门应当与委员会协商，颁布有关针灸执照最低标准的规定，并为针灸实践实施执照方案。在颁布第16515（1）条的规定时，监管部门在征询委员会意见后，可参考国家认证机构委员会认可的认证计划颁布的专业标准。在颁布第16515（2）（b）条的规定时，监管部门在征询委员会意见后，应考虑申请人是否已完成包括针灸现场讲座、示范和受监督的临床培训在内的系统针灸教育。

（2）2020年3月3日生效的关于针灸师注册的规则持续有效，直至第（1）款颁布的规则生效日期。

第333.16529条　第三方补偿或劳工补偿

根据本条规定，不要求执业针灸师承担新的或额外第三方补偿以及强制性补偿。

密歇根州针灸行政法①

第一节 总 则

第 R338.13001 条 定义

（1）下列定义适用于本法：

（a）"委员会"系指根据《公共卫生法》第 16521 条（MCL333.16521）创建的密歇根州针灸委员会。

（b）"法典"系指《公共卫生法》1978 PA 368，第 MCL333.1101 条至第 333.25211 条。

（c）"部门"系指许可和监管事务部（以下简称监管部门）。

（2）法典中定义的术语在本法中使用时具有相同的含义。

第 R338.13002 条 识别人口贩运受害者的培训标准及要求

（1）根据法典第 16148 条（MCL333.16148），申请、注册执照或者已经通过注册获得执照的个人应当完成识别符合以下标准的人口贩运受害者的培训：

（a）培训内容包括：

（i）了解美国境内人口贩运的类型和场所。

（ii）在卫生保健机构查明人口贩运的受害者。

（iii）识别成人和未成年人卫生保健机构中贩运人口的警告标识。

（iv）报告疑似人口贩运受害者的信息。

（b）可接受的培训机构或者培训方法包括：

（i）由国家或者州认可的卫生保健机构提供的培训。

（ii）由州或者联邦机构提供或联合提供的培训。

（iii）在经委员会批准的、针对初次获得执照或者注册的培训计划，或者由学院或者大学批准的培训计划。

（iv）阅读一篇符合本条第（a）项规定的、发表在同行评审期刊、卫生保健期刊或者专业或科学期刊上的关于识别贩运人口受害者的文章。

（c）可接受的培训方式包括：

（i）电话会议或者网络会议。

（ii）在线演示。

（iii）现场演示。

（iv）印刷或电子媒体。

（2）监管部门可以在所有成员中任选一名，审核其所提供的材料，并要求其提供完成培训的证明文件。经部门审核后，当事人须提供可接受的完成培训证明，包括下列任何一项：

---

① 根据《密歇根州行政法典》第 338 卷"针灸—总则"专章译出。

（a）培训机构出具的完成证书证明,包括日期、培训机构名称、培训名称和个人姓名。

（b）个人声明。该声明必须包括有关人士的姓名及下列任何一项:

（i）根据本条第(1)(b)(i)项至第(iii)项完成的培训,需要说明培训的日期、培训提供者以及培训计划的名称。

（ii）根据本条第(1)(b)(iv)项完成的培训,需要说明文章的标题、作者、同行评审期刊、卫生保健期刊或者专业或科学期刊的出版物名称,以及出版物的日期、卷数和发行(视情况而定)。

（3）根据法典第 16148 条(MCL333.16148),本条第(1)款中规定的要求适用于 2018 年 7 月 2 日开始的执照续期申请人和 2021 年 4 月 22 日开始的初始执照申请人。

第 R338.13003 条　远程医疗

（1）针灸师在根据法典第 16284 条(MCL 333.16284)提供远程医疗服务前,须取得同意。

（2）提供远程医疗服务的针灸师,应当符合以下两项规定:

（a）在其执业范围内行事。

（b）采用与传统现场医疗服务相同的卫生保健标准。

第 R338.13004 条　采用标准

国家针灸与东方医学认证委员会(NCCAOM)关于针灸和东方医学的国家能力标准的文件《NCCAOM 认证手册》于 2019 年 1 月 1 日生效,该标准由委员会批准并引用。该文件可以在执照及监管事务部查阅及分发,每页收费十美分,地址:密歇根州兰辛市渥太华西街 611 号,邮政信箱 30670,邮编 48909,也可以登录 NCCAOM 免费网址 www.nccaom.org 查看。

第二节　颁 发 执 照

第 R338.13005 条　密歇根州注册针灸师执照的颁发及要求

自本法颁布之日起,在颁布后的三十六个月内,该部门应向除符合本法的所有要求外,同时满足以下两项要求的申请人颁发执照:

（a）用监管部门提供的表格递交填妥的申请,随附所需费用。

（b）目前在本州注册为针灸师。

第 R338.13006 条　非 NCCAOM 认证的针灸师执照;要求

（1）在本法颁布后的三十六个月内,监管部门应当为符合本法典要求,填妥表格并且提交所需费用的申请人颁发执照。

（2）申请人须向委员会证明,其已经具备根据法典第16515条及第16525条(MCL 333.16515 和 333.16525)规定的获取执照所需的教育、培训及经验。申请人须符合下列各项规定:

（a）申请人应当通过提交其教育记录、培训记录或者申请人教育和培训的其他可验证的证明,包括现场讲座、演示和受监督的针灸临床培训,以证明其完成了至少一千二百四十五学时的系统针灸教育,该术语的定义见法典第 16501(1)(v)条(MCL 333.16501)。

（b）申请人须证明获得针灸和东方医学学院委员会的洁针技术认证。

（c）申请人应当通过提交或者同时提交患者病历、账单记录,以证明在执照申请日期之前的四年内,每年平均为 50 名或者更多的患者提供针灸服务。申请人应当确保患者所提交的每一份文件均妥善地保护了患者隐私。

（3）如果根据本条提交的文件是英文以外的语言,则必须提交原始的正式译文。

第 R338.13007 条　NCCAOM 认证的针灸执照颁发及要求

自本法颁布之日起,监管部门向除满足法典的所有要求外,同时符合以下要求的申请人颁发执照:

（a）用监管部门提供的表格递交填妥的申请,并随附所需费用。

（b）提交给监管部门可接受的证明,证明其目前已被 NCCAOM 认证为针灸文凭或者东方医学文凭。

第 R338.13008 条　受限执照相关要求及限制

（1）自本法颁布之日起三十六个月内,监管部门应当向符合法典规范要求和下列条件的申请人颁发受限执照:

（a）申请人提供文件证明,在 2020 年 3 月 4 日之前,其在法典第 170 节(MCL 333.17001 至 333.17097)或法典第 175 节(MCL 333.17501 至 333.17556)授权的医生的监督下从事针灸实践至少两年。

（b）申请人提交一份由部门提供的表格,其中包含督导医生的姓名和签名,确认承担了法典第 16109(2)条(MCL 333.16109)规定的监督责任。

（c）申请人在申请时持有《医疗卫生法典》第 16105(2)条(MCL 333.16105)所定义的从事其他医疗卫生职业的执照。

（2）受限执照持证人应当遵守下列规定:

（a）仅在根据本条第(1)(b)项认定的医生的监督下从事针灸实践。

（b）如根据本条第(1)(b)项认定的医生不再愿意或者不能监督受限执照持证人,应当通知监管部门。

（i）如果督导医生不再愿意或者不能监督受限执照持证人,则受限执照持证人不得提供针灸服务,直至根据法典第 170 节或第 175 节持有执照的新督导医生进行担保,并且新督导医生已符合本条第(1)(b)项的要求,且已向部门提交表格,表格中包含督导医生的姓名和签字,并确认承担该守则第 16109(2)条(MCL 333.16109)所规定的监督责任。

（ii）如果根据法典第 170 节或者 175 节取得执照的督导医生身份不明,则受限执照不能续期。

（c）受限执照持证人不得就针灸执业范围内的服务向保险人收取费用。

第 R338.13010 条　以背书方式颁发执照及要求

（1）以背书方式申请针灸执照的申请人,除满足法典规定以外,还须填妥由监管部门提供的表格,随附所需的费用,并须同时符合以下两项条件:

（a）在提出执照申请之日,以背书方式向监管部门证明其持有来自另一州的信誉良好的执业执照或注册资格。

（b）向监管部门提交其目前被 NCCAOM 认证为针灸或者东方医学文凭的证明。

（2）申请人信誉良好的执照或注册资格,应当由执照或者注册证书颁发的州执照或注册机构验证。如条件允许,验证材料应包含对申请人采取或尚未决定的纪律处分的相关记录。

第 **R338.13015** 条　接受未经审核的培训的申请人及要求,已撤销

第 **R338.13020** 条　针灸师注册的续期及要求,已撤销

第 **R338.13025** 条　针灸师重新注册的申请及要求

执照失效的申请人可以在提交下列文件后,重新获得执照:

	(1) 密歇根州执照已失效,现持有另一个州或者加拿大执照的针灸师	失效 0~3 年	失效 3 年以上
(a)	以部门提供的表格提交填妥的申请,并附上所需的费用	√	√
(b)	确定其具有 1974 年 PA381 节第 1 至 7 条(MCL338.41 至 338.47)所定义的良好品德	√	√
(c)	根据法典第 16174(3)条[MCL333.16174(3)]的要求提交指纹		√
(d)	提交在申请前的两年内,按照第 R338.13026 条和第 R338.13028 条完成三十个学时的继续教育的证明	√	√
(e)	申请人的执照或注册必须经过州执照或注册机构的验证,且申请人在该州持有或曾经持有针灸执照或者注册。如条件允许,验证材料应当包括对申请人采取的纪律处分或者尚未决定的纪律处分的相关记录	√	√
	(2) 密歇根州执照已失效,且目前没有另一个州或者加拿大执照的针灸师	失效 0—3 年	失效 3 年以上
(a)	按部门提供的表格提交填妥的申请,并随附所需的费用	√	√
(b)	确定其具有 1974 年 PA381 节第 1 至 7 条(MCL338.41 至 338.47)所定义的良好品德	√	√
(c)	根据法典第 16174(3)条[MCL333.16174(3)]的要求提交指纹		√
(d)	提交在申请前的两年内,按照第 R338.13026 条和第 R338.13028 条完成三十个学时的继续教育的证明	√	√
(e)	持有 NCCAOM 认证的现行有效的针灸文凭或者东方医学文凭		√
(f)	申请人的执照或者注册必须经过州执照或注册机构的验证,且申请人在该州持有或曾经持有针灸执照或者注册。如条件允许,验证材料应当包括对申请人采取的纪律处分或者尚未决定的纪律处分的相关记录	√	√

第三节　执照续期,受限执照的续期以及继续教育

第 **R338.13026** 条　针灸师执照的续期、续期受限执照的要求、限制及豁免请求

(1)根据法典第 16517 条(MCL 333.16517),执照或者受限执照的续期申请人应当根据

本条,在执照到期前的两年期间内,累计接受经过委员会的批准的三十个学时与针灸服务相关的继续教育。

（2）根据法典第 16204（2）条和第 16517（2）条（MCL 333.16204 和 333.16517）,执照或者受限执照的续期申请人,应当在每个执照周期内积累至少五个学时与针灸服务相关的疼痛和症状管理所需的继续教育学时数。

（3）续期受限执照的申请人,除满足本条第（1）和（2）款的要求外,还应当满足下列所有条件：

（a）根据法典第 16517（3）条（MCL 333.16517）,申请人在申请时应当持有法典第 16105条（MCL 333.16105）所定义的从事其他卫生职业的执业执照,作为续期其受限执照的条件。

（b）除为续期其他卫生职业执照而累积的继续教育学分外,申请人还须累积本条第（1）款和第（2）款所规定的继续教育学分。

（c）申请人应当提交一份由监管部门提供的表格,其中包含其督导医生的姓名和签字,确认该医生在前一个执照周期内履行了第 16109（2）条（MCL 333.16109）所要求的监督责任,并同意在下一个执照周期内履行这些监督责任。

（4）提交续期申请视作申请人遵守本条的证明。申请人应当自申请执照续期之日起保留符合本条要求的文件,期限为四年。委员会可以要求申请人提交证据以证明其遵守了本条规则。未遵守本条规则即构成违反第 16221（h）条（MCL 333.16221）的规定。

（5）在执照到期日前,监管部门必须收到根据法典第 16205 条（MCL 333.16205）的规定提出的豁免申请。

（6）在一个执照周期内获得的继续教育学分,不得延续到下一个执照周期。

（7）申请人在同一执照周期内完成同一活动两次,无法获得继续教育学分。

第 R338.13028 条　可接受的继续教育及要求

（1）委员会将获 NCCAOM 批准的一项课程或活动,作为一次专业拓展活动（PDA）。一个 PDA 学分相当于一个学时的继续教育学分,可累计计算以符合第 R 338.13026 条的要求。

（2）根据法典第 16517（1）条（MCL 333.16517）,符合 NCCAOM 继续教育标准的个人符合执照续期的继续教育要求。

（3）如果申请人不符合本条第（2）款的要求,其应当通过参加 NCCAOM 批准的课程或者活动,以积累不少于 30 个继续教育学分。

第 R338.13030 条　教育计划标准及采用参考,已撤销

第 R338.13035 条　委托代理及监督

针灸师应当根据法典第 16104 条、第 16109 条和第 16215（3）条[MCL 333.16104、333.16109和 333.16215（3）]的规定,在对抗疗法医师或者整骨疗法医师和外科医师的授权下执业。

第 R338.13040 条　病历的保留、处置及保密——已撤销

第 R338.13045 条　禁止的行为——已撤销

明 尼 苏 达 州

明尼苏达州针灸法[①]

第 147B.01 条　定义

1. 适用性。本条中的定义适用于本章。

2. 穴位按压。"穴位按压"系指按压穴位。

3. 针灸实践。"针灸实践"系指运用东方医学理论和其独特的诊疗方法,形成的一套完整的医疗保健体系。它的治疗技术包括将针灸针插入皮肤以及使用其他生物物理方法进行穴位刺激,包括使用热疗,推拿,电刺激,草药补充疗法,膳食指南,呼吸技巧,和基于东方医学原理的功法。

4. 针灸针。"针灸针"系指专门以针灸为目的而设计的针。针灸针有实心的针体,锥形的针尖,厚度为 0.12 毫米到 0.45 毫米。由不锈钢、金、银或者其他经委员会批准的材料制成,这些材料应当按照国家疾病控制和预防中心的建议进行消毒。

5. 穴位。"穴位"系指根据公认的针灸参考文献所定义的具体解剖学描述的位置。相关信息列在国家针灸与东方医学认证委员会认证考试的学习指南中。

6. 针灸医师。"针灸医师"系指根据本章获得针灸执照的人员。

7. 委员会。"委员会"系指医疗服务委员会及其指定机构。

8. 本条根据 2002 年立法的第 375 章第 3 条第 11 款的规定废止。

9. 呼吸技巧。"呼吸技巧"系指作为治疗计划的一部分,教给患者的东方呼吸功法。

10. 拔罐。拔罐疗法系指使用一个罐子形状的器械附着在皮肤上,通过使用吸力产生负压。

11. 刮痧。"刮痧"系指使用表面光滑、无尖端,且可以消毒的,或者一次性使用的工具,配合使用外用药膏在皮肤表面摩擦。

12. 针灸学位证书。"针灸学位证书"系指认可 NCCAOM 的道德规范,并经 NCCAOM 认证,达到 NCCAOM 规定的能力标准,并拥有现行有效的 NCCAOM 证书的人。现行有效

[①]　根据《明尼苏达州议会法》注释版第 147B 章"针灸执业者"译出。

的 NCCAOM 证书表明顺利完成了继续教育的专业发展,并且已经满足了 NCCAOM 的要求。

13. 电刺激。"电刺激"系指用 0.001 至 100 毫安的电流或者委员会批准的其他电流刺激穴位的方法。电刺激可以通过将设备连接到针灸针上来使用,也可以在不穿透皮肤的情况下经皮使用。

14. 中草药疗法。"中草药疗法"系指在患者的治疗过程中使用中草药作为补充的疗法。

15. 本条根据 2002 年立法的第 375 章第 3 条第 11 款的规定废止。

16. NCCAOM。"NCCAOM"系指美国国家针灸及东方医学认证委员,一个根据《国内税收法典》第 501(c)(4)条组织的非营利性法人机构。

16(A)NCCAOM 认证。"NCCAOM 认证"系指 NCCAOM 授予达到 NCCAOM 认证的针灸或者东方医学的能力标准的人。

17. 晕针。"晕针"系指一种短暂的恶心和头晕的状态,这是针头插入时的一个潜在副作用,当针被取出时就会完全恢复。

18. 东方医学。"东方医学"系指一种医疗体系,它将身体能量的循环和平衡视为个人健康的基础,是一种通过专门的方法,分析人体能量状态,并运用针灸等相关方法对人体进行治疗,以强身健体、改善能量平衡、维持或者恢复健康、改善生理功能、减轻疼痛为目的的理论。

第 147B.02 条　执照

1. 执照要求。除本条第 4 款另有规定外,任何无有效执照的人员在 1997 年 6 月 30 日以后从事针灸实践都是非法的。每位执业针灸医师须在执业地点的显著位置展示该执照。

2. 称号。根据本章获得执照的人员,在各种形式的广告、专业文献及账单中,可以在其姓名后附加执业针灸师或者 L.Ac. 的头衔。任何未根据本条获得执照的人员,在从事与针灸实践或与其姓名有关的职业或者专业时,不得使用"执业针灸师""明尼苏达州执业针灸师"或者任何其他词语、字母、缩写,或者表明或暗示其是针灸师。参加针灸培训计划的学生必须被认定为见习针灸师。

3. 处罚。违反本条规定的人将被判轻罪,并根据第 147.09 条的规定受到惩戒。

4. 免责条款。(a)下列人员可以在没有针灸执照的情况下在其执业范围内从事针灸实践:

(1)根据第 147 章获得执照的医师。

(2)根据第 147 章获得执照的骨科医师。

(3)根据第 148 章获得执照的脊医。

(4)正在修读第 147B.05 条设立的针灸咨询委员会批准的正式课程或者辅导制实习计划的人员,前提是该人的针灸实践在执业针灸师或者根据第(5)条获豁免的人员的监督下进行。

(5)在明尼苏达州高等教育局注册的学校内,以教学为唯一目的在教学环境中从事针灸实践的客座针灸师,可以无照执业一年,并允许两个为期一年的续期。

(6)在州内的客座针灸师,其来访的唯一目的是在一年内提供不超过 30 日的辅导或者研讨会。

(b)本章不禁止没有针灸师执照的人员从事特定的非侵入性技术,例如穴位按压,这些技术属于第 147B.06 条第 4 款规定的执业范围。

5. 本条被 2004 年法律的第 279 章第 3 条第 3 款废止。

6. 互惠原则。如果委员会确定其他司法管辖区的认证满足或者超过明尼苏达州的执照要求,并收到该司法管辖区的信函证明针灸师在其司法管辖区内信誉良好,则委员会应当向持有其他司法管辖区现行执照或者证书的针灸师颁发针灸执照。

7. 执照要求。

(a)在 1997 年 6 月 30 日后,执照申请人必须:

(1)填写并提交一份由委员会提供的执照申请,表格必须包括申请人的姓名和记录地址,并须公开。

(2)除非根据第 5 或者第 6 部分获得执照,否则须提交经过公证的现行 NCCAOM 认证复印件。

(3)就申请人所知所信,签署一份声明,说明申请书中的信息真实无误。

(4)连同申请一并提交所需的所有费用。

(5)签署一份弃权书,授权委员会查阅申请人在本州或任何申请人从事针灸实践的州的记录。

(b)委员会可以要求申请人提供任何必要的额外资料,以确保申请人能够以合理的技能及安全的方式为公众提供针灸服务。

(c)委员会可以调查申请人所提供的资料是否准确及完整。委员会须通知申请人就该申请所采取的行动,以及如被拒发执照,则须告知拒发执照的理由。

8. 执照到期。根据本条颁发的执照每年到期。

9. 续期。

(a)申请人必须:

(1)每年(或者根据委员会的决定)在委员会提供的表格上填写续期申请。

(2)提交续期费。

(3)提供现行有效的 NCCAOM 认证文件。

(4)如根据第 5 或第 6 款获得执照,须达到 NCCAOM 规定的、与根据第 7 款获得执照者相同的专业拓展活动要求。

(b)申请人须提交委员会要求的任何补充信息,以阐明在续期申请中提交的信息。有关信息必须在委员会提出申请后三十日内提交,否则将取消续期申请。

(c)申请人必须与委员会保持正确的邮寄地址,以便接收委员会的资讯、通知和执照续期文件。将执照续期申请以美国普通邮件方式邮寄给申请人最后告知的地址,并支付邮费,即构成有效服务。未能收到续期文件并不免除申请人遵守本条规定的义务。

(d)在本条要求的期限内未提交完整的执照续期申请、年度执照费用或者逾期申请费(如适用)的申请人的姓名,应当从续期期间授权从事针灸实践的人员名单中删除。如果申请人的执照恢复,应当将其列入授权从事针灸实践的人员名单中。

10. 执照续期通知。在执照续期日前至少三十日,委员会应当向执照持有人最后已知的地址发出续期通知。该通知必须包括续期申请和续期所需费用的通知。若持证人未收到续期通知,则持证人仍须符合本条规定的注册续期要求。

11. 续期的最后期限。续期申请及费用的信件必须加盖续期当年 6 月 30 日或者之前,或者由委员会决定的日期的邮戳。

12. 非执业状态。

(a) 在向委员会提出申请并支付非执业状态费用后,可以将执照置于非执业状态。如果执照已经失效,且在两年内没有续期执照,委员会不得续期或者恢复该执照。

(b) 非执业执照可以由持证人向委员会申请后重新激活。如果持证人的执照因不能续期而被取消,则必须通过申请执照并满足在明尼苏达州行医的初始针灸执照的所有要求来获得新的执照。该项申请必须包括:

(1) 现行有效的 NCCAOM 认证文件。

(2) 证书持有人缴付非执业状态费用的证据。

(3) 年费。

(4) 自上次续期以来的所有逾期费用。

(c) 根据本条第5款获得执照的人,如果将执照置于非执业状态,必须获得 NCCAOM 认证。

12a. 执照状态失效后的执照持有人及转换条件。(a) 2020 年 1 月 1 日之前,因第 4 款导致持证人执照失效,并且在 2020 年 1 月 1 日之后寻求重新恢复执业状态的,仅为制定执照续期计划之目的,应视为首次获得执照,且不受第 147B.09 条中执照周期转换条款的约束。

(b) 本款将于 2022 年 7 月 1 日到期。

13. 临时许可证。只有在完成执照申请,符合本条所有要求,并已缴付委员会规定的不可退还费用的情况下,委员会才可以向符合本条要求的申请人颁发临时针灸许可证。该许可证有效期至针灸师的申请在委员会会议上作出决定前。

第 147B.03 条　NCCAOM 的专业拓展活动要求

1. NCCAOM 要求。除非根据第 147B.02 条第 6 款获得执照,否则每个持证人都必须满足 NCCAOM 专业拓展活动要求,以达到 NCCAOM 认证的要求。这些要求可以通过委员会批准的继续教育计划实现。

2. 委员会批准。如果继续教育计划符合以下要求,委员会应当批准该计划:

(1) 直接与针灸实践有关。

(2) 每位教员均持有教育机构颁发的学位或者证书,在传统东方医学方面具有可以证实的经验,或者在该学科领域接受过专门培训,从而显示其在该学科领域的专长。

(3) 面授学时不少于一学时。

(4) 有明确的书面目标,为参与者描述项目的目标。

(5) 计划发起人保存四年的出勤记录。

3. 继续教育主题。

(a) 继续教育计划的主题可能包括但不限于东方医学理论和技术,包括推拿;东方营养学;东方草药与膳食疗法;东方功法;西方科学包括解剖学、生理学、生物化学、微生物学、心理学、营养学、医学史等;以及医学术语或者编码。

(b) 本条不包括实践管理课程。

4. 查证。委员会应当定期随机挑选一名针灸师,并要求针灸师出示已完成 NCCAOM 专业拓展活动要求的证明。无论是针灸师、州还是保持继续教育记录的国家机构,都可以向委员会提供继续教育计划文件。

第 147B.04 条　委员会对申请采取的行动

1. 核实申请信息。根据第 147B.05 条成立的委员会或者针灸咨询委员会,在获得委员会的批准后,可以核实根据第 147B.02 条提出的执照申请所提供的信息,确定该信息是否准确和完整。

2. 委员会行动通知。委员会须在收到申请后一百二十日内,以书面形式通知每名申请人就该申请需做的准备。

3. 申请人的听证请求被拒绝。被拒绝颁发执照的申请人必须被告知有关决定及理由,并可以在收到委员会的通知后二十天内,向委员会提交一份有关问题的书面陈述,要求就有关决定进行听证。在听证后,委员会须以书面形式通知申请人其决定。

第 147B.05 条　针灸咨询委员会

1. 创建。针灸医疗服务委员会的咨询委员会由委员会任命的七名成员组成,任期三年。其中,四名成员必须是执业针灸师,一名成员必须是执业医师或者同时从事针灸实践的骨科医生,一名成员必须是经 NCCAOM 认证的执业脊医,一名成员必须是接受过由 NCCAOM 认证的针灸师使用针灸治疗过的普通民众。

2. 管理、补偿、注销、法定人数。咨询委员会受第 15.059 条的管理。

3. 职责。咨询委员会应当:

(1) 就颁发、拒发、续期、吊销、撤销或限制针灸执照,或为执照附加条件向委员会提供建议。

(2) 就有关接受、调查、举行听证会及针对针灸师的投诉采取规范行动的事宜,向委员会提供建议。

(3) 保存根据第 147B.02 条获得执照的针灸师名册。

(4) 保存咨询委员会的所有行动记录。

(5) 规定注册申请表、执照申请表、协议表格和其他必要的表格。

(6) 审核申请人在过渡期提交的患者就诊记录。

(7) 就针灸师的标准向委员会提出建议。

(8) 发放针灸实践标准的信息。

(9) 审查控诉。

(10) 就继续教育计划向委员会提出建议。

(11) 审查对控诉报告的调查,并向委员会建议是否应当采取惩戒措施。

(12) 按照委员会的指示,履行咨询委员会根据第 214 章授权的其他职责。

第 147B.06 条　职业行为

1. 实践标准。

(a) 在对患者进行治疗前,针灸师应询问患者是否已经由第 145.61 条第 2 款定义的执业医师或者其他专业人员就其疾病或者损伤进行过检查,并应审查该报告诊断结果。

(b) 医生应当在患者首次就诊前或就诊时以书面形式提供并告知患者以下信息,以取得患者的知情同意：

（1）执业资格，包括：

（i）教育。

（ii）执照信息。

（iii）明尼苏达州针灸师执业范围概述。

（2）副作用可能包括：

（i）治疗区域疼痛。

（ii）轻微擦伤。

（iii）感染。

（iv）晕针。

（v）断针。

（c）如果患者的情况需要或者患者选择针灸治疗，则针灸师应取得患者的书面确认，确认其已建议患者就针灸治疗咨询其初级保健医生。

（d）针灸师应当询问患者是否有心脏起搏器或者出血障碍。

2. 消毒设备。针灸师应当使用符合国家疾病控制和预防中心标准消毒过的设备。

3. 国家和城市公共卫生制度。就相关公共卫生，针灸师应当遵守所有适用的国家和市政的要求。

4. 针灸执业范围。针灸的执业范围包括但不限于：

（1）运用东方医学理论对患者进行评估和诊断。

（2）运用东方医学理论制定治疗方案。可以选择的治疗技术包括：

（i）通过皮肤插入无菌针灸针。

（ii）针灸刺激包括但不限于电刺激或者热疗。

（iii）拔罐。

（iv）刮痧。

（v）穴位按压。

（vi）草药疗法。

（vii）传统中医膳食指导。

（viii）呼吸技巧。

（ix）按照东方医疗原则进行锻炼。

（x）推拿。

5. 病历。针灸师须为每一位接受治疗的患者保存病历，包括：

（1）知情同意书副本。

（2）与患者面谈的有关患者病史和当前身体状况的证据。

（3）传统针灸检查诊断的依据。

（4）治疗记录，包括治疗穴位。

（5）针对患者的评估和指导。

6. 转诊给其他卫生保健从业者。当针灸师看到潜在严重疾病的患者时，需要转诊给其

他卫生保健从业者,这些疾病包括但不限于:

(1)心脏疾病,包括高血压失控。

(2)急性、剧烈腹痛。

(3)急性、未确诊的神经学变化。

(4)在不到三个月的时间内,不明原因的体重减轻或者增重超过15%。

(5)疑似骨折、脱位。

(6)疑似全身感染。

(7)严重的未确诊的出血性疾病。

(8)无既往病史的急性呼吸窘迫。

针灸师应当向有潜在严重疾病的患者要求由执业医师出具的咨询或书面诊断。

7. 数据服务。针灸师保存针灸患者的资料受第144.336条的规定的约束。

第147B.07条 规范和报告

为本章之目的,针灸师持证人及申请人须受第147.091条至第147.162条规定的约束。

第147B.08条 费用

第1款至第3款已经被2017年7月1日生效的法律的第一卷第6章第11条56(a)款所废止。

4. 针灸师申请和执照费用。

(a)委员会可收取下列不可退还的费用:

(1)针灸师申请费一百五十美元。

(2)针灸师每年的注册续期费一百五十美元。

(3)针灸师临时注册费六十美元。

(4)针灸师非执业状态费五十美元。

(5)针灸师滞纳金五十美元。

(6)执照副本费二十美元。

(7)认证费二十五美元。

(8)教育或者培训计划批准费一百美元。

(9)报告创建和生成费,每小时六十美元。

(10)核实费二十五美元。

(b)委员会可以按比例分配初始年度执照费。所有持证人必须在续期时支付全部费用。收费产生的收入必须存入州政府专项收入基金账户。

第147B.09条 执照续期周期转换

1. 一般情况。执业针灸师的执照续期周期转换为每年一次,在持证人出生月份的最后一日到期。本条规定的转换从2020年1月1日开始。本条适用于2019年12月31日之前持证人的续期程序。转换续期周期是指2020年1月1日后首次执照续期后的续期周期。转换执照期为转换续期周期的执照期。转换执照期为六至十七个月,截至2020年或者2021年持证人出生月份的最后一日,如第2款所述。

2. 现行持证人转换执照续期周期。对于截至2019年12月31日执照仍处于有效状态的持证人,其转换期从 2020 年 1 月 1 日开始,至当年持证人出生月份的最后一日结束。对于出生月份为 1 月、2 月、3 月、4 月、5 月或者 6 月的持证人,续期周期将于 2021 年持证人出生月份的最后一日结束。

3. 失效执照持有人的执照续期周期。这一款的规定适用于在 2019 年 12 月 31 日之前获得执照,但是截至 2019 年 12 月 31 日执照失效的人员。执照失效人员在 2020 年 1 月 1 日后首次续期时,转换续期周期从个人申请续期之日开始,到当年持证人出生月份的最后一日结束。但是,如果此人出生月份的最后一日是该个人申请续期之日后不足六个月的,则在下一年该人出生月份的最后一日结束续期。

4. 后续的续期周期。在执照持有人根据第 2 款或者第 3 款规定的转换续期周期之后,后续的续期周期为每年一次,自持证人出生月份的最后一日开始。

5. 转换期和费用。

（a）持有 2020 年 1 月 1 日之前颁发的执照,并根据第 2 款或者第 3 款续期该执照的持证人,应当按照本款的要求支付续期费。

（b）应当向持证人收取第 147B.08 条中列出的执照续期年费。

（c）对于转换执照期限为六至十一个月的持证人,应当调整在转换执照期限后收取的首个年度执照费,以抵扣在转换执照期限内支付的超额费用。金额的计算方法为:（1）12 个月减去持证人转换执照期限的月数;（2）将第（1）条的结果乘以年费的十二分之一后四舍五入的美元数值。

（d）对于转换执照期为 12 个月的持证人,在转换执照期后收取的首个年度执照费不作调整。

（e）对于转换执照期为十三至十七个月的持证人,应当调整转换执照期后收取的第一笔年度执照费,以增加未包含在转换执照期支付的年度执照费中的月份的年度执照费。额外付款的计算方法是:（1）从执照持有人的转换执照期限的月数中减去十二;（2）将第（1）条的结果乘以年费的十二分之一后四舍五入的美元数值。

（f）对于转换执照期后的第二次和所有后续执照续期,持证人的年度执照费按照第 147B.08 条的规定收取。

6. 到期。本条将于 2022 年 7 月 1 日到期。

明尼苏达州针灸行政法[①]

脊医执业资格及针灸

第 2500.3000 条　针灸

（1）灭菌;废弃处置。使用非一次性针头进行针灸时,针灸针必须通过以下方式消毒:

---

① 根据《明尼苏达州行政法典》第 2500 章"脊医执照颁发与服务"之"针灸"一节译出。

A. 高压灭菌器。

B. 干热灭菌。

C. 环氧乙烷杀菌。

每位患者的针灸针必须为单独包装。单独包装的针灸针必须在治疗患者后丢弃,或者在使用非一次性针灸针时按照上述消毒方法进行消毒。

针灸针必须根据《传染性废物控制法》《明尼苏达州议会法》第116.75条至第116.83条的规定处置。此外,所有要丢弃的针灸针在处置前必须经过消毒,并放置在坚硬的防刺穿容器中。必须使用无腐蚀的针灸针。必须向卫生部提交一份传染性废物处置计划。

(2)资格和费用。获得执照的脊医必须在委员会注册,才能从事针灸实践。首次注册前,脊医必须完成不少于一百个学时的学习,再从事针灸实践。委员会应接受由认证学校、国家针灸师协会提供的课程或者研讨会,或者根据第2500.1200条至第2500.1600条由委员会单独批准的课程或者研讨会。脊医必须提交经过批准的课程结业证明,以及一百美元的注册费。此外,申请人还必须顺利完成国家脊医审查委员会针灸考试或者国家针灸与东方医学认证委员会(NCCAOM)考试。

正在根据第2500.0800条的规定申请执照的脊医,如果无法证明自己已遵守上述的规定,可以向委员会提供下列事项的宣誓书,以符合有关规定:

A. 脊医在提交本申请前,已从获得委员会批准的教育机构获得不少于一百学时的针灸相关教育。

B. 脊医在申请注册前至少三年每年接受不少于五百次针灸疗法相关的患者就诊。

脊医在向注册委员会申请注册时,除须缴纳一百美元的注册费外,还必须提交宣誓书。申请人必须每年续费五十美元,以维持在委员会的注册身份。

(3)继续教育。脊医在获得注册续期批准前,必须符合注册委员会第2500.1200条所设定的继续教育规定。

(4)卫生室或者诊所。使用不卫生或不安全的设备是违反职业道德的行为,因为这涉及针灸的使用。

(5)注册证书。在收到委员会的注册证书后,脊医可以使用针灸脊椎矫正的准备或补充。

(6)豁免。任何根据《明尼苏达州法规》第147B编单独注册的脊医,都不受本条第(2)款和第(5)款的限制。

(7)续期。针灸注册续期日到期后十四日内,委员会须通过邮寄的方式通知尚未完成注册的申请人。

任何在到期后超过三十日未续期的注册申请人,如果希望续期,必须在提供针灸服务前重新申请注册,支付初始注册费以及第2500.1150条所规定的罚款。

任何超过一年但未满五年未续期的注册申请人,如果希望续期,必须在提供针灸服务前重新申请注册,支付初始注册费以及第2500.1150条所规定的罚款,并完成未续期注册的每年十个学时的针灸相关继续教育。

任何超过五年未续期的注册申请人,如果希望续期,必须在提供针灸服务之前重新申请注册,支付初始注册费以及第 2500.1150 条所规定的罚款,并通过国家脊医审查委员会针灸考试或者 NCCAOM 考试。

未经授权而继续提供针灸服务的人员,视为违反《明尼苏达州议会法》第 148.10 条的规定。

第 2500.3100 条　非执业状态的针灸注册

持有执照的明尼苏达州脊医,可以向委员会申请将其执照转换为非执业状态。非执业状态针灸注册适用于将在其他地方积极执业的脊医。在申请批准后,委员会将修改年度针灸注册证书,以表明非执业注册状态。

第 2500.3200 条　每年续期非执业状态的针灸注册

注册申请人必须完成年度的续期申请,并根据《明尼苏达州议会法》第 148.108 条的授权缴纳非执业针灸注册的年度续期费用。

第 2500.3300 条　非执业状态的针灸注册恢复

(1)一般情况。非执业状态针灸注册可以根据下列 A 至 C 项恢复为执业状态针灸注册:

A. 完成获委员会批准的恢复申请。

B. 根据《明尼苏达州议会法》第 148.108 条的授权支付恢复费用。

C. 每年注册均为非执业状态的,提交一份医生出具的公证声明,声明注册申请人已经获得由委员会批准的两个学时的针灸或者针灸相关科目的继续教育学分。

(2)拒绝申请。如果医生不符合本条第 1 款 A 至 C 项的各项规定,委员会将拒绝批准恢复执业的申请。维持非执业状态针灸注册的人员将无须参加用于恢复执业的 NBCE 针灸考试。

第 2500.4000 条　根据 2014 年法典第 291 章第 4 条第 59 条废除

第 2500.5000 条　根据 2010 年法典第 329 章第 1 条第 24 条废除

内布拉斯加州

内布拉斯加州针灸法[①]

第 38－2006 条　针灸及其定义

针灸系指根据针灸理论,在人体的特定穴位或者经络上刺入、操作和取出针灸针,并通过针灸针进行手法、器械、温针、电针和电磁治疗,以促进、维持和恢复健康并治疗疾病。针灸可能包括推荐治疗性运动、膳食指南和营养支持,以提高针灸治疗的有效性。针灸不包括脊柱推拿、活动或者调整、脊柱外推拿或者医学营养疗法服务。

第 38－2007 条　针灸师及其定义

针灸师系指专门从事针灸实践的人员。

第 38－2057 条针灸及豁免

《医学和外科实践法案》中与针灸相关的规定不适用于下列情形:

(1) 根据《统一资格认证法案》获得认证的、在其专业范围内执业的任何其他卫生保健从业者。

(2) 根据《统一资格认证法案》将针灸作为部门批准的研究课程的一部分,并在获得针灸执照的人的监督下从事针灸实践的学生。

(3) 在本州核准的针灸或者专业组织赞助的教育研讨会上,由根据《统一资格认证法案》获得针灸执照的人直接监督的任何其他司法管辖区的持证人或者受认证的人从事针灸实践。

第 38－2058 条　针灸、执照及护理标准

除针灸师是根据《统一资格认证法案》从事针灸实践外,在本州从事针灸实践是非法的。根据《统一资格认证法案》执业的针灸师,应当与根据该法案提供医学和外科,或者与整骨相关的医学和外科实践者采用相同的医疗护理标准。在患者的问题超出针灸师的培训、经验或者能力范围时,针灸师应当将其转诊给适当的执业者进行处理。

第 38－2059 条　针灸需征得同意

针灸实践应当在服务对象自愿和知情同意的情形下实施。与获得其知情同意有关的信

---

① 根据《内布拉斯卡州州议会》法注释版第 38 卷第 20 章"医学和外科服务法案"译出。

息应当包括但不限于以下内容：

（1）针灸实践与医学疗法的区别和辨别。

（2）披露针灸师未获准予行医或者对患者的疾病或者状况作出医学诊断，在作出此类医学诊断时应当征询医生的意见。

（3）针灸治疗的性质和目的。

（4）与治疗有关的各种医疗或者其他风险。

第 38 - 2060 条　针灸及获得执照的条件

首次申请针灸执照时，申请人应当向州健康和人类服务规制与许可部提供以下证明：

（1）完成由州医学委员会批准的大学、学院或者针灸学院的正式的全日制针灸课程后毕业。该课程包括至少一千七百二十五学时的入门针灸教育，其中至少包括一千个教学学时和五百个临床学时。

（2）通过州医学委员会批准的针灸考试，包括针灸理论、诊疗技术、穴位等方面的综合笔试。

（3）顺利完成州医学委员会批准的洁针技术课程。

内布拉斯加州针灸行政法①

第 1 条　范围及权限

这些法规根据《内布拉斯加州修订法规》第 38 - 2001 条至第 38 - 2063 条，《医学和外科实践法案》和《统一资格认证法案》管理针灸执照。

第 2 条　定义

以下定义由《医学和外科实践法案》《统一资格认证法案》《内布拉斯加州行政法典》第 172 卷第 10 章以及本章规定。

（1）获批的针灸考试。美国国家针灸与东方医学认证委员会（NCCAOM）针灸综合笔试，是包括针灸理论、诊疗技术和国家针灸与东方医学认证委员会（NCCAOM）穴位考试在内的综合性笔试。

（2）获委员会批准的学校。一所大学、学院或者针灸学院的正式全日制针灸课程，包括至少一千七百二十五学时的入门针灸教育，其中至少一千个教学学时和五百个临床学时，经针灸和东方医学认证委员会认证或者候选认证，或者经美国教育部长认可的另一个认证机构认证。

（3）获批的洁针技术课程。由 NCCAOM 批准的洁针技术课程，或者由委员会批准的同等课程。

第 3 条　执照要求

针灸执照的申请人必须提交一份由部门提供的完整申请，提供文件证明申请符合《内布

---

① 根据《内布拉斯加州行政法典》"人类健康服务制度"第 172 卷第 89 章"针灸服务"译出。

拉斯加州议会法》修订版第 38－2060 条以及《内布拉斯加州行政法典》第 172 卷第 10 章的规定,并且符合以下要求:

（A）顺利完成获批学校针灸课程并毕业。

（B）顺利通过针灸考试。

（C）顺利完成经批准的洁针技术课程。

（D）提交下列文件至部门:

（i）官方机构向卫生部提交的成绩单。

（ii）达到及格分数通过针灸考试的官方文件。

（iii）证明顺利完成洁针课程要求的正式文件。

第 4 条　知情同意

持证人必须遵守《内布拉斯加州议会法》修订版第 38－2059 条规定,向每位接受治疗的患者提供一份《自愿和知情同意书》。每位接受治疗的患者必须在《知情同意书》上签字并注明日期,表明他们已阅读并理解《同意书》的信息,并且同意接受针灸治疗。在治疗结束后,《自愿和知情同意书》在每个患者的记录中必须保存至少五年。

第 5 条　执照续期、豁免继续教育,以及非执业状态

申请人必须满足《内布拉斯加州行政法典》第 172 卷第 10 章规定的要求。所有针灸执照在每个奇数年的 5 月 1 日到期。

第 6 条　继续教育

在到期日当日或者之前,在内布拉斯加州获得执照的针灸师,必须达到以下的继续教育要求之一,作为其执照续期的条件:

（A）经 NCCAOM 批准的五十个学时继续教育。

（i）继续教育学时数应当在到期日前二十四个月内获得,但在二十四个月的续展期内获得超过执照续展所需五十学时者,允许最多将二十五学时结转至下一个二十四个月之中。

（B）经持续性医学教育认证委员会（ACCME）或者美国骨科协会（AOA）批准的五十小时一类项目的继续教育。

（i）继续教育时数应当在到期日前二十四个月内获得,但在二十四个月的续展内获得超过执照续展所需五十学时者,允许最多将二十五学时结转至下一个二十四个月之中。

（C）在到期日前二十四个月内获得 NCCAOM 的文凭证书的有效认证或者有效再认证。

（1）证明。持证人必须向部门提交一份证明,证明其在到期日前二十四个月内满足了继续教育要求。

（2）继续教育证明。持证人负责保存记录,以证明其参加继续教育项目或者以其他方式满足继续教育要求。

第 7 条　违反职业道德的行为

违反职业道德的行为,根据《内布拉斯加州议会法修订版》第 38－179 条、《内布拉斯加州行政法典》第 172 卷第 88 章和本章确定。

（A）未能获得本章第 4 条规定的《自愿和知情同意书》。

（B）未能向患者提供与根据《统一资格认证法案》获得执业资格的从事医学和外科或者骨科医学和外科的人员提供的相同标准的护理。

第 8 条　执照的恢复

申请人必须满足《内布拉斯加州行政法典》第 172 卷第 10 章规定的要求。

第 9 条　费用

费用参见《内布拉斯加州行政法典》第 172 卷第 2 章的规定。

第 10 条　重新编排

第 11 条　重新编排

第 12 条　废止

第 13 条　重新编排

威 斯 康 星 州

威斯康星州针灸法[①]

第 451.01 条　定义

下列定义适用于本章:

(1)"针灸"系指基于治疗人体特定部位(即穴位或者经络)的东方医学传统观念,通过下列任何一种操作来促进、维持或者恢复健康,以及诊断、预防或者治疗疾病:

(a)刺入针灸针。

(b)艾灸。

(c)应当用手法、热或电刺激及任何其他辅助治疗技术。

(2)"针灸师"系指从事针灸实践的人。

第 451.02 条　适用性

下列各项,均不要求本章所规定的证书:

(1)持有第 441 章、第 446 章、第 447 章、第 448 章以及第 449 章规定的执照、许可证或者证书,以及根据第 448 章第 9 节或第 11 节规定的享有针灸契约特权的,在其执照、许可证、证书或者特权范围内从事针灸实践的个人。

(2)在针灸师监督下协助针灸师实践的个人。

(3)从事针灸实践作为针灸专业指导课程或者由院系批准的住院医师针灸培训项目的一部分的个人,如果其称谓或者头衔明确表明是该针灸师的学生或者实习生。

第 451.04 条　认证

(1)需要针灸师证书。除非得到安全与专业服务部的认证,否则任何人不得从事针灸服务或者使用"针灸师"以及任何类似的头衔。

(2)针灸师证书。安全与专业服务部应当向完成以下程序的个人授予针灸师执照:

(a)按安全与专业服务部规定的格式向管理安全与专业服务部提交证明申请。

(b)支付第 440.05(1)条中规定的费用。

---

① 根据《威斯康星州议会法》注释版第 451 章"针灸"译出。

(c)根据第 111 章第 321 条、第 322 条和第 335 条的规定,提交符合管理安全与专业服务部要求的凭证,证明本人无被逮捕或者被定罪的记录。

(d)根据第 451.08 条的规定,提交符合安全与专业服务部要求的证明,证明本人已完成符合安全与专业服务部规定的标准针灸学习和住院医师课程。

(e)根据第 451.08 条的规定,通过安全与专业服务部认证的考试,以确认其具有胜任针灸师的能力。

(3)证书发放。安全与专业服务部应当向满足第(2)项或者第 451.08 条要求的个人颁发证书,以证明持证人有权在此州从事针灸实践。持证人应当将证书摆放在其营业场所的显著位置。

(4)到期和续期。续期申请应当在第 440.08(2)(a)条规定的适用续期日期之前,以规定的格式提交给安全与专业服务部,并应当缴纳安全与专业服务部根据第 440.03(9)(a)条拟定的续期费。

第 451.06 条　考试

考试应当包括书面或者实践测试,主要考察申请人的基本服务能力和与针灸实践实质相关的知识。

第 451.08 条　互惠证书

申请并支付第 440.05(2)条规定的费用。如果安全与专业服务部确定申请人已经积极从事针灸实践超过五年,或者申请人符合其他州或者地区与第 451.04(2)条相近的认证或者执照要求,则应当向在美国其他州或者地区持有针灸师执照或者证书的申请人颁发针灸师证书。

第 451.10 条　于 1991 年根据第 39 号法案第 3386 条废除。有效期至 1991 年 8 月 15 日。

第 451.12 条　感染控制

安全与专业服务部应当公布有关预防感染、针灸针和其他能够传播传染病的设备或者材料的消毒以及对潜在传染性物质安全处置的规定。该规定应当要求在用高压灭菌器灭菌之前,先用抗菌溶液彻底清洁针灸针,并允许针灸师使用经过预先消毒的、预包装的一次性针灸针。

第 451.14 条　惩戒和处理

(1)在符合根据第 440.03(1)条发布的规则的前提下,安全与专业服务部可以进行调查或者举行听证会,以确定是否发生了违反本章或者根据本章所颁布的规则的情况。

(2)遵守根据第 440.03(1)条制定的规则,如果发现申请人或者认证针灸师有下列行为之一,安全与专业服务部可以根据本章申斥该针灸师以及拒绝颁发、限制、吊销或者撤销其证书:

(a)在申请证明书或者续期时作出重大错误陈述。

(b)从事针灸实践过程中明显缺乏应用专业原则及技能的知识和能力。

(c)根据第 111 章第 321 条、第 322 条和第 335 条的规定,作为认证针灸师期间因犯罪被逮捕或者定罪。

(d)以虚假,欺骗或者误导的方式刊登广告。

（e）冒用他人针灸师执业证书或者允许别人使用本人针灸师执业证书者。

（f）根据第 111 章第 321 条、第 322 条和第 34 条的规定，服用酒精或者药物影响针灸实践者。

（g）违反本章或者根据本章所颁布的规则的。

（3）除第（2）款中提到的谴责或者拒绝颁发、限制、吊销或者撤销证书之外，针对以上违规行为，安全与专业服务部可以对申请人或者认证针灸师进行评估，处一百美元以上一千美元以下的罚款。

第 451.16 条　处罚

违反本章或者根据本章所颁布的规则的人，可处一百美元以上一千美元以下的罚款，或处九十日以下的监禁处罚或两罪并罚。

威斯康星州针灸行政法[①]

第 70.02 条　定义

下列定义适用于《本州议会制定法》第 451 章、《行政法典》第 70 章至第 73 章：

（1）（a）"积极从事经认证的针灸实践"系指在执照、证书或注册的授权下，使用针灸作为患者的主要治疗手段，而不是辅助疗法，并且该治疗取决于对东方诊断理论和实践的透彻理解和应用。

（b）申请人向安全与专业服务部提供符合要求的证明，证明在申请之前的五年内在美国各州或者地区"积极从事经认证的针灸实践"。申请人无论是否获得执照、注册或证书从事另一种医疗技术，均应当向安全和专业服务部门提供符合要求的证明：

1. 基于东方诊断和治疗理论和实践使用针灸作为主要的治疗手段系指，在申请日前十二个月内有五百名患者就诊，至少为一百名患者治疗疾病，有病例或宣誓书展示。

2. 在所有就诊患者中，至少有百分之七十的患者进行一般保健，在不超过百分之三十的患者就诊中，进行专业保健，如麻醉剂、美容治疗、成瘾治疗或者体重控制。

3. 实践符合安全和专业服务部门批准的洁针技术课程标准。

（2）"针灸"系指使用手法刺激针灸穴位。

（3）"针灸"与《威斯康星州议会法》第 451.01（1）条的含义相同。

（4）"针灸师"系指在通过根据《威斯康星州议会法》认证的从事针灸实践者。

（5）"AIDS"系指获得性免疫缺陷综合征。

（6）"本部门"系指安全和专业服务部门。

（7）"草药"系指帮助达到或者保持健康状态或者缓解疾病症状的植物、动物和矿物质。

（8）"HIV"系指人类免疫缺陷病毒。

（9）"激光疗法"系指使用激光来刺激穴位。

---

① 根据《威斯康星州行政法典》"安全与职业服务卷""执业服务编"第 70 章与针灸服务有关条文编辑而成。

（10）"艾灸"系指将干燥的艾草燃烧产生的热量用于人体的特定部位,而不是直接在皮肤上燃烧艾草。

（11）"NCCAOM"系指美国国家针灸与东方医学认证委员会。

（12）"晕针"系指针灸治疗引起的恶心、头晕或者其他身体不适。

第 71.01 条　认证申请

从未从事针灸服务或者不符合本法第 71.03 条认证条件的,申请人应当向安全和专业服务部门提交以下材料:

（1）安全和专业服务部门提供的表格申请。

注:申请表可以向本部门索取,地址:威斯康星州麦迪逊市华盛顿东大街 1400 号,邮政信箱 8935,邮编 53708。

（2）费用详见《威斯康星州议会法》第 440.05（1）条。

（3）申请人从未受到任何专业机构或者许可证颁发机构惩戒的证明,并且符合《威斯康星州议会法》第 111.321 条、第 111.322 条和第 111.335 条的规定,且未触犯与针灸服务相关罪名。

（4）顺利完成国家针灸与东方医学认证委员会的针灸考试证明,通过分数由国家针灸与东方医学认证委员会确定。

（5）顺利完成学习与实习课程的证明,相当于在针灸与东方医学院校认证委员会或者国家针灸与东方医学认证委员会认证的学校,连续两年接受东方诊断和治疗理论与实践的全日制教育和临床工作。

（6）顺利完成获批的洁针技术课程的证明。

第 71.04 条　五年后的执照续期

针灸执业证书持有人未能在证书续期日期后五年内续期其证书,则应当在申请续期之日的一年内参加并通过本法第 71.01(5)条规定的考试,除非申请人提供在申请之前的五年内,申请人在美国任何其他州或者准州积极从事经认证的针灸实践的证明。

第 72.03 条　治疗程序

（1）在开始治疗之前,应当允许患者选择自费使用一次性针灸针进行治疗,一次性针灸针应当按照《威斯康星州议会法》第 451.12 条的规定进行消毒和包装,并根据本法第 72.02(7)条的规定进行维护。

（2）在治疗期间,针灸师应当在针灸程序前和接触血液、体液或者明显的环境污染物后,用肥皂或者抗菌产品彻底擦洗双手至少十秒。

（3）应当保持场地干净,以保护每位患者针灸治疗所用设备的无菌性。

（4）在刺入针头或者破坏皮肤的治疗之前,应当在该区域的皮肤表面局部消毒。

（5）无菌针头在刺入穴位之前应当保持无菌状态,其针体在刺入、定位或者其他操作过程中不得与手指接触。

第 72.07 条　安全实践

（1）针灸师不得从事任何违反良好和公认针灸规范标准的治疗,或者使用任何不卫生或者非无菌设备的治疗。

（2）针灸师需从每位患者处获取与其主诉相关的病史。

（3）当针灸师遇到患有潜在严重疾病的患者时，包括但不限于心脏疾病病情、未控制的高血压、急腹症、急性未诊断的神经病变、原因不明三个月内体重减轻或者增加超过体重的百分之十五，疑似骨折或者脱位，疑似全身性感染、传染病、任何严重的未诊断出血性疾病或者急性呼吸窘迫既往无病史或者诊断，针灸师应当：

（a）在非紧急情况下，如果在治疗过程中发现这种情况，在开始针灸治疗或者继续治疗之前，请求执业医师咨询或者作出书面诊断。

（b）在紧急情况下，为患者维持生命并将其运送到最近的合法医疗机构。

（4）针灸师应当为每位接受治疗的患者提供一份由患者和针灸师签署的书面确认书，确认已建议患者就其寻求针灸治疗的情况咨询医生。

第73.01条　拒绝认证或者处罚的理由

根据《威斯康星州议会法》第451.14（2）（b）条的规定，从事针灸实践时存在如下行为，表明缺乏应用专业原理或技能的知识或能力，包括但不限于：

（1）当能力因精神或者情绪障碍、身体残疾、酒精或者其他药物而受损时从事针灸实践。

（2）在与针灸或者其他医疗技术有关的情形下，违反、协助或者教唆违反任何法律。

（3）在不具备有效执照时从事针灸实践。

（4）基于《威斯康星州议会法》第451.14条或者本法第70条至第73条规定的相同原因，在另一个司法管辖区受到认证、注册或者发证机构的处罚。

（5）在本部门提出要求后，未能及时配合调查针对针灸师提出的控诉。如果针灸师超过三十日才对本部门的要求作出回应，本部门将会作出可反驳的推定，即该针灸师没有及时采取行动。

（6）在其授权范围之外欺诈性地从事针灸实践。存在严重不称职行为或者有重大过失，一次或者多次不称职，一次或多次疏忽，或者在超出其培训、教育或者经验范围或者与其不一致的情况下从事针灸实践或者任何二级治疗技术。

（7）仅基于某人的种族、肤色、年龄、性别、性取向、政治或者宗教信仰、残疾、婚姻状况或者国籍，拒绝向其提供专业服务。

（8）未能根据患者或者科室要求，提供病历副本。如果原始记录不是英文的，针灸师应当提供由合格翻译人员翻译的英文副本。获得译文的合理期限为三十日。

（9）在记录患者最近一次就诊后的七年内，或者患者达到成年年龄的时，未能完整准确地记录每次患者就诊，包括病史、检查总结、诊断和实施或开具的治疗，以及转诊给其他针灸师或者任何其他医疗从业者。

（10）未经患者知情同意进行针灸治疗。知情同意书需要：

（a）向患者解释所有备用可行的针灸治疗模式以及这些治疗的益处和风险，包括与使用以下药物相关的风险和益处：

1. 针灸针刺激穴位和经络，包括针刺某些穴位的具体风险。

2. 对穴位进行机械、磁或者电刺激，尤其是在对躯干主干或者心脏有病史的患者进行此类刺激的情况下。

3. 艾灸。

4. 草药。

5. 激光针疗法。

6. 针压法。

（b）应向患者解释以下副作用，包括：

1. 有痛感。

2. 轻微挫伤。

3. 感染和感染区域针刺的风险。

4. 晕针。

5. 断针。

第 73.02 条　头衔的使用

（1）根据《威斯康星州议会法》第 451 章的规定认证的从事针灸实践者，应当包括"针灸师""威斯康星州合法针灸师"或者针灸服务广告中的类似称谓。（2）根据《威斯康星州议会法》第 451 章的规定认证的从事针灸实践者被授予东方医学博士学位，除了在广告中使用"针灸师""威斯康星州合法针灸师"或者针灸服务广告中的类似称谓之外，还可以在广告中使用"东方医学博士"或者"D.O.M."的头衔向公众宣传其作为针灸师提供的服务。

第 73.03 条　虚假、欺骗性或者误导性广告

根据《威斯康星州议会法》第 451.14（2）（d）条的规定，虚假、欺骗性或者误导性广告包括：

（1）除非针灸师符合根据《威斯康星州议会法》第 448.03（3）（a）条的要求，否则不得使用包括"医学博士"或者缩写"M.D."头衔的针灸服务广告。

注：《威斯康星州议会法》第 448.03（3）条称谓的使用。（a）除非下列情况之一，否则任何人不得使用"医学博士"的头衔，或者在其姓名后附加字母"M.D."：

1. 该人是拥有博士学位的医生。

2. 根据本款规定，该人被授予医师执照，通过拥有联合国世界卫生组织认可和列出的医学院授予的医学学位，满足了第 448.05（2）条的学位要求。

（2）在针灸服务中使用"博士"或者缩写"Dr."或者"Ph.D."宣传针灸实践。除非针灸师拥有授权使用的执照或者证书，或者拥有针灸或者东方医学的博士学位。

伊利诺伊州

伊利诺伊州针灸法[①]

第1条　简称

本法案应称为《针灸服务法案》。

第5条　对象和目的

特此声明,在伊利诺伊州进行针灸实践会对公众健康、安全和福利产生影响,为了维护公众利益,应对针灸实践进行监管和控制。兹进一步宣布,符合本法案规定的针灸实践应得到公众的信任,且只有符合本法案规定的合格人员才有权在伊利诺伊州从事针灸实践,该事项关乎公众利益,且受到公众关注。本法案应作宽松解释,以促进上述目标和宗旨的实现。

第10条　定义

下列定义适用于本法案:

"针灸"系指插入预先消毒的一次性针头刺激身体某些穴位进行的评估或治疗,但医学上禁忌的除外。"针灸"包括但不限于热刺激,包括远红外线,或者冷敷、电流、电刺激或磁刺激、冷激光、振动、拔罐、刮痧、手法按压或其他方法,无论是否同时使用针头,均可以预防或者改变疼痛感,使生理功能正常化,或者治疗身体疾病或功能障碍,包括根据本法案第15条中所述的传统东亚原则和活动确定治疗方案,实施此类治疗方案不需要书面转诊。根据本条规定,被称为干针疗法或者肌肉内手法刺激的疗法,或旨在描述此类疗法的类似措辞被确定为符合针灸的定义、范围和疗法。针灸还包括根据东亚医学理论的传统和现代疗法进行评估或治疗,包括但不限于使用艾灸、草药、天然或者膳食补充剂、手法疗法、功法和饮食等方法,达到预防或者减缓疼痛感的目的,使生理功能正常化,实现治疗身体疾病或者功能障碍的作用,包括本法案第15条所述的无须书面转诊的活动。针灸不包括放射治疗技术、电外科技术、脊椎按摩技术、物理疗法、推拿技术,或者药物、疫苗的使用或者处方,以及鉴别诊断的确定。根据本法案获得执照的针灸师,如未同时根据《伊利诺伊州物理疗法法案》获得理疗师执照,则其无资格提供物理疗法或者理疗服务。

---

① 根据《伊利诺伊州议会法》注释版第225卷第2章"针灸服务法案"译出。

"针灸师"系指从事针灸实践(包括传统和现代疗法)并已获得监管部许可的人。在对患者进行评估或者治疗时,针灸师须将病情超出针灸师执业范围的患者转诊给执业医生或牙医。

"记录地址"系指监管部在申请人的申请文件或持证人的执照文件中记录的指定地址,该地址由监管部执照管理部门保存。

"委员会"系指由部长委任的针灸委员会。

"牙医"系指根据《伊利诺伊州牙科执业法案》获得执照的人。

"监管部"系指财务与职业监管部。

"邮箱地址"系指监管部在申请人的申请文件或持证人的执照文件记录的指定邮箱地址,该电子邮箱地址由监管部的执照管理部门保存。

"医生"系指根据 1987 年《医疗执业法》获得执照的人。

为本法案之目的,"书面转诊"系指经医生或者牙医签字证实的诊断确定患者的病情,并建议采用本法案中规定的针灸治疗。在医生或者牙医改变诊断之前,该诊断将持续有效。医生或者牙医可在转诊后通过明确指示继续管理患者。

"部长"系指金融和职业监管部部长。

"州/地区"包括:

(1)美国各州。

(2)哥伦比亚特区。

(3)波多黎各联邦。

第 12 条　记录地址和电邮地址

所有申请人和持证人应当:

(1)向金融和职业监管部提供有效的地址和电子邮件地址,分别作为申请或者续展执照的记录地址和电子邮件地址。

(2)记录地址或者电子邮件地址变更后的 14 日内,通过监管部网站或者联系监管部执照管理部门通知本监管部。

第 15 条　具有针灸执业资格的人

根据本法案获得执照的人不得使用本法案规定的针灸疗法以外的方法治疗人类疾病,并且只能按照本法案规定的方法,在获得执照的前提下从事针灸实践。在伊利诺伊州获得执照的医生或者牙医可以根据本法案或者 1987 年《医疗执业法》的规定,根据其接受的培训来进行针灸服务。在进行评估或者治疗时,针灸师须将应当被确定在针灸师执业范围之外的患者情况转介给具有执业资格的医生或者牙医。

本法案中关于使用膳食补充剂或者草药的各项规定,均不得解释为禁止根据其他法案在本州获得执照的人从事其被许可的行为。

第 16 条　中草药学及相关认证措施

依照本法案获得执照的人,未经国家针灸与东方医学认证委员会认证的东方医学文凭的证明或者监管部批准的实质同等地位的证明,或者不能证明其顺利通过国家针灸与东方医学认证委员会的中草药学考试或者经监管部认可的实质同等的考试,不得自称接受过中草药学培训。违反本条规定者将受到第 110 条所述的惩罚措施。

第 20 条　豁免行为

本法案并不禁止在本州获得执照的个人从事其被许可的行为。

第 20.1 条　特邀针灸讲师及职业教育

本法案的规定不禁止来自其他州或者国家已获得执照的针灸师,包括专业针灸协会、科学针灸基金会或者针灸培训计划的受邀嘉宾或者根据本法案获得监管部批准的继续教育提供者,通过讲座、诊所或者示范的形式进行专业教育,其前提是该针灸师由国家针灸与东方医学认证委员会或者经监管部认可的类似机构认证,具有另一个州或者国家的现行有效,并且未受过处分的执照。

本法案规定的持证人可以作为专业针灸协会或者科学针灸基金会或者针灸培训计划的受邀嘉宾或者根据本法案获得监管部批准的继续教育提供者,通过讲座、诊所或者示范进行专业教育。监管部可以制定有关本条的规则。

第 20.2 条　客座针灸师

本法案的规定并不禁止未获得本法案许可的另一州或者国家的针灸师在伊利诺伊州州长宣布于紧急状态期间在本州执业,前提是该针灸师具有另一个州或者国家现行有效的,未受过惩罚措施的执照,或者经国家针灸与东方医学认证委员会或者经监管部认可的类似机构认证为针灸师。这种做法仅限于宣布的紧急状态生效期间,并且每年不得超过连续两周或者总共三十日。

第 25 条　监管部的权力和职责

监管部应当根据本法案行使以下权力和职责:

(1)审核申请,以确定申请人的资格。

(2)在管理和执行上采用符合本法案规定的规则,并可以规定与本法案有关的形式。这些规则可以规定职业操守和规范的标准和准则。监管部在颁布规则时应当与委员会协商。

(3)随时就与本法案实施有关的各个事项向委员会和专家寻求建议和意见。

第 30 条　伊利诺伊州行政诉讼法

《伊利诺伊州行政诉讼法》特此明确通过并纳入本法案,同该法的所有条款均包含在本法案中效力相同,但《伊利诺伊州行政诉讼法》第 10 条至第 65(d)条的规定被明确排除在外。该条款规定,在听证会上,持证人有权证明其遵守有关保留、延续或者续期执照的所有合法要求。为本法案之目的,将《伊利诺伊州行政诉讼法》第 10 条至第 25 条要求的通知邮件邮寄到记录地址即可。

第 35 条　针灸委员会

部长应当委任一个由七人组成的针灸委员会,作为部长的顾问。其中,四名成员必须持有在本州从事针灸服务的执照。此外,一名成员应当是根据 1987 年《医疗服务法》获得执照的积极从事针灸服务的脊医,一名成员应当是在伊利诺伊州所有分支机构获得执业许可的医生,一名成员必须是没有根据本法案或者其他司法管辖区的类似法获得执照且与该职业没有任何关联的公众成员。

成员任期为四年,直至其继任者获得任命并合格。各个成员的任期不得超过连续两届。

任命填补空缺的方式应当与原任命填补空缺期间未届满部分的方式相同。初始条款应当自1997年修正法案生效之日起生效。

委员会可以每年选举一名主席和一名副主席,在主席缺席时由副主席主持会议。委员会的成员应当对于本州各地理区域具有代表性。部长可以因故终止各个成员的委任。部长可以适当考虑委员会的所有建议。当前任命的委员会成员过半数即构成法定人数。委员会成员的空缺,不得损害法定人数行使委员会权利和履行委员会职责的权利。委员会成员对基于纪律处分程序或者以委员会成员的身份善意开展的其他活动而采取的行动,不承担任何附加义务。

第40条 执照申请

针灸师执照的初次申请,应当按照监管部规定的表格以书面形式提交,并应当缴纳所需的费用,费用不予退还。

监管部可以向提交下列各项证明的申请人颁发执照:

(1)(A)毕业于针灸及东方医学认证委员会认可的学校或者经监管部批准的类似认证机构;或者(B)完成经监管部批准的综合教育项目。

(2)2019年12月31日或者之前提交申请的,应当通过国家针灸和东方医学认证委员会考试或者监管部批准的具有同等效力的考试;2020年1月1日或者之后提交申请的,应当向国家针灸与东方医学认证委员会提供针灸文凭或者东方医学文凭,或者具有经监管部批准的具有同等效力的证书。

申请人应当自申请之日起三年内完成申请手续。三年内未办结的,驳回申请,没收费用,申请人必须重新申请,并满足重新申请时的有效条件。

第45条 根据1997年7月3日生效的P.A.90-61第15条废除

第50条 禁止行为

除获得监管部根据本法案颁发有效的针灸师执照之外,任何人都不得使用"针灸师""执业针灸师""认证针灸师""针灸中医师""针灸和东方医学博士""针灸医师""东方医学从业者""东方执业医师""东方医学医师""东方医学执业医师""C.A.""Act.""Lic.Act.""Lic.Ac.""D.Ac.""DACM""DAOM"或者"O.M.D."的头衔和称谓,直接或者间接地做与其职业和业务有关的事项。根据本法案获得执照的人不得直接或者间接地在其职业或者业务中使用"医疗"这一称谓。但不能阻止医师使用"针灸师"的称谓。

未经本法案许可,任何人不得作为执业针灸师执业,或提供、尝试针灸实践,抑或是声称自己是执业针灸师。

本法案不禁止一个人在以下情况下,将针灸针、针灸疗法或者技术作为其教育培训的一部分:

(1)依照本法案规定,开展本州批准的针灸课程。

(2)毕业于针灸学院并参加研究生培训计划。

(3)毕业于针灸学院,为参加国家针灸与东方医学认证委员会考试做准备而复习课程。

(4)正在参加由本州批准的提供者提供的国家批准的继续教育课程。

针灸学校的学生和在伊利诺伊州没有执照的专业针灸师,可以依照本法案的规定,与其教育结合在一起进行针灸服务,但是不得开设诊所、在指定地点会见私人患者、向私人患者提供咨询或者以其他方式进行超出其教育要求的针灸服务。

第 55 条 背书

如果一名执照申请人是其他州的针灸师,其获得执照之日时法律规定的条件与本州当日所规定的法律具有等同性,或者申请者的个人认证证书等资料与本州规定相符,在缴纳相关费用后,监管部可以酌情决定该申请者不必经过考试而认定其为本州的执业针灸师。

申请人应当自申请之日起三年内完成申请手续。三年内未办结的,驳回申请,费用不予退还,申请人须重新申请,并满足重新申请时所规定的有效条件。

第 60 条 根据要求出示执照以及更改地址

在必要时,持证人应当向监管部的代表机构或者国人出示其执照。

第 70 条 续期或者恢复执照、继续教育以及服兵役后如何恢复执照

根据本法案颁发的执照有效期和续期应当依法设定。持证人可以在执照截止日期前一个月内支付必要的费用续期执照。

为了续期或者恢复执照,申请人应当提供符合监管部规定的继续教育证明。监管部批准的继续教育主办方不得利用个人进行临床示范,除非该个人根据本法案获得有效许可,或者根据本法案第 20.1 条的规定获得其他州或者国家的许可。

执照到期或者处于非执业状态的人可以通过向监管部提交申请、满足继续教育要求、提交监管部认可的证明文件来恢复执照,其中可以包括经宣誓的证据,证明在另一司法管辖区内的执业活动符合监管部要求,并应当缴纳所需的恢复费用。如该人在另一司法管辖区内没有保持符合监管部要求的活跃执业状态,则监管部应决定其是否适合恢复执业状态,并可能要求其通过相关考试。

任何执照到期的针灸师如(1)是在美国武装部队或州民兵服役或受训的联邦现役军人或(2)在美国预备服兵役初期的教育训练阶段,则其若在光荣终止服役、培训或者教育后的两年内,向监管部提供了充足的证据,证明其已经终止服役、培训或者教育,可在不支付任何续期费的情况下恢复其执照。

第 75 条 非执业执照

根据监管部的规定,持证人应当以监管部规定的书面形式,选择将其执照置于非执业状态,并在其书面通知监管部恢复之前,免于支付续展费用。持证人要求解除非执业状态的,应当支付当前的续期费用,符合继续教育要求,并应当按照本法案第 70 条的规定恢复其执照。

第 80 条 费用

监管部应当按照规则提供管理和执行本法案的费用表,包括但不限于初始执照、续期和恢复。所缴费用不予退还。

根据本法案收取的所有费用应当存入一般职业专项基金,并应当拨入监管部,作为监管部在执行本法案时的一般及或有开支。

根据 2017 年 8 月 25 日生效的 P.A.100－375 第 15 条已废除

第 100 条 广告

根据本法案获得执照的人可以在公共媒体或者提供此类专业服务的场所宣传专业服务

的可用性。此类广告应当限于以下信息：

（1）该人的姓名、职务、办公时间、地址和电话号码。

（2）该人的专业领域或者专业实践限制的信息。

（3）日常专业服务的常规费用信息,该信息应当包括由于复杂情况或者不可预见的情况可能会调整费用的通知。

（4）开业、变更、退出或者恢复营业的公告。

（5）专业注册人员增设或者删除的公告。

（6）商务或者预约卡的发放。

本法案不允许未获得执照的专业服务提供者进行专业服务的广告宣传。广告商不得使用包含虚假、欺诈性、迷惑性或者误导性材料或者保证成功的声明,不得使用利用公众虚荣心或者恐惧的声明,不得使用引发不公平竞争的声明。

第105条　无证开业及民事处罚

（a）未经许可擅自执业、有执业意愿、尝试执业或者试图以执业针灸师的身份执业者,除法律规定的其他罚款外,还应当就每项违法行为向本监管部缴纳民事罚款,罚款数额由监管部规定,不得超过一万美元。民事处罚应当由监管部在听证会后,按照本法案的规定关于对被许可人的惩罚措施进行听证的规定进行评估。

（b）该监管部有权力调查所有未经许可的活动。

（c）民事处罚应当自判处民事处罚的裁定生效之日起六十日内缴纳。该命令须构成一项判决,并可以与其他法庭判决的相同方式存档及执行。

第110条　处罚的依据

（a）基于下列原因,监管部可以拒绝颁发或者续期、处罚、吊销、撤销或者采取其他认为适当的惩罚措施或者非惩罚措施,包括对每次违法行为处以其认为适当的罚款（不超过一万美元）：

（1）违反本法案及其规则。

（2）根据美国任何司法管辖区的法律,属于不诚实或者与职业活动直接相关的(i)重罪或者(ii)轻罪,以认罪或者放弃答辩的方式定罪、裁定有罪、陪审团裁决、进入判决或者量刑阶段,包括但不限于定罪、先前的监督判决、有条件释放或者初犯缓刑。

（3）以取得执照为目的,进行谎报。

（4）协助他人违反本法案的规定或者规则者。

（5）监管部已通过挂号信或电邮的方式发送要求至持证人的记录地址,却在六十日之内未收到监管部要求提供的书面信息。

（6）如果该处罚的依据中至少有一项与本条规定相同或者实质上等同,则适用美国其他司法管辖区或者外国的惩罚措施。

（7）以本法案许可外的其他方式寻求专业服务。

（8）未按照患者的书面请求向其提供病历副本。

（9）针灸实践中的重大疏忽。

（10）对酒精、麻醉品、兴奋剂或者任何其他化学物质或者药物的习惯性或者过度使用或者成瘾,导致针灸师不能以合理的判断、技巧或者安全性从事针灸实践。

（11）认定以欺诈手段申请或者获得执照。

（12）表现出不具备能力或不适合从事本法规定的针灸实践的执业模式或其他行为。

（13）在儿童与家庭服务部根据《虐待和忽视儿童举报法》指定的报告中被指定为犯罪者,并且经过明确且令人信服的证据证明,持证人已导致儿童成为《虐待和忽视儿童举报法》所定义的受虐待儿童或者被忽视的儿童。

（14）故意不按照《虐待和忽视儿童举报法》的要求举报涉嫌虐待或者忽视儿童的案件。

（15）使用任何词汇、缩写、数字或者字母（例如"针灸师""执照针灸师""认证针灸师""针灸和中医医生""针灸和东方医学医生""针灸医生""东方医学从业者""东方执业医师""东方医学医生""东方医学执业者""C.A.""Act.""Lic.Act.""Lic.Ac.""D.Ac.""DACM""DAOM"或者"O.M.D."）或者在没有根据本法案颁发的有效针灸师执照的情况下,试图通过针灸和东方医学认证委员会使用的各个名称表明自己是一名有执照的针灸师执业。

当执业针灸师的名称被专业地用于口头、书面或者印刷的公告、专业卡片或者出版物中,供公众参考时,应当在头衔和姓名之后加上学位名称或者学位缩写。公告、专业卡或者刊物以书面或者印刷形式出现时,解释性文字、字形或者印文,尺寸应当不小于名称及头衔所用字体的二分之一。除本法案规定的有效执照持有人外,任何人都不得在其执业或者业务活动中直接或者间接地使用"针灸师"的头衔和称号。

（16）利用优质医疗服务的宣传来吸引公众,或者将其提供的服务与其他人士提供的针灸服务的费用进行比较。

（17）在未获授权的情况下提供专业服务的广告。包含虚假、欺诈性、欺骗性或者误导性材料或者保证成功的专业服务广告、利用公众虚荣心或者造成恐惧心理的声明,或促使造成不公平竞争的声明。

（18）用本法案规定的针灸以外的方法治疗疾病,或者根据医生或者牙医提供管理患者的处方医嘱以执业针灸师的身份治疗转诊患者的疾病,而没有通知作出诊断的医生或者牙医该患者正在接受针灸治疗。

（19）法律规定的不道德、未经授权或违反职业道德的行为。

（20）身体疾病、精神疾病或者其他损害导致不能以合理的判断能力、技巧和安全性从事该职业,包括但不限于随着年龄增长而恶化的精神疾病或者身体残疾。

（21）违反《卫生保健工作者自荐转诊法》。

（22）未能将病情在评估或者治疗时已确定超出针灸师执业范围的患者,转介给执业医生或者牙医。

（23）自称接受过中草药培训,但不能向本监管部提供经国家针灸和东方医学认证委员会认证的东方医学文凭身份证明或者经监管部认可的基本同等的身份证明,或者已通过国家针灸和东方医学认证委员会中草药考试或者经监管部批准的基本同等的考试的证明。

巡回法院根据《精神健康和发育障碍法案》发布命令确认,持证人应当接受强制收治或经司法程序收治,该执照自动吊销。在巡回法院裁定该患者不再受强制收治或经司法程序收治，并对患者发布出院的命令，且由委员会向监管部提出恢复执照的建议，执照才能恢复。如果有情况表明需要如此，委员会可以建议监管部在恢复被吊销的执照前进行审查。

监管部可以针对下述情形拒绝颁发或者续期执照：（i）未能提交报税表或者缴付报税表所列明的税款、罚款或者利息。（ii）未能按照本州税务局管理的税法要求，支付各项税务、罚款或者利息的最终评估，直到该税法的要求得到满足为止。

在执行本条时，如果发现可能存在的违规行为时，监管部可以强制对执照持有者和申请人进行精神、身体检查，费用由监管部支付。监管部可以要求检验医生对此检查活动提供证词。不得因任何与持证人或者申请人与检查医生之间的通讯有关的普通法或者法定特权而排除任何信息。检查医生由监管部指定。被检查者还可以在检查期间自主选择另一位医生，费用自付。如果一个人没有按照要求接受精神或者身体检查，且监管部在进行通知和听证后发现其拒绝接受检查没有合理理由，那么在该人接受检查之前，其执照将被吊销。

如果监管部发现个人由于本条所述原因无法执业，则可以求该人接受其批准、指定的医生的护理、咨询或者治疗，以此作为申请继续、恢复或续期执照的条件、条款或限制；或者，监管部可以提起诉讼，立即吊销、撤销或者以其他方式处罚该执照，以此代替护理、咨询或治疗。如果个人的执照是根据上述期限、条件或限制而被授予、继续、恢复、续期、处罚或者监督的，而该人没有遵守上述条款、条件或者限制，则应交由监管部部长决定是否应立即吊销该人执照，并等待监管部的听证会。

如果部长根据本条立即吊销某人的执照，则监管部必须在吊销后三十日内召开听证会，并在没有明显延误的情况下完成听证。在保护病历保密性的适用联邦法规和条例允许的范围内，监管部和委员会有权审查个人关于损害的治疗和咨询记录。

根据本法案获得执照并受本条约束的个人应当有机会向监管部证明，他或她可以按照执照规定，依据现行标准恢复执业。

第 117 条　未赔偿者吊销执照

根据法院命令证明未根据《伊利诺伊州公共援助法案》第 8A－3.5 条或者 1961 年《刑法》第 17－10.5 条或者 2012 年《刑法》第 46－1 条的规定向某人支付赔偿的，监管部可以未经进一步处理或者听证，吊销其执照或者其他授权。在全额赔偿之前，被吊销执照或其他授权者不得执业。

第 120 条　因资金不足而拒付给监管部的支票或者汇票

向监管部发出或者交付支票或者其他汇票的人，由于账户资金不足、账户被关闭或者已停止付款而两次没有被其提取的金融机构兑现支票或者其他汇票，除了支票或者其他汇票上的欠款外，还需向监管部加付五十美元费用。如果执照到期且未能使用支票或者其他汇票支付续期费或颁发执照费以及本节规定的五十美元费用，但是继续从事针灸实践的，应加收一百美元费用。本条规定加收的费用，是针对使用到期执照或者未续期执照执业的处罚规定的补充。如果在执照到期通知之日起三十日内，执照失效的人申请一个新执照，其应向监管部申请恢复执照，并向监管部缴纳所有相关费用。监管部可以制定执照恢复申请的费用，用于支付所有与处理该申请有关的费用及开支。部长在个别个案中如果认为根据本条应当缴付的费用是不合理的或者不必要的负担，可以豁免该等费用。

第 130 条　禁令、刑事犯罪及令行禁止

（a）如果个人违反本法案的规定，部长可以以伊利诺伊州人民的名义，通过伊利诺伊州的总检察长或者各州的州检察长，申请禁止违法的命令或者强制执行本法案令的命令。向法院提出申请时，法院应当发出临时限制令，不设任何通知或者条件，并可以预先永久禁止违法行为。如果确定某人已经或者正在违反禁令，法院可以以藐视法庭的罪名实施惩罚。本条规定的诉讼是对本法案规定的救济和处罚措施的补充，而不是替代。

（b）无论何时监管部认为某人违反本法规定，监管部都可以颁布规则，说明不应对该人发出停止令的理由。该规则应当清楚列明监管部的决策依据，并允许在该规则生效日起七日内提交令监管部满意的答复。未能作出令监管部满意答复的，监管部应立即发出停止令。

（c）除本法案第 20 条规定的情况外，在没有获得监管部颁发的有效执照的情形下，任何人作为针灸师从事针灸实践或者自称依据本法案拥有针灸执照，除部长外，各执业针灸师、利益相关方或者因此受到侵害的人都可以依据本条第（a）款的规定申请救济。

第 135 条　犯罪

个人在未经许可的情况下故意在本州从事或者企图从事针灸实践，应构成 A 类轻罪，此后每次定罪，应构成第四级重罪。除本法案另有其他规定外，监管部依据本条或者其他州或者联邦法规收取的所有形式罚款、金钱或者其他财产，包括但不限于依据《伊利诺伊州管制物品法案》第 505 条或者《甲基丙胺控制和社区保护法案》第 85 条没收的财产，应当存入专业监管证据基金。

第 140 条　调查；通告；听证

依据本法案规定，可以拒绝颁发、撤销、吊销或者以其他方式限制执照的使用。如果持证人的行为经证明后，根据本法案即构成拒绝颁发、续期或者吊销、撤销或者给予其他处分的理由，则监管部应当调查申请、持有或者声称持证人的行为。监管部可自行动议，或应其他人的申诉阐明事实。监管部应当在拒绝颁发或者续期、吊销、撤销，或者根据本法案第 110 条采取其他纪律处分之前，至少在确定听证会日期前三十日，以书面形式通知申请人或者持证人提出的任何指控，应当向申请人或者持证人提供亲自或者由律师就指控进行听证的机会。还应当指示其提交书面答复。未提交答复将被视为违约，其执照将会被吊销、撤销、列入察看期或者将受到其他纪律处分，处分包括部长认为适当的有关执业范围、性质或者程度的限制。书面通知可以由以下方式送达：

（1）亲自交付给申请人或者持证人。

（2）以挂号信的方式，将通知邮寄至申请人或者持证人最后一次向本监管部发出通知时所指明的记录地址或者营业地点。

（3）通过电子邮件向申请人或者执照持有人的电子邮件地址发送通知。如果此人在收到通知后未能提交答复，则监管部可以酌情决定吊销、撤销其执照或者将其执照列入察看状态，或者监管部可以采取任何适当的处罚措施，包括限制执业范围、性质或者程度，或者在没有听证的情况下处以罚款，前提是所指控的一项或者多项行为构成了根据本法案采取此类行为的充分理由。在通知中规定的时间和地点，监管部应当听取相关的指控，并且应当为申请人或者持证人以及申诉人提供足够的机会，亲自或者由律师提出任何可能与控罪或者其辩护有关的陈述、证词、证据及论点。监管部可以随时开展听证会。如果委员会未在通知中规定的时间和地点开会，或者未在听证会继续进行的时间和地点开会，则监管部可以在不超过三十日的期限内继续听证。

第 142 条　保密

监管部在审查或者调查持证人或者申请人过程中收集的所有资料，包括但不限于监管部对执照所提出的诉讼以及为调查该诉讼而收集的资料，应当严格保密，不得泄露。除执法人员、由监管部部长确定的监管机构或者向监管部提交合法传票的机构外，监管部不得向任何人披露该信息。向联邦、州、县或者地方执法机构披露的信息和文件，该机构不得以任何目的向各个其他机构或者个人披露。除法律另有禁止外，监管部对持证人或者申请人提出的正式诉讼均属公开记录。

第 145 条　正式听证会及保存相关记录

对于涉及拒绝颁发或续期执照或者处罚持证人的任何案件，监管部应自费保存正式听证的所有程序的记录。听证通知书、申诉书，以及在法律程序中提交的所有其他法律文书性质的文件和书面材料、证词记录、听证人员报告，以及监管部的命令均为法律程序的记录。

第 150 条　保密

在根据本法案第 140 条进行诉讼的监管部或其指定人员或者申请人或者持证人的申请下，各个巡回法院均可以发出命令，要求证人出席提供证词，并出示文件、报告、档案、账簿以及任何与调查或者听证有关的记录。法院可以以藐视法庭的罪名提起诉讼，强制当事人服从命令。

第 152 条　认证的记录

除非收到原告支付的提供及核证记录的费用，否则监管部无须向法院证实任何记录，也不需要在法庭上作出任何答复或者以其他方式参与司法复审程序。举证证据无须产生花费。原告没有向法院提交回执的，可以作为不起诉的理由。

第 154 条　令人信服的证据

在根据本法案第 140 条进行诉讼的监管部或其指定人员或者申请人或者持证人的申请下，各个巡回法院均可以发出命令，要求证人出席提供证词，并出示文件、报告、档案、账簿以及与任何与调查或者听证有关的记录。法院可以以藐视法庭的罪名提起诉讼，强制当事人服从命令。

第 155 条　传票及宣誓

在本州巡回法院的民事诉讼中，监管部有权传唤本州的任何人并将其带到法庭，按照法律在司法程序中所规定的相同费用和补贴，以同样的方式进行口头或者宣誓作证。监管部亦有权传唤提交与听证或者调查有关的文件、报告、档案、账簿以及记录。

部长及部长指定的听证官均有权在监管部根据本法案授权进行的听证会上要求证人宣誓，以及其他依本法案要求或者授权监管部执行的宣誓。

第 160 条　事实的裁决、法律结论和建议

在听证结束时，委员会须向部长提交一份书面报告，说明委员会对事实的裁决、法律结论及建议。该报告应当包含对被告是否违反本法案或者未能遵守本法案规定的裁决。委员

会须指明违反或者未能遵守规定的性质,并须向部长提出建议。

有关事实裁决的报告、法律结论和委员会建议的报告,可以作为是监管部命令的依据。如果部长对委员会的报告有任何异议,可以发出与报告不一致的指令。该裁决不能作为针对因违反本法案而被提起刑事诉讼的人的证据,但听证和裁决并不妨碍与本案相关的刑事诉讼。

第 165 条　听证官

部长有权任命在伊利诺伊州获得合法执照的任何一位律师为听证官,参与有关执照的处分程序。听证官在听证中拥有完整的权力。听证官须向委员会和部长报告其对事实的裁定、法律结论和建议。委员会应当复审听证官的报告,并将事实裁决、法律结论及建议提交部长。

第 170 条　送达报告、重审及命令

根据本法案有关送达听证通知的规定,在涉及拒绝颁发、续期或者处罚执照的情况下,监管部应当将委员会报告的副本送达被告。在送达听证书后二十日内,被告可以向监管部提出重审的书面申请,并指明重审的具体理由。如果在期限届满为提出申请时,或者复审申请被否决后,部长可以根据委员会的建议发出命令,但本法案第 175 条另有规定的除外。如果被告在提出复审的时间内向送达机构订购副本并支付费用,则可提出复审申请的二十日期限应自该副本交付给被申请人之日起开始计算。

第 175 条　伸张实质正义及复审

当部长认为撤销、吊销、拒绝颁发、恢复、续期执照或者其他涉及对持证人和申请人的处罚有失公允时,可以安排同一或者其他审查员重新听证。

第 180 条　命令或者核证副本作为初步证据

经监管部盖章并由部长签署的命令或者该命令的核证副本,应当作为初步证明:

(1) 该签名是部长的真实签名。

(2) 该部长已获正式委任且具备资格。

(3) 委员会及其成员有资格采取行动。

第 185 条　恢复执照

执照被吊销或者撤销后,监管部可以随时恢复执照。经调查和听证后,监管部认为恢复执照不符合公众利益的除外。若有吊销或者撤销的情况,监管部可要求被告在恢复其执照前对其进行检查。

第 190 条　交还执照

当执照被撤销或者吊销时,被告应当立即将执照交还监管部。逾期不办理的,监管部有权没收其执照。

第 195 条　对公众构成紧迫危险及暂时吊销的情况

如果部长发现其持有的证据表明继续从事针灸实践将对公众产生紧迫的危险,则部长可以不经听证吊销执照的使用,并与本法案第 140 条规定的听证程序同时进行。如果部长在没有举行听证会的情况下吊销执照,监管部的听证会必须在吊销执照发生后的三十日内举行,并在没有明显延迟的情况下完成听证。

第200条　行政复议法下的复核

监管部作出的所有最终行政决定,均按照《行政复议法》和《行政复议法》有关规定接受司法审查。"行政决定"一词的定义见《民事诉讼法》第3－101条。

司法审查程序应当在申请复核的当事人所在县的巡回法院提起;但是,如果当事人不是本州居民,则审理地点应当是桑加蒙县。

第205条　根据1997年7月3日生效的P.A.90－61第15条废除

第210条　违反及处罚

任何违反本法案的个人均属A类轻罪。一经定罪,其后再次出现类似行为将被判处第四级重罪。

2/999.　生效日期

本法案自公布之日起施行。

伊利诺伊州针灸行政法[①]

第1140.10条　定义

"法案"系指《针灸实践法》[225 ILCS 2]。

"ACAOM"系指针灸及东方医学教育审核委员会,它是美国教育部认可的机构,对针灸和东方医学领域的教育计划进行认证。

"针灸师"系指根据《针灸实践法》获准从事该法案中定义的针灸工作者。

"委员会"系指针灸委员会。

"CCAOM"系指针灸和东方医学院委员会。

"CE"系指继续教育。

"CNT课程"系指由CCAOM管理的洁针技术课程。

"监管部"系指金融和职业监管部。

"处长"系指金融和职业监管部职业监管处处长。

"处"是指金融和职业监管部职业监管处。

"NCCAOM"是指国家针灸与东方医学认证委员会,负责认证针灸文凭和东方医学文凭。

第1140.20条　收费

下列费用必须向职业监管处缴纳,且不予退还:

(a)申请费

(1)针灸师执照申请费为五百美元。

(2)申请成为继续教育机构的费用为二百五十美元。

(b)续期费

(1)针灸师执照续期费每年二百五十美元。

---

① 根据《伊利诺伊州行政法典》第68卷第7编B分编第1140章"针灸服务法案"译出。

（2）继续教育机构的续期费每两年二百五十美元。

（c）一般收费规则

（1）恢复非执业执照的费用为二十美元,同时缴纳执照失效期间断缴的续期费,上限不超过一千美元。

（2）任何用途的执照认证费为二十美元。

（3）在本州取得针灸执照的人员名册费用应根据编写该名册产生的实际成本收取。

第 1140.30 条　申请颁发执照

（a）针灸执照申请人应向职业监管处提交以下证明：

（1）教育背景

（A）毕业于经 ACAOM 认可的学校,或者经职业监管处认可的类似认证机构。

（B）完成职业监管处根据第 1140.40 条批准的综合教育培养计划。

（2）对于 2019 年 12 月 31 日或者之前提交的申请,通过 NCCAOM 举办的针灸考试或者职业监管处批准的同等考试。

（3）自 2020 年 1 月 1 日或者之后提交的申请,须提供已取得 NCCAOM 针灸文凭（三年制课程）或者东方医学文凭（四年制课程）,或者经职业监管处批准的同等学力的证明。

（4）提供顺利完成 CCAOM 开展的针灸洁针技术（CNT）课程的证明。

（5）缴纳第 1140.20 条所规定的费用。

（b）所有文档应使用英语提交至监管处。

（c）如申请人曾在其他司法管辖区取得执照,也需要根据职业监管处要求的格式,提交一份证明文件。证明文件必须由申请人曾经及当前取得执照的司法管辖区颁发。并且证明文件中必须载明：

（1）申请人在该司法管辖区获得执照的时间,包括执照的初始颁发日期。

（2）申请人在该司法管辖区参加的考试情况说明。

（3）申请人的档案是否载有任何违纪处分记录或者待处理违纪处分的记录。

（d）如因资料不足、所提供资料存在差异或者冲突,或者内容需要澄清而使职业监管处或者委员会对申请人所提交的任何文件或者经历的准确性提出质疑,则执照申请人需要：

（1）提供必要的资料。

（2）参加委员会组织的谈话,解释所提交资料的相关性或者充分性,澄清信息,或者澄清信息中存在的任何差异或者冲突。

第 1140.35 条　客座导师

（a）未获得本州针灸执业许可但由专业针灸协会、科学针灸基金会、针灸培训课程或者经职业监管处批准的继续教育提供者邀请的人员可以根据法案第 20.1 条之规定以讲座、门诊或者示范的形式提供专业教育。

（b）根据本条规定提供服务的个人,须根据职业监管处的书面要求提供下列材料：

（1）下列资料中的任何一种：

（A）NCCAOM 或者职业监管处批准的其他组织颁发的现行有效针灸文凭或现行有效东方医学文凭。

（B）在其他司法管辖区获得的针灸执照。

（2）由各针灸协会、科学针灸基金会、针灸培训课程或者经批准的继续教育机构出具的证明表明：

（A）此人已获邀请或者预约以讲座、门诊或者示范的方式教授针灸技法。

（B）申请人即将提供的教育服务的性质。

（C）邀请的期限或者合同的期限。

（3）申请人的最新简历复印件。

（c）客座导师可以以讲座、门诊和示范的形式教授针灸技法的应用，但不得开设诊所，设立会见私人患者的处所，为患者提供咨询服务，或者在提供讲座、门诊或者示范之外从事针灸实践。

（d）如根据本条之规定提供服务的个人，希望留在本州从事或者教授其专业，则其必须申请并获得相应的执照。对于根据本条规定提供服务的个人，允许其在本州申请并获得针灸执照。

第1140.40条　针灸课程

如果申请人的针灸方案符合（a）、（b）或者（c）的最低标准，则职业监管处应当认可申请人的针灸培训计划。

（a）申请人毕业的学校：

（1）所在地法律允许其授予针灸学位。

（2）拥有足够数量的师资队伍，能够确保完成教学任务。且教师必须具备专业学院或者机构颁发的、与其教学领域相对应的学位。

（3）永久保存学生档案，包括入学资格、考勤、成绩单和其他方面的表现记录。

（b）对于一个三年的课程，核心课程包括至少一千九百〇五个学时或者同等课程，时间不少于二十七个日历月。应当至少包括：

（1）七百九十五个学时（或者同等时间）的针灸理论与治疗技术及相关研究。

（A）课题应当包括但不限于下列内容：

（i）针灸的历史。

（ii）基本理论。内容包括但不限于基础阴阳理论、五行八法、脏器、腑器、奇恒之腑；经络理论与功能；气、血、津液；益气（补）镇静（泻）；病因，如六淫七情；病理学。

（iii）穴位与经络理论。内容包括但不限于：体表十四条经脉的名称和分布十二条正经、任脉和督脉。穴位的分类。穴位研究应当包括穴位的定位方法、解剖结构、穴位分类、功能、适应证和禁忌证。了解具体穴型，如五输穴、原穴、络穴、郄穴、背俞穴、募穴、交会穴、奇经八脉。

（iv）针灸治疗。内容包括但不限于特殊评价方法的运用、气与血、脏腑、经络理论等八大原则的辨证论治。根据患者病史和图表进行病例回顾。四诊合参。测量与记录生命体征和症状，制定治疗计划和预后。治疗的禁忌证。潜在危险的指征。是否有修改标准治疗方法的需要（如针对婴幼儿和孕妇）以及明显良性表现下可能存在的严重病因（如高血压、头痛）。

（v）针灸治疗。内容包括但不限于行针的深度、行针时间、具体操作和退针。气的出现。艾的直接与间接应用等。其他疗法（如放血、灸、拔火罐、刮痧、七星针法）。补泻手法。急慢性疾病的治疗、急救、镇痛、麻醉和电刺激相关的知识。安全问题。东方人体疗法（如推拿、指压按摩、阿玛按摩、穴位按压等）。某些疾病的禁忌证。

（vi）伦理与实践管理。内容包括但不限于知情同意。HIPPA 法案指南。了解实践范围。记录保存。法律要求。数据公布。将患者转诊给其他医生时涉及的道德与法律问题。专业行为与适当的人际行为。针灸实践相关的法律法规。患者期望的了解与说明。一般责任保险。法律要求。职业责任保险。风险管理和质量保证。实践的建立与管理，包括第三方报销的伦理与法律问题。职业发展。

（B）历史、道德和实践管理方面的学时不得超过九十学时。

（2）六百六十个学时（或者同等时间）的临床培训。

（A）该课程必须确保每位学员至少参加五百一十个学时受监督的针灸治疗。临床培训部分应当在经课程规定的导师指导下进行。在培训期间，学生必须完成二百五十例的治疗，包括开展患者访谈、参与治疗计划、开展适当的针灸治疗，并对患者对治疗的回应进行随访。

（B）导师指导下的临床实习必须能够让学生在患者治疗的所有阶段都能得到锻炼，并且必须在由该机构运营的教学门诊或者与该机构有官方附属关系的临床机构中进行。该机构的学术监督基本等同于对该机构的教学门诊进行的学术监督，其中：

（i）临床导师的资格应当符合学校的临床教学要求。

（ii）须对临床经验进行定期、系统的评估。

（iii）临床培训监督程序应当与该机构的教学门诊所采用的程序基本同等。学院必须接受来自不同临床教员的培训，以确保其能够接触到不同的实践方式和教学方法。

（C）该计划必须确保每个学生获得至少一百五十个学时的观察时间。

（3）生物医学临床科学的学时数为四百学时（或者同等时间）。

（A）生物医学临床科学。内容包括但不限于基础科学课程。生物医学与临床概念及术语。人体解剖学和生理学。病理学与生物医学模型。药理学。生物医学临床过程的性质，包括病史、诊断、治疗和随访。实验室和诊断试验和程序以及生物医学体检结果的相关性。以及生物医学体检结果。转诊和/或咨询的基础和需要。生物医学转诊资源的范围及其采用的方式。

（B）针灸洁针技术。内容包括但不限于传染病、消毒程序、针的处理与处置，以及与血源性和表面病原体相关的其他问题。

（c）对于一个四年的课程，核心课程包括不少于二千六百二十五个学时，或者同等课程，在不少于三十六个日历月内。应当至少包括：

（1）七百九十五个学时（或者同等时间）的针灸理论与治疗技术及相关研究。

（A）课题应当包括但不限于下列内容：

（i）针灸史。

（ii）基本理论。内容包括但不限于基础阴阳理论、五行八法、脏器、腑器、奇恒之腑。经络理论与功能。气、血、津液。益气（补）镇静（泻）。病因，如六淫七情。病理学。

（iii）穴位与经络理论。内容包括但不限于：体表十四条经脉的名称和分布十二条正经、任脉和督脉。穴位的分类。穴位研究应当包括穴位的定位方法、解剖结构、穴位分类、功能、适应证和禁忌证。了解具体穴型，如五输穴、原穴、络穴、郄穴、背俞穴、募穴、交会穴、奇经八脉。

（iv）针灸治疗。内容包括但不限于特殊评价方法的运用、气血、脏腑、经络理论等八大原则的辨证论治。根据患者病史和图表进行病例回顾。四诊合参。测量与记录生命体征和症状，制定治疗计划和预后。治疗的禁忌证。潜在危险的指征。是否有修改标准治疗方法的需要（如针对婴幼儿和孕妇）以及明显良性表现下可能存在的严重病因（如高血压、头痛）。

（v）针灸治疗。内容包括但不限于行针的深度、行针时间、具体操作和退针；气的出现；艾的直接与间接应用等；其他疗法（如放血、灸、拔火罐、刮痧、七星针法）；补泻手法；急慢性疾病的治疗、急救、镇痛、麻醉和电刺激相关的知识；安全问题；东方人体疗法（如推拿、静坐、按摩、指压等）；某些疾病的禁忌证。

（vi）伦理与实践管理。内容包括但不限于知情同意；HIPPA 法案指南；了解实践范围；记录保存；法律要求；数据公布；将患者转诊给其他医生时涉及的道德与法律问题；专业行为与适当的人际行为；针灸实践相关的法律法规；患者期望的了解与说明；一般责任保险；法律要求；职业责任保险；风险管理和质量保证；实践的建立与管理，包括第三方赔偿的伦理与法律问题；职业发展。

（B）历史、道德和实践管理方面的学时不得超过九十个学时。

（2）四百五十个学时（或者同等时间）的东方草药研究。

（A）主题应当包括但不限于以下内容：

（i）东方中药介绍，整个东方的中药医疗系统的发展，美国东方草药发展的历史，以及草药的法律和伦理考虑。

（ii）基本的中药理论。主题应当包括但不限于植物部分术语和使用意义；中药特性（例如中药类别概念、五味、四性、归经）；炮制方法（即干燥、蜜制）；服用方法（例如汤剂、局部、定时）；配伍方法，包括常见禁忌证、禁忌、预防措施；治疗方法（即汗法、清法、和法）。

（iii）东方的诊断和治疗模式。主题应当包括但不限于伤寒六个阶段、温病四个阶段、脏腑、中医内科学和外科学理论下的中药运用。

（iv）中药策略。主题应当包括但不限于规划、实施和评估治疗的方法和系统；根据中医原则对各种不协调模式的中药配方进行区分和修改；适用于生物医学诊断患者的中药方案。

（v）本草。包括至少三百种不同的中药的指导，主题包括但不限于功效和含义；视觉识别，包括不同的切割方法；四性、五味、归经；分类法和命名法；介绍植物中文名称；注重经典和新发展的功能和作用；每味中药的具体禁忌证；中药剂量的应用；个别中药研究的当前发展；濒危物种及其替代品。

（vi）中药配方。包括至少一百五十个配方中的说明，主题包括但不限于传统配方的类别、功能和含义;中国传统配方名称的含义;注重经典和新发展的功能和行动;每个配方的具体禁忌证;配方研究的当前发展;每个配方中个别草药的组成和比例;配方的主要修改;关于管理、潜在副作用、配方制备和储存的患者教育;准备好的草药配方,重点是修改和交付格式。

(vii)临床实习和中药药房。主题包括但不限于临床实习,学生采访、诊断和编写适当的草药配方,从完全监督到独立的配方开发;中药药房的清洁标准;中药的储存(生的和准备的配方),包括腐败和虫子的问题;在中药药房环境中填充草药配方;西方草药科学;植物学、非植物学和园艺(例如,由于环境因素而导致的草药特性的变化),因为它们属于草药;药物认知的一般原则;中药和天然物质的生化成分;参考当前文献的药物相互作用的考虑。

(3)八百七十个学时(或者同等时间)的综合针灸和草药临床培训。

(A)该课程必须确保每位学员至少参加七百个学时的患者针灸监督护理。临床培训部分应当在经课程规定的导师指导下进行。这部分的临床培训,在项目批准的监督人员的监督下进行,必须包括至少三百五十名学生进行的治疗,学生对患者进行面谈,进行诊断和治疗计划,进行适当的针灸治疗,并跟踪患者对治疗的反应。

(B)导师指导下的临床实习必须能够让学生在患者护理的所有阶段都能得到锻炼,并且必须在由该机构运营的教学门诊或者与该机构有官方附属关系的临床设施中进行。在该机构进行的学术监督实际上等同于对该机构的教学门诊进行学术监督,其中:

(i)临床导师的资格应当符合学校的临床教学要求。

(ii)须对临床经验进行定期、系统的评估。

(iii)临床培训监督程序应当与该机构的教学门诊所采用的程序基本上相同。学院必须接受来自不同临床教员的培训,以确保其能够接触到不同的实践方式和教学方法。

(C)该计划必须确保每个学生获得至少一百五十学时的观察时间。

(4)五百一十个学时(或者同等时间)在生物医学临床科学中。

(A)生物医学临床科学。内容包括但不限于基础科学课程;生物医学与临床概念及术语;人体解剖学和生理学;病理学与生物医学模型;药理学;生物医学临床过程的性质,包括病史、诊断、治疗和随访;实验室和诊断试验和程序以及生物医学体检结果的相关性;生物医学体检结果;转诊和/或者咨询的基础和需要;生物医学转诊资源的范围及其采用的方式。

(B)针灸洁针技术。内容包括但不限于传染病、消毒程序、针的处理与处置,以及与血源性和表面病原体相关的其他问题。

(C)课程工作不足的个人可以在地区认证的学院或者大学或者针灸和东方医学认证委员会认证的针灸学院完成必修课程。个人将被要求提交一份课程记录,表明顺利完成课程和课程描述。

第1140.50条 批准

(a)对于根据美国其他州或者准州法律获得执照或者在美国其他州或者准州注册的申请人,如果其希望在伊利诺伊州获得针灸执照,应当按照职业监管处提供的格式向其提出申

请,须提交的材料包括:

（1）下列资料中的任何一种:

（A）对于在 2001 年 12 月 31 日或者之前在其他州获得执照的申请人,须证明下列情况之一:

（i）顺利完成 NCCAOM 综合针灸考试或者经职业监管处批准的同等考试。

（ii）目前持有针灸文凭或者 NCCAOM 东方医学文凭。

（B）对于 2001 年 12 月 31 日以后在另一个州获得执照的申请人,证明:

（i）完成下列其中一个:

毕业于 ACAOM 认可的学校,或者经职业监管处认可的类似认证机构的正式成绩单。

完成职业监管处根据第 1140.40 条批准的综合教育培养计划的正式成绩单。

（ii）顺利完成 NCCAOM 综合针灸考试或者经职业监管处认可的同等考试的证明。

（C）对于 2020 年 1 月 1 日或者之后在其他州获得执照的申请人,目前具有针灸和东方医学学院的理事会的针灸或者东方医学文凭证书或者经职业监管处批准的同等证书。

（2）顺利完成由 CCAOM 管理的洁针技术课程的证明。

（3）由申请人的初始执照所属的州以及申请人目前以针灸师身份执业的州（如非初始执照所属的州）提供的证明,说明申请人的执照号、申请人在该州取得执照的时间、该司法管辖区执照考试的情况说明,以及申请人的档案中是否存在已经采取的或未决的任何纪律处分。

（4）缴纳 1140.20 条中所列费用。

（b）职业监管处应当对各批准申请书进行核查,以便确定颁证之日所在司法管辖区的要求和审查是否基本等同于法案载明的要求与审查,或者申请人是否具有基本同等的资格。

（c）职业监管处应当批准并向申请人颁发执照,或者以书面形式通知申请人不予批准的理由。

第 1140.60 条　执照续展与更换

（a）根据法案颁发的执照会在奇数年的 6 月 30 日到期。持证人可在执照有效期届满前一个月缴纳一定的费用办理换证手续。续期执照申请人需按照第 1140.90 条只要求接受三十个学时的继续教育。

（b）各持证人有责任向职业监管处报告其地址的变更情况。未能收到职业监管处发放的续期申请表,不构成未支付续期费或者未续期执照的借口。

（c）使用已过期执照执业的行为将被视为无照执业,且根据法案第 110 条之规定,其行为人应当受到相应处罚。

第 1140.70 条　停用执照

（a）执业针灸师可以使用职业监管处提供的申请表向其提出申请,将其执照转为非执业状态。执照在非执业期间不必缴纳续期费,直到其再次以书面形式通知职业监管处恢复其执照为止。

（b）如欲将执照从非执业状态恢复到执业状态,执业针灸师须按照本部第 1140.80 条之规定办理。

（c）执照处于非执业状态的针灸师不得在伊利诺伊州使用"针灸师"头衔或者法案第50条中所列的其他名称。任何违反本条规定的人均会被视为无证执业，并应当受到本法第110条规定的纪律处分。

第1140.80条　恢复执照

（a）执照已过期或者处于非执业状态五年以内的针灸师，可以通过支付本部第1140.20条规定的费用，并且按照本部第1140.90条之规定证明其已在提交恢复申请前的两年内参加过为期三十个学时的继续教育，将执照恢复到执业状态。进修时间必须按照第1140.90条的规定完成并保留记录。

（b）对于执照已到期或者置于非执业状态五年以上的针灸师，如欲将其执照恢复为执业状态，可以按职业监管处提供的格式向委员会提交恢复申请，并按本部第1140.20条之规定附具所需费用。进修时间必须按照第1140.90条的规定完成并保留记录。此外，申请人还应当提交：

（1）下列资料中的任何一种：

（A）在其他司法管辖区内继续执业的宣誓证明。此项证据应当包括其他司法管辖区内相应委员会或者执照发放机关的陈述，表明持证人被授权执业。

（B）依照法案第70条规定提供服兵役的宣誓书。

（C）NCCAOM出具的考试通过证明或者在恢复申请前两年内经职业监管处批准的其他同等考试的通过证明。

（D）证明完成与针灸临床相关的教育计划或者研究生课程，包括在针灸和东方医学审核委员会认证的针灸学院或者职业监管处批准的类似认证机构开设的课程、面向专业的继续教育课程以及特殊的研讨会，或者其他经委员会批准的类似课程。申请人完成这些课程的时间，不得早于提交恢复执照申请前的两年。

（i）对于执照已到期五至十年的申请人，应当提交九十个学时有关针灸临床教育计划或者课程的证明。

（ii）对于执照已到期十年或者以上的申请人，应当提交一百二十个学时有关针灸临床方面的教育计划或者课程的证明。

（2）提供其在过去的五年内顺利通过针灸和东方医学学院委员会开展CNT课程的证明。

（c）如果因信息不足、所提供信息存在差异或者冲突或者需要澄清，使得职业监管处或者委员会对申请人所提交资料的准确性或者课程/经验的相关性或者充分性提出质疑，则执照恢复申请人需要：

（1）提供必要的资料。

（2）参加委员会组织的谈话，解释所提交资料的相关性或者充分性，澄清信息，或者澄清信息中存在的任何差异或者冲突。

第1140.90条　继续教育

（a）继续教育学时要求

（1）每一位申请续展换证的执业针灸师应当在申请之前参加与针灸实践的专业技能和

科学知识为期三十个学时的继续教育。

（2）每个奇数年的 6 月 30 日前二十四个月为一个续期周期。

（3）每个继续教育学时应当等于一小时，其中教学内容不少于五十分钟。三十至四十九分钟的教学内容报告为半个继续教育学时，五十至六十分钟的教学内容报告为一个继续教育学时。

（4）在伊利诺伊州，首次续期执照的申请人可以不必满足继续教育的要求。

（5）持有伊利诺伊州执照但在其他州定居并执业的针灸师也应当按本条要求参加继续教育。

（6）如果在其他司法管辖区获得的继续教育学分满足伊利诺伊州有关继续教育的规定，则在伊利诺伊州同样适用。

（b）经认可的继续教育（CE）

（1）继续教育的学时应当按符合第（c）款规定的进修教主办机构所提供课程的出勤率（如出勤证明或者结业证明）进行计算，但（b）（3）、（4）、（5）和（6）所规定的活动除外。

（2）如果申请人参加符合第（c）款规定的继续教育机构提供的自学（包括在线、通信、音频或者视频）课程，在每次执照续展时可以获得最多二十三个学时的继续教育学分。且每门自学课程应当包含一次考试。

（3）在针灸和东方医学认证委员会认证的针灸学院或者该职业监管处批准的类似认证机构，顺利完成与针灸临床方面相关的研究生课程，最多可以获得三十个学时的继续教育学分。继续教育学分将按每学期十五个学时分配或每季度十个继续教育学时分配。

（4）在续期前的期限内，最多可获得十五个学时的继续教育学分，该等学分是由 ACAOM 或经 ACAOM 批准的类似认证机构认证，和/或由 ACAOM 根据（c）款批准的机构提供的继续教育讲师的针灸计划课程的一部分。应当按照每一个半教学学时一个学分的比率进行换算，但只有首次参加该课程才会计算学分（即重复参加同一课程时，不得对学分进行重复计算）。

（5）完成认证学院或者大学的课程和/或者完成本职业监管处批准的伊利诺伊州继续教育课程，可以在续期期限内获得五学时的继续教育学分。该课程或者计划材料必须与持证人在针灸实践中的专业技能和科学知识相关。

（6）在相关专业期刊或者书籍上发表论文，最多可以获得五个学时的继续教育学分。

（c）经批准的继续教育机构和继续教育课程

（1）本条所称的经批准的继续教育机构系指：

（A）美国针灸和东方医学协会或者其附属机构。

（B）亚美针灸学会，或者其附属机构。

（C）伊利诺伊州针灸和东方医学协会，或者其附属机构。

（D）伊利诺伊州韩美针灸协会，或者其附属机构。

（E）芝加哥韩美针灸协会，或者其附属机构。

（F）国家针灸与东方医学认证委员会（NCCAOM），以及 NCCAOM 批准提供针灸继续教育计划的个人和组织。

（G）美国针灸师协会，或者其附属机构。

（H）美国医学针灸学会。

（I）经委员会建议,职业监管处根据本条(c)(2)批准和授权的任何其他协调和提供继续教育课程或者计划的人士、公司、协会、法人或者团体。

（2）根据(c)(1)(I)之规定申请成为继续教育主办机构的单位应当提交继续教育主办机构申请、(c)(3)的继续教育计划样本、(c)(4)的样本评估,以及(c)(5)的出席证书样本以及第1140.20条规定的费用(伊利诺伊州的州立机构、州立学院和州立大学将免除支付此项费用)。申请人还应当证明下列事项:

（A）继续教育主办机构所提供的课程中的学分应当符合(c)(3)中的标准和本条中的所有其他标准。

（B）主办机构须负责每项课程计划的出勤情况,并提供按(c)(5)所载的出勤证明。

（C）按照职业监管处要求,主办机构还需提供相关证据材料(如出勤证明或者课程资料),以证明其符合本条之规定。如职业监管处有理由认为主办机构没能充分遵守相关法规和本部之规定,并且认为这些信息很有必要,则主办机构应当按要求提供相应证据材料。

（3）所有课程计划应当:

（A）有助于提升、拓展和提高职业资格授予人在针灸实践方面的专业技能和科学知识,包括患者的直接和间接治疗、针灸治疗、治疗技术、穴位位置及其理论,以及伦理。

（B）促进普通或者专业针灸实践的发展,提高其价值。

（C）由接受过相关教育和/或拥有相关经验的人员开展或者主持。

（D）明确课程目标、教学内容和教学方法。

（E）根据伊利诺伊州为执照续期之目的而开展的继续教育所设定的要求,明确继续教育的学时。

（4）每个继续教育计划应当为参与者提供一个评估计划和讲师的机制。

（5）主办机构应当负责向课程的每位参与者提供一份出勤或者参与证明。主办机构出具的出勤证明应当包括以下信息:

（A）主办机构的名称、地址和许可证号码。

（B）参与者的姓名和伊利诺伊州针灸执照号。

（C）课程主题的简短陈述。

（D）各课程计划的学时数。

（E）课程的授课日期与场所。

（F）主办机构的签名。

（6）主办机构应当负责确保每个参与者只根据参加计划的时间获得继续教育学分。

（7）主办机构须保留不少于五年的出勤记录。

（8）所有由经批准的主办机构提供的计划都应当向所有有执照的针灸师开放,而不限于单个组织或者团体的成员。

（9）经批准的主办机构可以与个人和组织分包,按照本条规定的标准提供计划。

（10）为了保持作为注册继续教育主办机构的批准,每个主办机构应当按照第1140.60

条的规定提交续期申请,以及第 1140.20 条中规定的续期费用。根据职业监管处的要求,主办机构应当提供其在续期前提供的每个计划的清单,包括计划的名称、主题的简要描述、可用的学时数、日期和地点。

(11)如果主办机构未能遵守上述任何要求,职业监管处在通知主办机构并听取了委员会的建议(参见《伊利诺伊州行政法规》第 68 条第 1111 款)后,应当拒绝接受参加或者参加任何主办机构的继续教育计划,直到职业监管处收到遵守本条的保证。

(12)尽管本条有任何其他规定,职业监管处或者委员会可以随时对任何经批准的继续教育计划的任何主办机构进行评估,以确保符合本条的要求。

(d)符合继续教育规定的证明

(1)每位续展申请人须在进行续展申请时证明其完全满足(a)和(b)所载之继续教育规定。

(2)职业监管处可能需要其他证据,证明申请人满足继续教育规定(如出勤证明)。职业监管处在审计时可能随时需要这些证据。每位续期执照申请人有责任保留或者以其他方式提供其符合规定的证据。

(3)如发现申请人不符合继续教育相关规定,应当以书面形式通知该申请人,且申请人可以要求与委员会会面。届时,委员会可以建议根据《伊利诺伊州行政程序法》第 10 - 10 - 65 条的规定,启动违纪调查程序。

(e)在其他司法管辖区内参加的继续教育

(1)如果持证人在另一个州进行继续教育且其声称该学时完全满足伊利诺伊州的相关规定,培训主办单位并未根据第(c)款规定获得职业监管处的认可,申请人应当在参加培训计划之前或者在其执照到期的九十日之前,提交在本州外的继续教育批准表、继续教育计划、导师资格的描述、注册或者出勤的证明,以及二十五美元的手续费。针灸委员会或者职业监管处应当根据本条规定的标准,审查并建议准许或者不准许该计划。

(2)如果某执照持有人未能在规定的时间内提交外州继续教育审批表,可以通过提交如下材料和费用获得延迟的批准:即州外继续教育批准表、继续教育计划的描述和时间表、导师资格描述、出勤证明,以及所需的费用。所需的费用应当为二十五美元的手续费,外加要求延迟审批的每小时十美元的滞纳金。滞纳金不得超过一百五十美元。委员会或者职业监管处应当使用本条中规定的标准,审查并建议批准或者不批准该计划。

(f)继续教育规定的豁免

(1)对于未完全遵守本继续教育规定而进行执照续期的申请人,应当向职业监管处提交一份续期申请,按本部第 1140.20 条之规定缴纳相应费用,同时提交一份有关未能遵守规定的声明,并根据事实提交一份全部或者部分继续教育要求的豁免请求书。应当在执照有效期届满前提出弃权申请。如职业监管处根据委员会的书面建议,从该等宣誓书或者提交的任何其他证据中发现,给予豁免存在极端困难,该司须放弃执行申请人已申请的执照续期的继续教育要求。

(2)委员会应当根据申请人的个人情况对极端困难进行界定,并将其定义为在申请人周期内由于以下原因无法投入足够的时间来满足继续教育的规定:

（A）在续期周期内的大部分时间里,申请人在美国武装部队中全职服役。

（B）由执业医师书面确认,申请人身患可以导致无行为能力的疾病。

（C）由执业医师书面确认,申请人具有无法抵达经批准的授课地点的身体残疾。

（D）其他类似情有可原的情形。

（3）在执照到期之前,如果续期执照申请人根据本条之规定提交了全部或者部分豁免的请求,则在职业监管处对该申请作出最后裁决之前,其应当被视为处于状态正常。

第 1140.100 条　违反职业道德的行为

（a）根据法案第 110 条之规定,针灸实践中存在的不道德、未经授权或者违反职业道德的行为应当包括但不限于:

（1）通过贿赂或者欺诈性谎报获得、企图获得执照或者续期执照。

（2）故意编造或者提交虚假报告或者记录,故意不提交所在州或者联邦法律要求的报告或者记录,或者故意妨碍或者妨害材料的提交或者唆使他人采取类似做法。

（3）传播不真实、欺诈性、欺骗性或者误导性广告。

（4）故意不检举违反法案或者本条规定的行为。

（5）故意或者屡次违反委员会或者职业监管处此前在违纪听证会上制定的合法命令。

（6）接受并履行持证人知悉或者应当知悉其不具备履行能力的专业职责。

（7）持证人知悉或者有理由知悉某人不具备履行其职责的培训、经验或者执照资格时,将职责委派给此人行使。

（8）严重或者多次玩忽职守,或未能达到一个合理谨慎的接受过类似培训的针灸师认为在类似的条件和情况下可接受的护理、技术和治疗水平。

（9）除与持证人一起接受转诊的医生或者与持证人一起工作的其他针灸师外,与其他人就并非实际或者亲自提供的专业服务而收取的任何费用、佣金、回扣或者其他形式的报酬进行分成的行为。本款并不禁止持有有效执照者依据本法在以下形式的单位中执业。包括合伙、有限责任合伙关系、有限责任公司,或者根据专业公司法设立的公司,也不禁止其参与联营、共享、分割或者分配其合伙或者公司收到的费用和款项。

（10）从事与持证人的执业行为有关的任何不道德行为。

（11）从事性虐待、不端性行为或者性剥削。

（b）职业监管处在此引用国家针灸和东方医学认证委员会的《伦理规范》,华盛顿特区 20036 号,西北大街 800 室(2016 年 1 月),此后无修订或者其他版本。

第 1140.110 条　允准差异

在下列情况下,处长允准个别案例与本章规定存在差异:

（a）允准存在差异的规定并非强制条款。

（b）任何一方均不会因允准差异而受到损害。

（c）在特定情况下,允准存在差异的规则属于不合理或者不必要的负担。

印 第 安 纳 州

印第安纳州针灸法[①]

第一章 定　　义

第 IC 25－2.5－1－1 条　定义的适用性

下列定义适用于本章的全部条款。

第 IC 25－2.5－1－2 条　"针灸"

"针灸"系指运用东方传统和现代医学理念、东方医学诊治与治疗手段、辅助疗法和诊断技术来促进、维持和恢复健康并预防疾病的一种保健形式。

第 IC 25－2.5－1－2.1 条　"针灸师"

"针灸师"系指根据第 IC25－2.5－2 条的规定获得印第安纳州针灸执照的人员。

第 IC 25－2.5－1－2.5 条　"机构"

"机构"系指根据第 IC 25－1－5－3 条规定的印第安纳州专业资格许可机构。

第 IC 25－2.5－1－3 条　"委员会"

"委员会"系指医疗许可委员会。

第 IC 25－2.5－1－4 条　被 2006 年 3 月 24 日生效的 P.L.1－2006，SEC.588 废除

第 IC 25－2.5－1－5 条　"针灸实践"

"针灸实践"系指以东方医学诊断为主要治疗方式，在人体特定部位插入针灸针、应用艾灸，以及本章规定的其他针灸应用方法。

第二章　执照和资格条件

第 IC 25－2.5－2－1 条　获得针灸执照的条件

除本节第 3 条的规定外，个人必须符合下列条件才能获得本章规定的执照：

（1）根据委员会所采用的规则，妥善填写有关执照的申请书。

---

① 　根据《印第安纳州法典》注释版第 25 卷第 2.5 章"针灸师"译出。

120

（2）缴纳委员会规定的各项费用。

（3）未被判有由委员会裁定与申请人执业能力直接相关的罪行。

（4）未因申请人不能安全从事针灸实践而被委员会或者其他州或者司法管辖区的专业资格许可机构做出针对申请人或者申请人执业资格的纪律处分。此项纪律处分的事由由委员会或者国家认证机构认定。

（5）向委员会证明申请人：

（A）拥有由国家针灸与东方医学认证委员会（NCCAOM）颁发的针灸文凭；

（B）顺利完成为期三年的高等教育培训课程或者针灸学院课程，且该课程：

（i）经国家针灸与东方医学学院认证委员会认证。

（ii）属于国家针灸与东方医学学院认证委员会认证的候选课程。

（iii）符合国家针灸与东方医学学院认证委员会制定的标准。

（C）顺利完成 NCCAOM 批准的洁针技术课程。

第 IC 25‑2.5‑2‑2 条　执照的颁发

除本节第 4 条的规定外，委员会应当向下列个人颁发执照：

（1）符合本节第 1 条规定的条件。

（2）根据本章规定具有符合获颁执照的其他情形。

第 IC 25‑2.5‑2‑3 条　获得在其他州执照或者具有相关领域执照的申请人

（a）申请人在缴纳委员会规定的费用之后，如满足下列要求，则可以获发执照：

（1）申请人向委员会提交符合要求的证据，证明申请人已在其他州或者国家获得针灸执照。

（2）申请人符合本第 1 条第（1）款至第（4）款所列的要求。

（3）申请人向委员会出示的证据表明：

（A）申请人已顺利完成与委员会认定的国家针灸协会批准的洁针技术课程基本同等的课程。

（B）申请人已顺利完成为期三年的高等教育培训课程或者针灸学院课程，且该课程与由委员会认定的国家针灸协会对三年高等教育培训课程或者针灸学院课程所规定的标准基本同等。

（C）申请人已通过了相应考试，该考试与由委员会认定的国家针灸协会举办的考试基本同等。

（b）如申请人向委员会提交符合要求的证据，证明其是：

（1）根据第 IC 25‑10 条执业的脊椎按摩师。

（2）根据第 IC 25‑14 条执业的牙医。

（3）根据第 IC 25‑29 条执业的足科医生。

且曾经接受过至少二百学时的针灸培训。

（c）委员会应当：

（1）至少每两年编制一份课程和机构清单，此类课程和机构的设立目的是使个人根据第（b）款的规定获得专业执照。

(2) 根据第(b)款的规定,针对培训的逐案审批程序制定规则。

(d) 如果第(b)(1)项,第(b)(2)项或者第(b)(3)项所述的个人执照因负责管理个人职业的委员会对该个人采取纪律处分而受到限制,则其针灸执照也应当受到同样的限制。

(e) 如果第(b)(1),第(b)(2)项或者第(b)(3)项所述的个人执照被吊销,则根据第(b)款颁发给该人的执照也应当被吊销。

(f) 如果第(b)(1)(2)项或者第(3)项所述的个人执照被撤销,则根据第(b)款颁发给该人的执照也应当被撤销。

(g) 根据(b)款规定获得专业执照的个人,其针灸实践仅限于第(b)(1)(2)项或者第(3)项规定的个人执照执业范围。

第 IC 25-2.5-2-4 条　拒绝颁发执照

如果出现下列情形,委员会可拒绝向申请人颁发执照:

(1) 在执照申请过程中,如果委员会认定申请人发生违纪行为时已在印第安纳州获得执照,则该申请人将受到本章第 1 条第(4)款规定的惩罚措施。

(2) 申请人的执照因触犯第 IC 25-1-1.1 条的规定而被撤销。

第 IC 25-2.5-2-5 条　执照有效期与续期、恢复失效执照

生效日期:2018 年 7 月 1 日。

(a) 委员会颁发的执照的到期日期(每偶数年)由机构根据第 IC 25-1-5-4 条规定。

(b) 如果需要续期执照,针灸师应:

(1) 在执照到期前缴纳续期费。

(2) 提交由国家针灸与东方医学认证委员会出具的现行有效的针灸证书证明。

(c) 如果个人未能在执照到期日或者之前缴纳续期费,则无须委员会采取进一步措施,该执照会自动失效。

(d) 如果个人持有的执照已失效,但不超过三年,且符合第 IC 25-1-8-6 条第(c)款的规定,则委员会应当恢复其执照。

(e) 如果执照失效已超过三年,持证人可通过满足 IC 25-1-8-6(d)中列明的执照恢复条件后申请恢复其执照。

第 IC 25-2.5-2-6 条　拒绝颁发、吊销或者撤销执照

如果申请人或者执业针灸师存在以下任一行为,则委员会可拒绝颁发、吊销或撤销其执照,要求其参加补救教育,或者对其发出谴责信:

(1) 从事与针灸实践不符的虚假或者欺诈行为,包括:

(A) 就执照申请或者委员会开展的调查作出谎报。

(B) 试图提前收费。

(C) 虚假广告,包括承诺针灸疗法可以治愈疾病。

(D) 主动向转诊患者的人分摊或同意分摊针灸服务费。

(2) 未能适当控制自己的执业行为,如:

(A) 协助无证人士从事针灸实践。

(B) 在针灸师知情或应当知情的情况下,将专业职责委托给不具备资格的人员。

（C）对于与针灸师一同参与针灸实践工作的无执照人员,未能实施充分的监督。

（3）未能以适当的方式保存记录,如:

（A）未保存各患者治疗过程的书面记录。

（B）在患者提出要求的情况下,拒绝向其提供为患者准备的记录或患者付费记录。

（C）未经患者同意,泄露患者的个人身份信息,但法律另有规定的情形除外。

（4）未能对患者实施适当的医疗行为,包括:

（A）在没有为连续护理做出合理安排的情况下放弃或忽视患者。

（B）针灸师在与患者接触期间实施或者企图实施不良行为,向患者提出性要求,或者以发生性行为作为治疗的条件。

（5）表现出药物滥用或精神障碍,且足以影响其提供安全有效治疗的能力。

（6）在提供不当针灸实践的指控中被判有罪,承认有罪或者不予抗辩。

（7）由于疏忽而在执业过程中未能以专业认可的技术水平从事针灸实践。

（8）故意违反本条或委员会的任何规定。

（9）在另一司法管辖区,因任何原因而被拒绝颁发、吊销或撤销执照,且相关行为根据本条也应受到同样处理。

第 IC 25－2.5－2－7 条　耳穴疗法

（a）不得将本法解释为禁止执业针灸师实施耳穴疗法。

（b）非根据本条规定获得执业资格的个人,如果符合以下情形,可以为治疗酗酒、药物滥用或者药物依赖而实施耳穴疗法:

（1）向委员会提供证明,表明其已顺利完成委员会批准的针对针灸治疗酗酒、药物滥用或者药物依赖的培训计划,且该项目达到或者超过国家针灸戒毒协会规定的培训标准。

（2）向委员会提供证明,表明其已顺利完成洁针技术课程。

（3）在州、联邦或者委员会批准的酗酒、药物滥用或者化学依赖项目范围内,在执业针灸师的指导下提供耳穴疗法服务。

（4）遵守本条和委员会制定的道德标准。

第三章　非　法　执　业

第 IC 25－2.5－3－1 条　本章适用性

本章不适用于下列情形:

（1）在医疗保健专业执照、证书或者注册范围内执业的医疗保健人员。

（2）在执业针灸师的直接监督下从事针灸实践的学员,其实践为委员会批准的针灸学习课程内容。

第 IC 25－2.5－3－2 条　针灸师头衔的使用

除非是根据本法案的规定取得的针灸执照,否则个人不得使用"执业针灸师"的称号。

第 IC 25－2.5－3－3 条　无针灸执照行医

（a）除本章第 1 条另有规定外,未根据本条取得针灸执照而从事针灸实践属于违法行为。

（b）如果执业针灸师在获得第 IC25－22.5 章规定的执业医师的书面转诊信或者书面诊

断后对患者进行治疗,则该医师应当免于承担因患者或者针灸师使用其诊断或者因转诊而产生的民事责任,但构成重大过失、故意或者不加节制的不端行为或者疏忽除外。

第 IC 25－2.5－3－4 条　违规行为

违反本条规定的行为均构成 B 类轻罪。

印第安纳州针灸行政法[①]

第一节　定　义

第 844IAC13－1－1 条　适用范围

下列定义适用于本法。

第 844IAC13－1－2 条　"针灸"

（a）"针灸"系指除医学禁忌外,通过插入预消毒的一次性针头,以刺激体表或体内的某个穴位或多个穴位,对受影响的人进行评估和治疗（不论是否使用热、电刺激或者手法按压）,以防止或者改变疼痛感,使生理功能正常化,或者用于治疗某些疾病或者身体机能失调。

（b）该术语不包括:

（1）放射、电子外科、脊椎按摩技术、物理治疗、使用或者开具任何毒品、药物、血清或者疫苗。

（2）对抗疗法鉴别诊断的确定。

第 844IAC13－1－3 条　"针灸师"

"针灸师"系指在印第安纳州获得针灸执照的个人,包括执业针灸师和专业针灸师。

第 844IAC13－1－4 条　"ADS"

（a）"ADS"系指指针灸戒毒专家。

（b）ADS 是:

（1）仅限于使用国家针灸戒毒协会（NADA）规定的五个穴位。

（2）为了治疗第 IC25－2.5－2－7 条定义的酗酒、药物滥用或者化学依赖。

（c）ADS 系指以下人员:

（1）符合第 844IAC13－3－1 条规定的最低要求。

（2）与委员会颁发执照的医生或针灸师有依赖关系。

（3）在其监督下执行一项任务或者多项任务,而这些任务通常是根据法律在化学依赖治疗方案中执行的,目的是治疗酗酒、药物滥用或者化学依赖。

第 844IAC13－1－5 条　"委员会"

"委员会"系指印第安纳州医疗许可委员会。

---

① 根据《印第安纳州行政法典》第 844 卷第 13 章"针灸师"译出。

第 844IAC13－1－6 条　"专业针灸师"

（a）"专业针灸师"系指第 IC25－2.5－2－3（b）条规定的专业执照持证人。

（b）专业针灸师系指：

（1）根据第 IC 25－10 条执业的脊椎按摩师。

（2）根据第 IC 25－14 条执业的牙医。

（3）根据第 IC 25－29 条执业的足科医师。

具有经委员会批准的至少两百个学时的针灸实践时长。

第 844IAC13－1－7 条　"执业针灸师"

"执业针灸师"系指根据第 IC25－2.5－2－1 条或者第 IC25－2.5－2－3（a）条规定的持证人。

第 844IAC13－1－8 条　"NADA"

"NADA"系指全国针灸戒毒协会。

第 844IAC13－1－9 条　"针灸导师"

"针灸导师"系指经委员会批准的,监督并负责某一特定针灸戒毒专家的医生、骨科医生、专业针灸师或者执业针灸师。在同一个时间,针灸导师监督 ADS 的总数不得超过二十名。

第 844IAC13－1－10 条　"在执业针灸师的指导和监督下"

本节有关针灸戒毒专家的规定提及"在执业针灸师的指导和监督下",系指在针灸戒毒专家提供服务时,其督导医师或关联执业针灸师应合理安排时间,始终对该针灸戒毒专家的行为负责。患者的护理应当始终由督导医师或关联执业针灸师负责。

第二节　执 照 颁 发

第 844IAC13－2－1 条　申请

针灸执照申请人应当提交下列资料：

（1）以委员会规定的形式和方式提出的申请。

（2）申请人的两张近期护照照片,大约两英寸乘以两英寸大小,底部用黑色墨水签字。

（3）本节第 6 条规定的费用。

（4）国家针灸认证委员会现行有效的针灸证书原件或者核验证明。

（5）经国家针灸和东方医学院校认证委员会批准的三年的高等教育培训课程或者针灸学院培训课程的成绩单。

（6）经国家针灸与东方医学认证委员会批准的洁针技术课程结业证明的公证件。

（7）来自申请人曾经或者当前持有执照的所有州的核验证明,该证明应包含申请人是否曾受到任何纪律处分。

（8）其他方面符合第 IC25－2.5－2－1 条的要求。

第 844IAC13－2－2 条　在另一州持有执照或在另一国家获得授权

在另一州持有执照或在另一国家获准从事针灸实践的申请人,应当提交下列资料：

（1）以委员会规定的形式和方式提出的申请。

（2）申请人的两张近期护照照片，大约两英寸乘以两英寸大小，底部用黑色墨水签字。

（3）本节第 6 条规定的费用。

（4）申请人当前或曾经获得执照或授权，在另一个州或者国家从事针灸实践的，由该州或国家出具证据，证明其资格条件与本节第 1 条中的规定相同。

（5）国家针灸认证委员会现行有效针灸文凭的公证副本或者原始证明。

（6）经国家针灸和东方医学院校认证委员会批准的或与之基本同等的三年高等教育培训课程或者针灸学院培训课程的成绩单，须提供源语言和译本。

（7）经国家针灸与东方医学认证委员会批准的洁针技术课程结业证明的公证件。

（8）来自申请人曾经或当前持有执照的所有州的核验证明，该证明应包含申请人是否曾受到任何纪律处分。

（9）其他方面满足第 IC25‑2.5‑2‑1 条的要求。

第 844IAC13‑2‑3 条　通过培训计划获得执照（已过期）

第 844IAC13‑2‑4 条　关联专业人员针灸执照

申请人如根据第 IC25‑10 章的规定取得脊椎按摩师执照，或者根据第 IC25‑14 章的规定取得牙医执照，或者根据第 IC25‑29 章的规定取得足科医生执照，可在提交下列材料后颁发专业执照：

（1）以委员会规定的形式和方式提出的申请。

（2）申请人的两张近期护照照片，大约两英寸乘以两英寸大小，底部用黑色墨水签字。

（3）本节第 6 条规定的费用。

（4）经美国教育部批准的认证机构认可的学院或者大学出具的学校或课程的官方证书，证明申请人完成了两百个学时的针灸培训。

（5）来自申请人曾经或当前持有执照的所有州的核验证明，该证明应包含申请人是否曾受到任何纪律处分。

（6）此外，须提交在印第安纳州的脊椎按摩师、足科医生或牙医现行执照证明。

第 844IAC13‑2‑5 条　提供专业人员执照培训的课程和机构清单

（a）委员会应当通过卫生专业局提供一份课程和机构清单，列出为获得关联专业人员针灸执照之目的而批准的培训。

（b）如果某项计划或者课程未被列出，委员会应逐项审查各项计划。

（c）上述材料应提交委员会审查。

第 844IAC13‑2‑6 条　费用

委员会应当收取以下费用：

执照申请费	150 美元
关联专业人员执照	150 美元
ADS 认证申请费	10 美元

续　表

针灸执照续期费(不适用于申请针灸专业执照)	100 美元/两年
专业人员执照续期费(主要执照续期时需支付的额外费用)	100 美元
针灸戒毒专家续期费	20 美元/两年
未续期罚款	150 美元
执照副本费	10 美元
执照核验费	10 美元

第三节　监　　督

第 844IAC13 - 3 - 1 条　认证针灸戒毒专家

(a) 申请人可以在经州、联邦或者委员会批准的酒精、药物滥用或化学依赖治疗方案的范围内,在针灸导师的监督下实施针灸戒毒方案。

(b) 针灸戒毒专家应向委员会提供以下文件:

(1) 以委员会规定的形式和方式提出的申请。

(2) 必须年满十八周岁。

(3) 申请人的两张近期照片,照片质量等同于护照质量。

(4) 第 844IAC13 - 2 - 6 条中规定的费用。

(5) 高中文凭或者普通教育发展文凭的公证副本。

(6) 完成了符合或者超过国家针灸戒毒协会培训标准的、经委员会批准的针灸治疗酒精中毒、药物滥用或者化学依赖性培训方案的公证文件副本。

(7) 经国家针灸与东方医学认证委员会或者国家针灸戒毒协会批准的洁针技术课程结业证明的公证副本。

(8) 所有监督人员名单。

(9) 其他方面符合第 IC25 - 2.5 - 2 - 7 条的要求。

第 844IAC13 - 3 - 2 条　针灸解毒专家的监督流程

(a) 在针灸戒毒专家治疗患者时,针灸导师应在现场或者随时待命。

(b) 如果执业针灸师有意监督针灸戒毒专家,须在开始监督前,以表格的方式向委员会登记。针灸导师应在委员会提供的表格上填写以下信息:

(1) 针灸导师或医生的姓名、营业地址和电话号码。

(2) 针灸师或者医生的现行执照号码。

(3) 在针灸导师或者医生指导下的执业状况描述,包括针灸导师或者医生的专业特长(如有)。

(4) 由针灸导师或者医生作出以下声明:

(A) 根据第 IC25 - 27.5 - 6 条和本节对针灸戒毒专家进行持续监督。

（B）每月一次审查针灸戒毒专家履行职责的状况，并始终保存适当文档资料。导师必须签署患者的病历并注明日期。

（C）在任何时候，承担对针灸戒毒专家提供服务的专业和法律责任。

（5）详细描述针灸师、专业针灸师或者医生的监督过程，以评估针灸戒毒专家的治疗。

（c）针灸导师、专业针灸师或者医生应在十五日内，将终止与针灸戒毒专家的监督关系的原因通知委员会。

（d）如果因任何原因，针灸戒毒专家不再受到医生、专业针灸师或者具有针灸戒毒专家身份的执业针灸师的指导，上述人员应在十五日内将这一情况书面通知委员会，针灸戒毒专家受监督的执业资格随之终止。该终止持续有效，直到委员会批准的同一名或另一名医生、专业针灸师或执业针灸师提出与其建立新的监督关系。医生、专业针灸师、执业针灸师和针灸戒毒专家，应当在书面报告中告知委员会该针灸戒毒专家不再开展执业的具体原因，以及/或者不再受到医生或执业针灸师监督的原因。

第四节 执 照 续 期

第 844IAC13－4－1 条　执照续期

（a）应当在每一偶数年的 9 月 30 日或者之前，使用表格的方式向办事处提交续期申请。

（b）申请书应当附有第 844IAC13－2－6 条所要求的续期费。

（c）持证人应当在办事处提供的续期申请上签字，确认申请人目前持有由国家针灸与东方医学认证委员会颁发的执照的有效性。

（d）执业针灸师应当按照第 IC25－2.5－2－5 条的要求每两年续期一次。

（e）在执照到期后三年内未续期的，不得续期。此后不得恢复、补发或者复原，但满足所有要求的，可以申请并取得新的执照。

第 844IAC13－4－2 条　专业针灸执照的续期

（a）脊椎按摩师、牙医及足科医生的续期申请，须于原执照续期当日或者之前向办事处提交。因此，续期要求如下：

（1）脊椎按摩师的针灸执照应当在每年偶数年的 7 月 1 日或者之前，与脊医执照的续期同时提交办事处。

（2）牙医的针灸执照应当在每年偶数年的 3 月 1 日或者之前，与牙医执照的续期同时提交办事处。

（3）足科医生的针灸执照应当在第四个奇数年 6 月 30 日或者之前，与足科医师执照的续期同时提交办事处。

（b）续期费不包括原执照的续期费。

（c）必须签署续期申请，表明执业医生目前在印第安纳州被许可为脊医、牙医或者足医。

第 844IAC13－4－3 条　针灸戒毒专家证书的续期

（a）应当在每一偶数年的 9 月 30 日或者之前，以卫生专业局提供的表格向其提交续期申请。申请须随附第 844IAC13－2－6 条要求的续期费。

(b) 持有针灸戒毒专家证书的人必须按照第 IC25－2.5－2－5 条的要求每两年续期一次。

第 844IAC13－4－4 条　地址和名称的变更

（a）每名执业针灸师、专业针灸师或者经认证的针灸戒毒专家须在地址或名称变更后十五日内，以书面形式通知委员会所有变更地址或者名称的情况。

（b）执业针灸师、专业针灸师或者经认证的针灸戒毒专家，因未能通知委员会地址或者姓名更改而未收到续期通知，不构成委员会或卫生专业局的错误，不应免除或者原谅其续期执照的责任。

第五节　职业行为标准

第 844IAC13－5－1 条　针灸师的职责

（a）针灸师在进行治疗时，应当遵守本节中的职业行为标准。

（b）针灸师应当对患者相关的知识和信息进行保密，包括但不限于针灸师与患者建立关系的过程中获知或以其他方式被告知的，有关患者的诊断、治疗和预后，以及与之有关的所有记录。针灸师应当在法律要求或者经患者或者负责患者治疗的人员授权时，才能披露有关患者的信息。

（c）针灸师应当如实、坦率和合理完整地向患者或者负责患者治疗的人员说明患者的状况。除非针灸师能够合理地确定，该信息将损害患者、未成年人、无行为能力者或者负责患者治疗的人员的身心健康。

（d）当针灸师不再负责该病例时，针灸师应当向积极关注自己病情的患者或者负责患者治疗的人员发出合理的书面通知，以便患者或者负责其治疗人员可以雇用另一名针灸师。针灸师不得抛弃患者。本条所称"积极关注自己病情的患者"，系指针灸师在退休、停止针灸服务或者离开社区前两年内为其进行检查、治疗或者以其他方式为其提供咨询的人。

（e）除紧急情况外，针灸师退出针灸师治疗时，应根据患者的书面请求，向患者提供由针灸师保管、拥有或控制的所有记录、检验结果、病史、诊断、文件和信息，或上述文件的复印件。

（f）针灸师应当根据经批准的科学原则、方法、疗法、专业理论和实践，对患者进行合理的治疗，勤加诊断和治疗患者。

（g）针灸师不得陈述、宣传、声明或表明其拥有任何学位可作为获得针灸执照的依据，除非该针灸师已在本州或者其执业的州基于该学位获得了执照。

（h）针灸师应在患者或者负责患者治疗的人员提出要求时提供咨询。

（i）针灸师个人有合理理由认为另一位针灸师在针灸实践中从事违法、违规、不称职或者欺诈行为的，应立即向委员会报告。此外，针灸师如果知悉某人在未经授权的情况下从事或者试图从事针灸实践，须立即向委员会报告该等行为。

第 844IAC13－5－2 条　服务费

（a）针灸师因其专业服务而收取的费用，应当只补偿针灸师实际提供的服务。

（b）针灸师不得与不是专业公司合伙人、雇员或者股东的另一从业者分割专业服务费

用,除非:

(1)患者在充分披露费用分割后同意雇用其他从业者。

(2)费用的分割与每个从业者实际提供的服务和承担的责任成比例。

(c)针灸师不得因转诊患者而支付或者收取从业者的报酬。

第844IAC13-5-3条　雇员的责任

针灸师应当对针灸师雇用的每个人员在其与针灸师雇用关系存续期间的每个行为或不作为承担责任。但针灸师对其雇用的与针灸实践没有直接关系的人员的行为不承担责任。

第844IAC13-5-4条　转诊

(a)执业针灸师只能在执业医生或者骨病医生转诊时提供服务。本款不适用于专业针灸师。

(b)针灸师可以在其认为对患者有益时,将患者送往或者转诊给有资质的特定卫生保健提供者。然而,在进行任何此类转诊之前,针灸师应当检查和/或咨询患者,以合理确定患者转诊是否符合特定卫生保健提供者的执业范围。

第844IAC13-5-5条　停止针灸实践

(a)针灸师退休、停止针灸实践或者离开社区后,应当以书面形式,每周一次,连续三周在社区普遍发行的报纸上出版,通知所有在院患者,其打算停止在社区从事针灸实践,并应当鼓励其患者寻求其他执业针灸师的服务。停止执业的针灸师应当与在院患者作出合理安排,将其病历或者其副本移交给继任医生或者经委员会批准的针灸协会。

(b)本条中的任何规定均不妨碍、禁止或者阻止针灸师出于利益考虑,将其患者的病历出售、传送或者转让给其他持证从业者,但须按本条规定向患者发出书面通知。

第844IAC13-5-6条　广告

(a)针灸师不得代表其本人、合伙人、协作者,或者与针灸师有关联的任何其他从业者或者特定卫生保健提供者,使用或者参与使用含有虚假、欺诈、实质性误导或者欺骗性陈述或者主张的任何形式的公共通信。

(b)为便于公众做出知情选择,针灸师可以通过公共媒体宣传其服务,包括但不限于电话簿、针灸师名录、报纸或者其他期刊、电台或者电视,或者通过不涉及当面接触的书面通信。

(c)如果该广告是通过无线电、有线或者电视向公众传播的,则应当预先录制,由针灸师批准播出,并由针灸师自最后一次播出之日起,保留实际传播的录音和备份三年。

(d)如果针灸师在广告中提及针灸材料、服务、治疗、咨询、检查或者其他项目的费用,针灸师提供上述材料、服务或项目收取的费用不得超过所宣传的收费标准。

(e)除非广告中另外强调说明,针灸师在每月出版超过一次的刊物上发表或者传达收费信息,应当受该刊物发表日期后三十日内所作任何陈述的约束。针灸师在每月出版一次或者不经常出版的出版物中发表或者交流收费信息,应当受其中所作的任何陈述的约束,直到下一期出版为止,除非广告中明确规定了较短的时间。针灸师在没有固定出版日期的刊物上发表或者传达收费信息,须受该刊登载后一年的约束,除非广告中明显指明较短的时间。

(f)除广告另有规定外,用无线电、有线或者电视广播收费信息的针灸师,应当在广播后九十日内受其约束。

（g）针灸师使用公司名称或者商标名称发布广告,须指明提供针灸服务的地点。须在该地点标明提供服务的针灸师姓名。

第 844IAC13‑5‑7 条　未遵守规定的处置

未遵守专业行为标准和合格的针灸实践,可能导致对违规针灸师的纪律处分。所有在印第安纳州获得执照的针灸师有责任知悉第 IC25‑2.5 章所规定的行为标准及合规操作的知识。

第六节　撤销或吊销执照

第 844IAC13‑6‑1 条　撤销执照及持证人的义务

执照被撤销的从业者,应做到下列事项:

（1）以委员会规定的方式和方法,迅速通知当时正在接受其治疗的所有患者或负责患者治疗的人员,其执照被撤销且以后无法以专业身份为他们服务。该通知应建议所有患者自行选择另一名信誉良好的执业针灸师的服务。

（2）立即通知或者要求通知所有该从业者享有特权的卫生保健机构,并附上一份当时由该从业者治疗的所有患者的名单。

（3）以一类邮件书面通知下列组织和政府机构其执照已撤销:

（A）印第安纳州公共福利部门。

（B）社会保障管理局。

（C）为其颁发针灸执照的各州委员会或者同等机构。

（D）国家针灸与东方医学认证委员会。

（4）与持证人的患者作出合理安排,将所有患者病历、研究和检验结果或者其副本转交给患者雇用的继任医生或者负责患者治疗的人员。

（5）在撤销执照之日起三十日内,该从业者应向委员会提交一份宣誓书,证明其遵守了撤销令的规定,并向委员会提交了第 844IAC7 号宣誓书,委员会可以延长该期限。宣誓书还应当说明该从业者仍然持有执照的所有其他司法管辖区。

（6）证明遵守本条规定是申请恢复执照的先决条件。

第 844IAC13‑6‑2 条　吊销执照;持证人的义务

（a）在执照被吊销的情况下,该人应当在发出吊销令之日起三十日内向委员会提交一份宣誓书,说明如下:

（1）按照委员会规定的方式和方法,通知所有接受该从业者治疗的患者暂停治疗,因为其无法以专业身份为他们服务。该通知应当建议患者自行选择另一位良好信誉的从业者的服务。

（2）向所有医疗卫生机构告知吊销令,并停止该针灸师享有特权的权利。

（3）作出合理安排,将患者记录、研究和检验结果或者其副本转交给患者雇用的继任医生或者负责患者治疗的人员。

（b）证明遵守本条规定是申请恢复执照的先决条件。

第 844IAC13－6－3 条　恢复执照(已过期)

第 844IAC13－6－4 条恢复执照申请;申请费(已过期)

第七节　执业地点的相关告知

第 844IAC13－7－1 条　专业标牌;公共通知;设施要求

(a) 从业者有义务和责任在针灸诊所成立时,设有公众明显可见的标牌,标明在该执业地点的所有从业者的姓名。专业标牌上的最低要求是包含从业人员的姓名和头衔。

(b) 从业者的头衔可以做如下提示:

(1) 如果从业者根据本节获得执照,该从业者可以自称为针灸师或者执业针灸师。

(2) 如果从业者是专业人员,从业者可使用以下称谓:

(A) 博士学位的首字母,如 D.C.、D.D.S 或者 D.P.M。

(B) 针灸师。

(c) 标志不得误导公众。

(d) 从业者有义务和责任在成立针灸诊所时,保持设施的安全和卫生,并配备足够的设备提供针灸服务。

Iowa

Iowa Code Annotated

Chapter 148E. Acupuncture (Refs&Annos)

148E.1. Definitions

As used in this chapter, unless the context otherwise requires:

1. "Acupuncture" means a form of health care developed from traditional and modern oriental medical concepts that employs oriental medical diagnosis and treatment, and adjunctive therapies and diagnostic techniques, for the promotion, maintenance, and restoration of health and the prevention of disease.

2. "Acupuncturist" means a person who is engaged in the practice of acupuncture.

3. "Board" means the board of medicine established in chapter 147.

4. "Practice of acupuncture" means the insertion of acupuncture needles and the application of moxibustion to specific areas of the human body based upon oriental medical diagnosis as a primary mode of therapy. Adjunctive therapies within the scope of acupuncture may include manual, mechanical, thermal, electrical, and electromagnetic treatment, and the recommendation of dietary guidelines and therapeutic exercise based on traditional oriental medicine concepts.

148E.2. License required — renewal

1. In order to obtain a license to practice acupuncture, an applicant shall present evidence to the board of all of the following:

a. Current active status as a diplomate in acupuncture of the national commission for the certification of acupuncturists.

b. Successful completion of a three-year postsecondary training program or acupuncture college program which is accredited by, in candidacy for accreditation by, or which meets the standards of the accreditation commission for acupuncture and oriental medicine.

c. Successful completion of a course in clean needle technique approved by the national certification commission for acupuncture and oriental medicine.

2. Notwithstanding subsection 1, a license to practice acupuncture shall be granted by the board to a resident of this state who has successfully completed an acupuncture degree program approved by the board, or an apprenticeship or tutorial program approved by the board, on or before July 1, 2001.

3. A license granted pursuant to this section shall be renewed every two years. Renewal shall require evidence of current active membership in the national commission for the certification of acupuncturists.

148E.3. Scope of chapter

This chapter does not apply to the following:

1. A person otherwise licensed to practice medicine and surgery, osteopathic medicine and surgery, chiropractic, podiatry, or dentistry who is exclusively engaged in the practice of the person's profession.

2. A student practicing acupuncture under the direct supervision of a licensed acupuncturist as part of a course of study approved by the board.

148E.4. Standard of care

A person licensed under this chapter shall be held to the same standard of care as a person licensed to practice medicine and surgery or osteopathic medicine and surgery.

148E.5. Use and disposal of needles

An acupuncturist shall use only presterilized, disposable needles, and shall provide for adequate disposal of used needles.

148E.6. Display of certificate and disclosure of information to patients

An acupuncturist shall display the license issued pursuant to section 148E.2 in a conspicuous place in the acupuncturist's place of business. An acupuncturist shall provide to each patient upon initial contact with the patient the following information in written form:

1. The name, business address, and business telephone number of the acupuncturist.

2. A fee schedule.

3. A listing of the acupuncturist's education, experience, degrees, certificates, or credentials related to acupuncture awarded by professional acupuncture organizations, the length of time required to obtain the degrees or credentials, and experience.

4. A statement indicating any license, certificate, or registration in a health care occupation which was revoked by any local, state, or national health care agency.

5. A statement that the acupuncturist is complying with statutes and rules adopted by the board, including a statement that only presterilized, disposable needles are used by the acupuncturist.

6. A statement indicating that the practice of acupuncture is regulated by the board.

7. A statement indicating that a license to practice acupuncture does not authorize a person

to practice medicine and surgery in this state, and that the services of an acupuncturist must not be regarded as diagnosis and treatment by a person licensed to practice medicine and must not be regarded as medical opinion or advice.

148E.7. Duties of board

The board shall adopt rules consistent with this chapter and chapter 147 which are necessary for the performance of its duties.

148E.8. License revocation or suspension

In addition to the grounds for revocation or suspension referred to in section 147.55, a license to practice acupuncture shall be revoked or suspended when the acupuncturist is guilty of any of the following acts or offenses:

1. Failure to provide information as required in section 148E.6 or provision of false information to patients.

2. Acceptance of remuneration for referral of a patient to other health professionals.

3. Offering of or giving of remuneration for the referral of patients, not including paid advertisements or marketing services.

4. Failure to comply with this chapter, rules adopted pursuant to this chapter, or applicable provisions of chapter 147.

5. Engaging in sexual activity or genital contact with a patient while acting or purporting to act within the scope of practice, whether or not the patient consented to the sexual activity or genital contact.

6. Disclosure of confidential information regarding the patient.

148E.9. Accident and health insurance coverage

This chapter shall not be construed to require accident and health insurance coverage for acupuncture services under an existing or future contract or policy for insurance issued or issued for delivery in this state, unless otherwise provided by the contract or policy.

148E.10. Repealed by Acts 2000 (78 G.A.) ch.1053, § 14

Iowa Administrative Code

653 – 17.1 (148E). Purpose.

The licensure of acupuncturists is established to ensure that practitioners are qualified to provide Iowans with safe and healthful care. The provisions of Iowa Code chapters 147, 148E and 272C authorize the board of medicine to establish examination requirements for licensure; evaluate the credentials of applicants for licensure (147.2, 148E.3); grant licenses to qualified applicants (148E. 2); institute continuing education requirements (272C. 2); investigate complaints and reports alleging that licensed acupuncturists violated statutes and rules governing the practice of acupuncture (147.55, 148E.6); make available participation in the Iowa physician health program (272C.3); and discipline licensed acupuncturists found guilty of infractions as provided in state law and board rules (147.55, 148E.6).

653 - 17.2 (148E). Scope of chapter.

The rules in this chapter shall only apply to individuals licensed under Iowa Code chapter 148E. In accordance with Iowa Code section 148E.3, the rules in this chapter shall not apply to the following:

1. A person otherwise licensed by the state to practice medicine and surgery, osteopathic medicine and surgery, chiropractic, podiatry, or dentistry who is exclusively engaged in the practice of the person's profession.

2. A student practicing acupuncture under the direct supervision of a licensed acupuncturist as part of a course of study approved by the board.

653 - 17.3 (148E). Definitions.

"*Accreditation Commission for Acupuncture and Oriental Medicine*" or "*ACAOM*" means the United States-based accreditation commission that certifies acupuncture and oriental medicine training programs and colleges. The ACAOM oversees all professional oriental medicine and acupuncture degree programs in the United States. The ACAOM was formerly known as the National Accreditation Commission for Schools and Colleges of Acupuncture and Oriental Medicine.

"*Acupuncture*" means a form of health care developed from traditional and modern oriental medical concepts that employs oriental medical diagnosis and treatment, and adjunctive therapies and diagnostic techniques, for the promotion, maintenance, and restoration of health and the prevention of disease.

"*Acupuncture needle*" means a solid-core instrument including but not limited to acupuncture needles, dermal needles, intradermal needles, press tacks, plum blossom needles, prismatic needles, and disposable lancets.

"*Acupuncture point*" means a specific anatomical location on the human body that serves as the treatment site for the use of acupuncture.

"*Applicant*" means a person not otherwise authorized to practice acupuncture under Iowa Code section 148E.3 who applies to the board for a license.

"*Ashi acupuncture point*" means an acupuncture point that is located according to tenderness upon palpation. An ashi acupuncture point is also known as a trigger point.

"*Board*" means the board of medicine established in Iowa Code chapter 147.

"*Committee*" means the licensure committee of the board with oversight responsibility for administration of the licensure of acupuncturists.

"*Department*" means the Iowa department of public health.

"*Disclosure sheet*" means the written information licensed acupuncturists must provide to patients on initial contact.

"*Disposable needles*" means presterilized needles that are discarded after initial use pursuant to Iowa Code section 148E.5.

"*License*" means a license issued by the board pursuant to Iowa Code section 148E.2.

"*Licensee*" means a person holding a license to practice acupuncture issued by the board pursuant to Iowa Code chapter 148E.

"*National Certification Commission for Acupuncture and Oriental Medicine*" or "*NCCAOM*" means the United States-based commission that validates entry-level competency in the practice of acupuncture and oriental medicine through professional certification.

"*Practice of acupuncture*" means the insertion of acupuncture needles and the application of moxibustion to specific areas of the human body based upon oriental medical diagnosis as a primary mode of therapy. Adjunctive therapies within the scope of acupuncture may include manual, mechanical, thermal, electrical, and electromagnetic treatment, and the recommendation of dietary guidelines and therapeutic exercise based on traditional oriental medicine concepts.

"*Service charge*" means the amount charged by the board for making a service available online and is in addition to the actual fee for a service itself. For example, one who renews a license online will pay the license renewal fee and a service charge.

653 – 17.4 (147, 148E).   Eligibility for licensure.

17.4 (1) *Eligibility requirements.* To be licensed to practice acupuncture by the board, a person shall meet all of the following requirements:

a. Fulfill all the application requirements, as specified in 17.5 (147, 148E).

b. Hold current active status as a diplomate in NCCAOM or, after June 1, 2004, hold current active status as a diplomate in acupuncture or oriental medicine from NCCAOM.

c. Demonstrate sufficient knowledge of the English language to understand and be understood by patients and board and committee members.

(1) An applicant who passed the NCCAOM written and practical examination components in English may be presumed to have sufficient proficiency in English.

(2) An applicant who passed NCCAOM written or practical examination components in a language other than English shall pass the Test of Spoken English (TSE) or the Test of English as a Foreign Language (TOEFL) examinations administered by the Educational Testing Service. A passing score on TSE is a minimum of 50. A passing score on TOEFL is a minimum overall score of 550 on the paper-based TOEFL that was administered on a Friday or Saturday (formerly special or international administration), a minimum overall score of 213 on the computer-administered TOEFL, or a minimum overall score of 79 on the Internet-based examination.

d. Successfully complete a three-year postsecondary training program or acupuncture college program which is accredited by, in candidacy for accreditation by, or which meets the standards of the Accreditation Commission for Acupuncture and Oriental Medicine.

e. Successfully complete a course in clean needle technique approved by the NCCAOM.

f. The applicant's license is not denied by the board due to the commission of a disqualifying offense, as provided in 653 — subrule 9.3(3).

17.4(2) *Waiver prohibited.* Provisions of this rule are not subject to waiver pursuant to 653 — Chapter 3 or any other provision of law.

653 ‒ 17.5 (147, 148E). Application requirements.

17.5(1) *Application for licensure.* To apply for a license to practice acupuncture, an applicant shall:

a. Submit the completed application form provided by the board, including required credentials and documents, a completed fingerprint packet and a sworn statement by the applicant attesting to the truth of all information provided by the applicant;

b. Pay the nonrefundable initial application fee identified in 653 — paragraph 8.2(2) "*a*"; and

c. Pay the fee identified in 653 — paragraph 8.2(2) "*e*" for the evaluation of the fingerprint packet and the national criminal history background checks by the Iowa division of criminal investigation (DCI) and the Federal Bureau of Investigation (FBI).

17.5(2) *Contents of the application form.* Each applicant shall submit the following information on the application form provided by the board:

a. The applicant's full legal name, date and place of birth, home address, mailing address, principal business address, and personal e-mail address regularly used by the applicant or licensee for correspondence with the board;

b. A photograph of the applicant suitable for positive identification;

c. A chronology accounting for all time periods from the date the applicant entered an acupuncture and oriental medicine training program or college to the date of the application;

d. The other jurisdictions in the United States or other nations or territories in which the applicant is authorized to practice acupuncture, including license, certificate of registration or certification numbers, and date of issuance;

e. Full disclosure of the applicant's involvement in civil litigation related to the practice of acupuncture in any jurisdiction of the United States, other nations or territories. Copies of the legal documents may be requested if needed during the review process;

f. A statement disclosing and explaining any informal or nonpublic actions, warnings issued, investigations conducted, or disciplinary actions taken, whether by voluntary agreement or formal action, by a medical, acupuncture or professional regulatory authority, an educational institution, a training or research program, or a health facility in any jurisdiction;

g. A statement disclosing and explaining any charge of a misdemeanor or felony involving the applicant filed in any jurisdiction, whether or not any appeal or other proceeding is pending to have the conviction or plea set aside;

h. The NCCAOM score report verification form submitted directly to the board by the NCCAOM;

i. An NCCAOM certificate that demonstrates that the applicant holds current active status as a diplomate in acupuncture or oriental medicine from the NCCAOM;

j. Proof of successful completion of a course in clean needle technique approved by the NCCAOM;

k. A statement of the applicant's physical and mental health, including full disclosure and a written explanation of any dysfunction or impairment which may affect the ability of the applicant to engage in the practice of acupuncture and provide patients with safe and healthful care;

l. A description of the applicant's clinical acupuncture training, work experience and, where applicable, supporting documentation;

m. A copy of the applicant's acupuncture degree issued by an educational institution. If a copy of the acupuncture degree cannot be provided because of extraordinary circumstances, the board may accept other reliable evidence that the applicant obtained an acupuncture degree from a specific educational institution;

n. A complete translation of any diploma not written in English. An official transcript, written in English and received directly from the educational institution, showing graduation from an acupuncture training program or an educational institution is a suitable alternative;

o. A sworn statement from an official of the educational institution certifying the date the applicant received the acupuncture degree and acknowledging what, if any, derogatory comments exist in the institution's record about the applicant. If a sworn statement from an official of the educational institution cannot be provided because of extraordinary circumstances, the board may accept other reliable evidence that the applicant obtained an acupuncture degree from a specific educational institution;

p. An official transcript sent directly from an acupuncture training program or an educational institution attended by the applicant and, if requested by the board, an English translation of the official transcript;

q. Proof of the applicant's proficiency in the English language, when the applicant has not passed the English version of the NCCAOM written and practical examinations;

r. Verification of an applicant's hospital and clinical staff privileges and other professional experience for the past five years if requested by the board; and

s. A completed fingerprint packet to facilitate a national criminal history background check. The fee for evaluation of the fingerprint packet and the DCI and FBI criminal history background checks will be assessed to the applicant.

17.5(3) *Disclosure sheet.* Rescinded IAB 2/15/17, effective 3/22/17.

17.5(4) *Application cycle.* If the applicant does not submit all materials, including a completed fingerprint packet, within 90 days of the board's initial request for further information, the application shall be considered inactive. The board office shall notify the applicant of this change in status.

a. To reactivate the application, an applicant shall submit a nonrefundable reactivation of application fee identified in 653 — paragraph 8.2(2) "*b*" and shall update application materials if requested by the board. The period for requesting reactivation is limited to 30 days from the date the applicant is notified that the application is inactive, unless the applicant is granted an extension in writing by the committee or the board.

b. Once the application reactivation period is expired, applicants must reapply and submit a new, nonrefundable initial application fee and a new application, including required documents and credentials.

17.5(5) *Applicant responsibilities.* An applicant for licensure to practice acupuncture bears full responsibility for each of the following:

a. Paying all fees charged by regulatory authorities, national testing or credentialing organizations, health facilities, and educational institutions providing the information specified in 17.5(2);

b. Providing accurate, up-to-date, and truthful information on the application form including, but not limited to, that specified under 17.5(2) related to prior professional experience, education, training, examination scores, diplomate status, licensure or registration, and disciplinary history; and

c. Submitting English translations of documents in foreign languages bearing the affidavit of the translator certifying that the translation is a true and complete translation of the foreign language original. The applicant shall bear the expense of the translation.

17.5(6) *Licensure application review process.* The process below shall be utilized to review each application. Priority shall be given to processing a licensure application when a written request is received in the board office from an applicant whose practice will primarily involve provision of services to underserved populations, including but not limited to persons who are minorities or low-income or who live in rural areas.

a. An application for initial licensure shall be considered open from the date the application form is received in the board office with the nonrefundable initial application fee.

b. After reviewing each application, staff shall notify the applicant about how to resolve any problems identified by the reviewer. An applicant shall provide additional information when requested by staff or the board.

c. If the final review indicates no questions or concerns regarding the applicant's qualifications for licensure, staff may administratively grant the license. The staff may grant the license without having received a report on the applicant from the FBI.

d. If the final review indicates questions or concerns that cannot be remedied by continued communication with the applicant, the executive director, the director of licensure and the director of legal affairs shall determine if the questions or concerns indicate any uncertainty about the applicant's current qualifications for licensure.

(1) If there is no current concern, staff shall administratively grant the license.

(2) If any concern exists, the application shall be referred to the committee.

e. Staff shall refer to the committee for review matters which include but are not limited to: falsification of information on the application, criminal record, malpractice, substance abuse, competency, physical or mental illness, or professional disciplinary history.

f. If the committee is able to eliminate questions or concerns without dissension from staff or a committee member, the committee may direct staff to issue the license administratively.

g. If the committee is not able to eliminate questions or concerns without dissension from staff or a committee member, the committee shall recommend that the board:

(1) Request an investigation;

(2) Request that the applicant appear for an interview;

(3) If an applicant has not engaged in active practice in the past three years in any jurisdiction of the United States, require an applicant to:

1. Successfully complete continuing education or retraining programs in areas directly related to the safe and healthful practice of acupuncture deemed appropriate by the board or committee;

2. Successfully pass a competency evaluation approved by the board;

3. Successfully pass an examination approved by the board; or

4. Successfully complete a reentry to practice program or monitoring program approved by the board;

(4) Issue a license;

(5) Issue a license under certain terms and conditions or with certain restrictions;

(6) Request that the applicant withdraw the licensure application; or

(7) Deny a license.

h. The board shall consider applications and recommendations from the committee and shall:

(1) Request an investigation;

(2) Request that the applicant appear for an interview;

(3) If an applicant has not engaged in active practice in the past three years in any jurisdiction of the United States, require an applicant to:

1. Successfully complete continuing education or retraining programs in areas directly related to the safe and healthful practice of acupuncture deemed appropriate by the board or committee;

2. Successfully pass a competency evaluation approved by the board;

3. Successfully pass an examination approved by the board; or

4. Successfully complete a reentry to practice program or monitoring program approved by

the board;

(4) Issue a license;

(5) Issue a license under certain terms and conditions or with certain restrictions;

(6) Request that the applicant withdraw the licensure application; or

(7) Deny a license. The board may deny a license for any grounds on which the board may discipline a license.

17.5(7) *Grounds for denial of licensure.* The board, on the recommendation of the committee, may deny an application for licensure for any of the following reasons:

a. Failure to meet the requirements for licensure specified in rule 653 − 17.4 (147, 148E) as authorized by Iowa Code section 148E.2 or of this chapter of the board's rules.

b. Pursuant to Iowa Code section 147.4, upon any of the grounds for which licensure may be revoked or suspended as specified in Iowa Code sections 147.55 and 148E.8 or in rule 653 − 17.12 (147, 148E, 272C).

17.5(8) *Preliminary notice of denial.* Prior to the denial of licensure to an applicant, the board shall issue a preliminary notice of denial that shall be sent to the applicant by regular, first-class mail at the address provided by the applicant. The preliminary notice of denial is a public record and shall cite the factual and legal basis for denying the application, notify the applicant of the appeal process, and specify the date upon which the denial will become final if it is not appealed.

17.5(9) *Appeal procedure.* An applicant who has received a preliminary notice of denial may appeal the denial and request a hearing on the issues related to the preliminary notice of denial by serving a request for hearing upon the executive director not more than 30 calendar days following the date when the preliminary notice of denial was mailed. The applicant's current address shall be provided in the request for hearing. The request is deemed filed on the date it is received in the board office. If the request is received with a USPS nonmetered postmark, the board shall consider the postmark date as the date the request is filed. The request shall specify the factual or legal errors and that the applicant desires an evidentiary hearing and may provide additional written information or documents in support of licensure.

17.5(10) *Hearing.* If an applicant appeals the preliminary notice of denial and requests a hearing, the hearing shall be a contested case and subsequent proceedings shall be conducted in accordance with 653 − 25.30 (17A).

a. License denial hearings are contested cases open to the public.

b. Either party may request issuance of a protective order in the event privileged or confidential information is submitted into evidence.

c. Evidence supporting the denial of the license may be presented by an assistant attorney general.

d. While each party shall have the burden of establishing the affirmative of matters asserted, the applicant shall have the ultimate burden of persuasion as to the applicant's qualification for licensure.

e. The board, after a hearing on license denial, may grant or deny the application for licensure. The board shall state the reasons for its decision and may grant the license, grant the license with restrictions, or deny the license. The final decision is a public record.

f. Judicial review of a final order of the board denying licensure, or issuing a license with restrictions, may be sought in accordance with the provisions of Iowa Code section 17A.19, which are applicable to judicial review of any agency's final decision in a contested case.

17.5(11) *Finality.* If an applicant does not appeal a preliminary notice of denial in accordance with 17.5(9), the preliminary notice of denial automatically becomes final. A final denial of an application for licensure is a public record.

17.5(12) *Failure to pursue appeal.* If an applicant appeals a preliminary notice of denial in accordance with 17.5(9) but the applicant fails to pursue that appeal to a final decision within one year from the date of the preliminary notice of denial, the board may dismiss the appeal. The appeal may be dismissed only after the board sends a written notice by first-class mail to the applicant at the applicant's last-known address. The notice shall state that the appeal will be dismissed and the preliminary notice of denial will become final if the applicant does not contact the board to schedule the appeal hearing within 30 days of the date the letter is mailed from the board office. Upon dismissal of an appeal, the preliminary notice of denial becomes final. A final denial of an application for licensure under this rule is a public record.

17.5(13) *Waiver prohibited.* Provisions of this rule are not subject to waiver pursuant to 653 — Chapter 3 or any other provision of law.

653 – 17.6 (147, 148E). Display of license and disclosure of information to patients.

17.6(1) *Display of license.* Licensed acupuncturists shall display the license issued by the board in a conspicuous place in their primary place of business.

17.6(2) *Distribution and retention of disclosure sheet.* Pursuant to Iowa Code section 148E.6, the licensee shall distribute a disclosure sheet on initial contact with patients and retain a copy, signed and dated by the patient, for a period of at least five years after termination of treatment. The disclosure sheet shall include the following:

a. The name, business address, and business telephone number of the acupuncturist.

b. A fee schedule.

c. A listing of the acupuncturist's education, experience, degrees, certificates, or credentials related to acupuncture awarded by professional acupuncture organizations and the length of time required to obtain the degrees or credentials and experience.

d. A statement indicating any license, certificate, or registration in a health care occupation that was revoked by any local, state, or national health care agency.

e. A statement that the acupuncturist is complying with statutes and rules adopted by the board, including a statement that only presterilized, disposable needles are used by the acupuncturist.

f. A statement indicating that the practice of acupuncture is regulated by the board.

g. A statement indicating that a license to practice acupuncture does not authorize a person to practice medicine and surgery in this state and that the services of an acupuncturist must not be regarded as diagnosis and treatment by a person licensed to practice medicine and must not be regarded as medical opinion or advice.

653 – 17.7 (147, 148E, 272C). Biennial renewal of license required.

Pursuant to Iowa Code section 148E.2, a license expires on October 31 of even-numbered years and can be renewed for the fee identified in 653 — paragraph 8.2(2) "*c.*" The applicant for renewal shall provide an NCCAOM certificate that demonstrates that the applicant holds current active status as a diplomate in acupuncture or oriental medicine from the NCCAOM.

17.7(1) *Expiration date.* Certificates of licensure to practice acupuncture shall expire on October 31 in even years.

17.7(2) *Prorated fees.* The first renewal fee for a license shall be prorated on a monthly basis according to the date of issue.

17.7(3) *Renewal requirements and penalties for late renewal.* Each licensee shall be sent a renewal notice at least 60 days prior to the expiration date. The licensee is responsible for renewing the license prior to its expiration. Failure of the licensee to receive the notice does not relieve the licensee of responsibility for renewing that license.

a. When online renewal is used, the licensee must complete the online renewal prior to midnight on December 31 in order to ensure that the license will not become inactive. The license becomes inactive and invalid at 12:01 a.m. on January 1.

b. Upon receipt of the completed renewal application, staff shall administratively issue a license that expires on October 31 of even-numbered years. In the event the board receives adverse information on the renewal application, the board shall issue the renewal license but may refer the adverse information for further consideration.

c. Every renewal shall be displayed in connection with the original certificate of licensure.

d. If the licensee fails to submit the renewal application and renewal fee prior to the expiration date on the current license, a \$50 penalty shall be assessed for renewal in the grace period, a period up until January 1 when the license becomes inactive if not renewed.

17.7 (4) *Inactive license.* Failure of a licensee to renew by January 1 will result in invalidation of the license and the license will become inactive.

a. Licensees are prohibited from engaging in the practice of acupuncture once the license is lapsed.

b. Having an acupuncturist license in lapsed status does not preclude the board from taking disciplinary actions authorized in Iowa Code section 147.55 or 148E.8.

653 – 17.8 (147 , 272C).   Reinstatement of an inactive license.

17.8(1) *Reinstatement requirements.* Licensees who allow their licenses to go inactive by failing to renew may apply for reinstatement of a license. Pursuant to Iowa Code section 147.11, applicants for reinstatement shall:

a. Submit upon forms provided by the board a completed application for reinstatement of a license to practice acupuncture. The application shall include the following information:

(1) The applicant's full legal name, date and place of birth, home address, mailing address, principal business address, and personal e-mail address regularly used by the applicant or licensee for correspondence with the board.

(2) Every jurisdiction in which the applicant is or has been authorized to practice, including license numbers and dates of issuance.

(3) Full disclosure of the applicant's involvement in civil litigation related to the practice of acupuncture in any jurisdiction of the United States, other nations or territories. Copies of the legal documents may be requested if needed during the review process.

(4) A statement disclosing and explaining any warnings issued, investigations conducted or disciplinary actions taken, whether by voluntary agreement or formal action, by a medical, acupuncture or professional regulatory authority, an educational institution, a training or research program, or a health facility in any jurisdiction.

(5) A statement of the applicant's physical and mental health, including full disclosure and a written explanation of any dysfunction or impairment which may affect the ability of the applicant to engage in practice and provided patients with safe and healthful care.

(6) Verification of an applicant's hospital and clinical staff privileges and other professional experience for the past five years if requested by the board.

(7) A chronology accounting for all time periods from the date of initial licensure.

(8) A statement disclosing and explaining any charge of a misdemeanor or felony involving the applicant filed in any jurisdiction, whether or not any appeal or other proceeding is pending to have the conviction or plea set aside.

b. Submit a completed fingerprint packet to facilitate a national criminal history background check. The fee identified in 653 — paragraph 8.2(2) "*e*" for the evaluation of the fingerprint packet and the DCI and FBI criminal history background checks will be assessed to the applicant.

c. Pay the reinstatement fee of $400 plus the fee identified in 653 — paragraph 8.2(2) "*e*" for the evaluation of the fingerprint packet and the DCI and FBI criminal history background checks.

d. Provide an NCCAOM certificate which demonstrates that the applicant holds current active status as a diplomate in acupuncture or oriental medicine from the NCCAOM.

e. Meet any new requirements instituted since the license lapsed.

17.8(2) *Reinstatement restrictions.* Pursuant to Iowa Code section 272C.3(2) "*d*", the committee may require an applicant who has not engaged in active practice in the past three years in any jurisdiction of the United States to meet any or all of the following requirements prior to reinstatement of an inactive license:

a. Successfully complete continuing education or retraining programs in areas directly related to the safe and healthful practice of acupuncture deemed appropriate by the board or committee;

b. Successfully pass a competency evaluation approved by the board;

c. Successfully pass an examination approved by the board; or

d. Successfully complete a reentry to practice program or monitoring program approved by the board.

653 - 17.9 (272C). Continuing education requirements.

Licensees shall demonstrate that they hold current active status as a diplomate from the NCCAOM. The NCCAOM requires 60 points of professional development activity every four years. Active NCCAOM certification satisfies the continuing education requirements established in Iowa Code section 272C.2.

653 - 17.10 (147, 148E, 272C). General provisions.

17.10(1) *Diagnostic and treatment modalities.* Diagnostic and treatment modalities used by licensees under this chapter may include one or more of the following acupunctural services:

a. The stimulation or piercing of the skin with an acupuncture needle for any of the following purposes:

(1) To evoke a therapeutic physiological response, either locally or distally to the area of insertion or stimulation.

(2) To relieve pain or treat the neuromusculoskeletal system.

(3) To stimulate ashi acupuncture points to relieve pain and dysfunction.

(4) To promote, maintain, and restore health and to prevent disease.

(5) To stimulate the body according to auricular, hand, nose, face, foot or scalp acupuncture therapy.

(6) To use acupuncture needles with or without the use of herbs, electric current, or application of heat.

b. The use of oriental medical diagnosis and treatment, including:

(1) Moxibustion, cupping, thermal methods, magnets, gua sha scraping techniques, acupatches, herbal poultices, hot and cold packs, electromagnetic wave therapy, light and color therapy, sound therapy, or therapy lasers.

(2) Massage, acupressure, reflexology, shiatsu and tui na massage, or manual stimulation, including stimulation by an instrument or mechanical device that does not pierce the skin.

(3) Herbal medicine and dietary supplements, including those of plant, mineral, animal, and nutraceutical origin.

c. Any other adjunctive service or procedure that is clinically appropriate based on the licensee's training as approved by NCCAOM or ACAOM.

17.10(2) *Use and disposal of needles.* A licensee shall use only presterilized, disposable needles and shall provide for the disposal of used needles in accordance with the requirements of the department.

17.10(3) *Standard of care.* A licensee shall be held to the same standard of care as persons licensed to practice medicine and surgery or osteopathic medicine and surgery. Pursuant to Iowa Code section 272C.3, any error or omission, unreasonable lack of skill, or failure to maintain a reasonable standard of care in the practice of acupuncture constitutes malpractice and is grounds for the revocation or suspension of a license to practice acupuncture in this state.

17.10(4) *Title.* An acupuncturist licensed under this title may use the words "licensed acupuncturist" or "L. Ac." to connote professional standing after the licensee's name in accordance with Iowa Code section 147.74 (18).

17.10(5) *Change of contact information.* Licensees shall notify the board of changes in home address, address of the place of practice, home or practice telephone number, or personal e-mail address regularly used by the applicant or licensee for correspondence with the board within one month of the change.

17.10(6) *Delegation of responsibilities.* A licensee shall perform all aspects of acupuncture treatment that involve penetration of the skin of a patient. The licensee may delegate other aspects of treatment to staff and patients who are properly trained by the licensee. It is permissible for appropriately trained staff and patients to remove acupuncture needles from the patient's body. The licensee is responsible for establishing and maintaining written training standards for staff.

17.10(7) *Change of full legal name.* A licensee shall notify the board of any change in the licensee's full legal name within one month of making the name change. Notification requires a notarized copy of a marriage license or a notarized copy of court documents.

17.10(8) *Deceased.* A licensee's file shall be closed and labeled "deceased" when the board receives a copy of the licensee's death certificate or other reliable information of the licensee's death.

653 – 17.11 (147, 148E, 272C). General disciplinary provisions.

The board is authorized to take disciplinary action against any licensee who violates the provisions set forth in state law and administrative rules pertaining to the safe and healthful practice of acupuncture. This rule is not subject to waiver pursuant to 653 — Chapter 3 or any other provision of law.

17.11(1) *Methods of discipline.* The board may impose any of the following disciplinary sanctions:

a. Revocation of a license;

b. Suspension of a license until further order of the board;

c. Nonrenewal of a license;

d. Restrict permanently or temporarily the performance of specific procedures, methods, acts or techniques;

e. Probation;

f. Additional or remedial education or training;

g. Reexamination;

h. Medical or physical evaluation, or alcohol or drug screening within a specific time frame at a facility or by a practitioner of the board's choice;

i. Civil penalties not to exceed $1,000;

j. Citations and warnings as necessary; and

k. Other sanctions allowed by law as deemed appropriate.

17.11(2) *Discretion of the board.* The board may consider the following factors when determining the nature and severity of the disciplinary sanction to be imposed:

a. The relative seriousness of the violation as it relates to assuring the citizens of Iowa a high standard of professional care.

b. The facts of the particular violation.

c. Any extenuating circumstances or other countervailing considerations.

d. Number of prior violations or complaints.

e. Seriousness of prior violations or complaints.

f. Whether remedial action has been taken.

g. Such other factors as may reflect upon the competency, ethical standards and professional conduct of the licensee.

653 – 17.12 (147, 148E, 272C). Grounds for discipline.

The board may impose any of the disciplinary sanctions set forth in 17.11(1) upon determining that a licensee is guilty of any of the following acts or offenses:

17.12(1) *Fraud in procuring a license.* Fraud in procuring a license is the deliberate distortion of facts or use of deceptive tactics in the application for licensure to practice acupuncture including, but not limited to:

a. Making false or misleading statements in obtaining or seeking to obtain licensure;

b. Failing to disclose by deliberate omission or concealment any information the board deems relevant to the safe and healthful practice of acupuncture pursuant to Iowa Code chapters 147 and 148E;

c. Misrepresenting any fact or deed to meet the application or eligibility requirements established by this chapter; or

d. Filing or attempting to file a false, forged or altered diploma, certificate, affidavit, translated or other official or certified document, including the application form, attesting to the applicant's eligibility for licensure to practice acupuncture in Iowa.

17.12(2) *Professional incompetence.* Professional incompetence includes, but is not limited to:

a. Substantial lack of knowledge or ability to discharge professional obligations within the scope of the acupuncturist's practice;

b. Substantial deviation by the licensee from the standards of learning or skill ordinarily possessed and applied by other acupuncturists when acting in the same or similar circumstances;

c. Failure by an acupuncturist to exercise in a substantial respect the degree of care which is ordinarily exercised by the average acupuncturist when acting in the same or similar circumstances; or

d. Willful or repeated departure from or the failure to conform to the minimal standard of acceptable and prevailing practice of acupuncture.

17.12(3) *Fraud in the practice of acupuncture.* Fraud in the practice of acupuncture includes, but is not limited to, any misleading, deceptive, untrue or fraudulent representation in the practice of acupuncture, made orally or in writing, that is contrary to the acupuncturist's legal or equitable duty, trust or confidence and is deemed by the board to be contrary to good conscience, prejudicial to the public welfare, and potentially injurious to another. Proof of actual injury need not be established.

17.12(4) *Unethical conduct.* The Code of Ethics (2008) prepared and approved by the NCCAOM shall be utilized by the board as guiding principles in the practice of acupuncture in this state. Unethical conduct in the practice of acupuncture includes, but is not limited to:

a. Failing to provide patients with the information required in Iowa Code section 148E.6 or providing false information to patients;

b. Accepting remuneration for referral of patients to other health care professionals;

c. Offering or providing remuneration for the referral of patients, excluding paid advertisements or marketing services;

d. Engaging in sexual activity or genital contact with a patient while acting or purporting to act within the scope of the acupuncture practice, whether or not the patient consented to the sexual activity or genital contact;

e. Disclosing confidential information about a patient without proper authorization; or

f. Abrogating the boundaries of acceptable conduct in the practice of acupuncture established by the profession that the board deems appropriate for ensuring that acupuncturists provide Iowans with safe and healthful care.

17.12(5) *Practice harmful to the public.* Practice harmful or detrimental to the public in the practice of acupuncture includes, but is not limited to:

a. Failing to possess and exercise the degree of skill, learning and care expected of a reasonable, prudent acupuncturist acting in the same or similar circumstances;

b. Practicing acupuncture without reasonable skill and safety as the result of a mental or physical impairment, chemical abuse or chemical dependency;

c. Prescribing, dispensing or administering any controlled substance or prescription medication for human use; or

d. Performing any treatment or healing procedure not authorized in Iowa Code chapter 148E or this chapter.

17.12(6) *Habitual intoxication or addiction.* Habitual intoxication or addiction to the use of drugs includes, but is not limited to, the inability to practice acupuncture with reasonable skill and safety as a result of the excessive use of alcohol, drugs, narcotics, chemicals or other substances on a continuing basis, or the excessive use of the same in a way which may impair the ability to practice acupuncture with reasonable skill and safety.

17.12(7) *Felony conviction.* A felony conviction related to the practice of acupuncture or that affects the ability to practice the profession includes, but is not limited to:

a. Any conviction for any public offense directly related to or associated with the practice of acupuncture that is classified as a felony under the statutes of any jurisdiction of the United States, the United States government, or another nation or its political subdivisions; or

b. Any conviction for a public offense affecting the ability to practice acupuncture that is classified as a felony under the statutes of any jurisdiction of the United States, the United States government, or another nation or its political subdivisions and that involves moral turpitude, civility, honesty, or morals.

A copy of the record of conviction or plea of guilty or nolo contendere shall be conclusive evidence of the felony conviction.

17.12(8) *Misrepresentation of scope of practice by licensees.* Misrepresentation of a licensee's scope of practice includes, but is not limited to, misleading, deceptive or untrue representations about competency, education, training or skill as a licensed acupuncturist or the ability to perform services not authorized under this chapter.

17.12(9) *False advertising.* False advertising is the use of fraudulent, deceptive or improbable statements in information provided to the public. False advertising includes, but is not limited to:

a. Unsubstantiated claims about the licensee's skills or abilities, the healing properties of acupuncture or specific techniques or treatments therein;

b. Presenting words, phrases, or figures which are misleading or likely to be misunderstood by the average person; or

c. Claiming extraordinary skills that are not recognized by the acupuncture profession.

17.12(10) *General grounds.* The board may also take disciplinary action against an acupuncturist for any of the following reasons:

a. Failure to comply with the provisions of Iowa Code chapter 148E or the applicable provisions of Iowa Code chapter 147, or the failure of an acupuncturist to comply with rules adopted by the board pursuant to Iowa Code chapter 148E;

b. Failure to notify the board of any adverse judgment or settlement of a malpractice claim or action within 30 days of the date of the judgment or settlement;

c. Failure to report to the board any acts or omissions of another acupuncturist authorized to practice in Iowa that would constitute grounds for discipline under 17.12 (147, 148E, 272C) within 30 days of the date the acupuncturist initially became aware of the information;

d. Failure to comply with a subpoena issued by the board;

e. Failure to adhere to the disciplinary sanctions imposed upon the acupuncturist by the board; or

f. Violating any of the grounds for revocation or suspension of licensure listed in Iowa Code chapter 147 or 148E.

653 – 17.13 (272C). Procedure for peer review.

Rule 653 — 24.3 (272C) shall apply to peer review procedures in matters related to licensed acupuncturists.

653 – 17.14 (272C). Reporting duties and investigation of reports.

653 — Chapters 22 and 24 shall apply to certain reporting responsibilities of licensed acupuncturists and the investigation of malpractice cases involving licensed acupuncturists.

653 – 17.15 (272C). Complaints, immunities and privileged communications.

653 — Chapter 24 shall apply to matters relating to licensed acupuncturists.

653 – 17.16 (272C). Confidentiality of investigative files.

653 — subrule 24.9(2) shall apply to investigative files relating to licensed acupuncturists.

653 – 17.17 to 17.28. Reserved

653 – 17.29 (17A, 147, 148E, 272C). Disciplinary procedures.

653 — Chapter 25 shall apply to disciplinary actions against licensed acupuncturists.

653 – 17.30 (147, 148E, 272C). Waiver prohibited.

Fees in this chapter are not subject to waiver pursuant to 653 — Chapter 3 or any other provision of law.

North Dakota

North Dakota Century Code Annotated

§ 43 – 61 – 01. Definitions

As used in this chapter, unless the context otherwise requires:

1. "Acupuncture" means an East Asian system of health care that maintains and restores the health of patients through treatments that include patient education, botanical medicine, qi gong, tai qi, or the stimulation of a certain point or points on or below the surface of the body, including traditional meridian points and ashi trigger points by the insertion of presterilized, filiform, disposable needles with or without electronic stimulation or by utilizing manual or thermal techniques.

2. "Acupuncturist" means an individual licensed to practice acupuncture under this chapter.

3. "Approved acupuncture program" means a board-approved graduate level educational program that is offered by an institution of higher education and accredited by a national or regional agency recognized by the United States department of education, or another such equivalent program approved by the board which:

a. Is accredited, has the status of candidate for accreditation, or meets the standards of an organization approved by the board, such as the accreditation commission of acupuncture and oriental medicine.

b. Has been approved by the board after an investigation that determines that the college or program meets education standards equivalent to those established by the accrediting agency under subdivision a and complies with the board's rules.

4. "Board" means the state board of integrative health care created under chapter 43 – 57.

§ 43 – 61 – 02. Exemptions

Some of the therapies used by an acupuncturist, such as the use of botanical medicine, foods, and such physical forces as needling and touch are not the exclusive privilege of acupuncturists. This chapter does not restrict or apply to the scope of practice of any other profession licensed, certified, or registered under the laws of this state.

§ 43 – 61 – 03.   License required — Title restrictions

1. Effective January 1, 2016, an individual may not practice any form of acupuncture without a current acupuncture license issued by the board.

2. An acupuncturist may use the title "Licensed Acupuncturist" and the abbreviation "LAc" when used to reflect that title. Effective January 1, 2016, an individual who uses these terms or initials as identification without having received an acupuncture license under this chapter is engaging in the practice of acupuncture without a license.

§ 43 – 61 – 04.   Qualifications for licensure

To obtain a license to practice acupuncture in this state, an application must be made to the board. The application must be upon the form adopted by the board and must be made in the manner prescribed by the board.

§ 43 – 61 – 05.   Application for licensure

1. An applicant for acupuncture licensure shall file an application on forms provided by the board showing to the board's satisfaction that the applicant is of good moral character and satisfied all of the requirements of this chapter and chapter 43 – 57, including:

a. Successful completion of an approved acupuncture program;

b. Successful completion of an examination prescribed or endorsed by the board, such as the national certification commission for acupuncture and oriental medicine;

c. Physical, mental, and professional capability for the practice of acupuncture in a manner acceptable to the board; and

d. A history free of any finding by the board, any other state licensure board, or any court of competent jurisdiction of the commission of any act that would constitute grounds for disciplinary action under this chapter and chapter 43 – 57. The board may modify this restriction for cause.

2. The application must be accompanied by the board-established license fees and application fees and by the documents, affidavits, and certificates necessary to establish that the applicant possesses the necessary qualifications.

§ 43 – 61 – 06.   Initial applications — Education testing exception

Notwithstanding the education and examination requirements for licensure under subdivisions a and b of subsection 1 of section 43 – 61 – 05, if an applicant was a bona fide resident of the state from January 1, 2015, through December 31, 2015, was practicing acupuncture in this state immediately preceding January 1, 2016, was required to apply for licensure under this chapter in order to continue that practice, and does not meet the educational or examination requirements or both, the board may issue a license or limited license to that applicant if, following an examination of the applicant's education and experience, the board determines the applicant has sufficient education and experience to prepare the applicant to practice acupuncture.

§ 43 – 61 – 07.　Licensure granted without examination to individuals licensed in other states

1. The board may issue an acupuncture license by endorsement to an applicant who complies with licensure requirements and who passed an examination given by a recognized certifying agency approved by the licensing agency if the board determines the examination was equivalent in every respect to the examination required under this chapter.

2. The board may enter reciprocal agreements with licensing agencies of other states providing for reciprocal waiver of further examination or any part of the examination.

3. If an applicant is exempt from the examination required under this chapter, the applicant shall comply with the other requirements for licensure. The board may adopt rules allowing for temporary and special licensure to be in effect during the interval between board meetings.

§ 43 – 61 – 08.　Practice of acupuncture

1. An acupuncturist may practice acupuncture as a limited practice of the healing arts as exempted under section 43 – 17 – 02. An acupuncturist may not:

a. Prescribe, dispense, or administer any prescription drug; or

b. Claim to practice any licensed health care profession or system of treatment other than acupuncture unless holding a separate license in that profession.

2. An acupuncturist may prescribe and administer for preventive and therapeutic purposes the following therapeutic substances and methods:

a. Patient education, botanical medicine, qi gong, and tai qi; and

b. The stimulation of a certain point or points on or below the surface of the body, including traditional meridian points and ashi trigger points by the insertion of presterilized, filiform, or disposable needles with or without electronic stimulation or by utilizing manual or thermal techniques.

§ 43 – 61 – 09.　Public health duties

An acupuncturist has the same duties as a licensed physician with regard to public health laws, reportable diseases and conditions, communicable disease control and prevention, and local boards of health, except that the authority and responsibility are limited to activities consistent with the scope of practice established under this chapter and chapter 43 – 57.

§ 43 – 61 – 10.　Employment by hospitals

A hospital may employ an acupuncturist in the same manner as provided under section 43 – 17 – 42.

North Dakota Administrative Code

Chapter 112 – 04 – 01. Admission to Practice Acupuncture

112 – 04 – 01 – 01. Definitions.

Unless specifically stated otherwise, all definitions found in North Dakota Century Code chapter 43 – 61 are applicable to this title. In this title, unless the context or subject matter otherwise requires:

1. "Accreditation commission" means the accreditation commission for acupuncture and oriental medicine (ACAOM) or its successor. The successor must be an accrediting agency recognized by the United States department of education.

2. "Certification commission" means the national certification commission for acupuncture and oriental medicine or its successor.

3. "In accordance with acupuncture and oriental medicine training" means the practice of acupuncture and oriental medicine by means that are consistent with the education of an approved acupuncture school, are generally recognized as safe and effective, and generally considered to be within the accepted practice standards for the acupuncture profession.

4. "National board examinations" means the diplomate of acupuncture or the diplomate of oriental medicine certification examinations established by the certification commission, or its successor.

5. "Oriental medicine" means a system of healing arts that perceives the circulation and balance of energy in the body as fundamental to the well-being of the individual. It implements the theory through specialized methods of analyzing the energy of the body and treating with needle acupuncture or other oriental treatment modalities for the purpose of strengthening the body, improving energy balance, maintaining or restoring health, improving physiological function, and reducing pain. The definition of acupuncture in North Dakota Century Code section 43 – 61 – 01 includes aspects of oriental medicine which are appropriate for acupuncturists to include in their practice.

6. "Prescription drug" means a legend drug as defined by section 503 (b) of the Federal Food, Drug and Cosmetic Act [21 U.S.C. 353 et seq.] and under its definitions its label is required to state "Rx only".

112 – 04 – 01 – 02. Approval of schools.

1. The board shall approve an acupuncture school that meets the following criteria:

a. Is accredited or a candidate for accreditation by the accreditation commission; and

b. Offers a residential graduate degree program with a curriculum of at least 1905 hours/105 credits.

2. Foreign schools may be considered for board approval if the requirement subdivision b of subsection 1 is met and graduates are approved to take the national board examination by the certification commission.

3. The board shall maintain an updated list of approved acupuncture schools in the United States and make it available upon inquiry.

112 - 04 - 01 - 03.   Applications for licensure.

Application shall be made on the official form issued by the board.

1. Applicants seeking licensure pursuant to the regular application procedure in North Dakota Century Code section 43 - 61 - 05 shall be considered when all of the following have been received:

a. A signed and dated completed official application form.

b. An official transcript of the national board examinations sent directly to the board from the certification commission verifying satisfactory passage of the national board examinations.

c. An official complete transcript sent directly to the board from the approved acupuncture school from which the applicant graduated verifying date of graduation and completion of clinical training.

d. The application fee and the initial license fee.

2. Applicants seeking a license or limited license pursuant to the grandfathering procedure in North Dakota Century Code section 43 - 61 - 06 shall submit the following documents for consideration:

a. A signed and dated completed official application form.

b. An official transcript from the certification commission verifying status as a certified diplomate.

c. Documentation of practical postgraduate clinical experience, including dates, clinic contact information, and supervisor contact information for verification purposes.

d. Documentation of North Dakota residency throughout calendar year 2015.

e. Documentation of the practice of acupuncture in North Dakota in 2015.

f. The application fee and the licensing fee.

112 - 04 - 01 - 04.   Licensure by endorsement.

An application for license by endorsement will be considered by the board if the following conditions are met:

1. The candidate has graduated from and holds a degree from an approved acupuncture school.

2. The candidate holds a current valid license in good standing to practice as an acupuncturist in another state or jurisdiction. Official written verification of licensure status must be received

by the board from the other state or jurisdiction.

3. The examination requirements of the other state or jurisdiction are substantially similar as in North Dakota.

4. The candidate has filed with the board an official application for licensure by endorsement, a copy of the diploma from an approved acupuncture school, a copy of the current valid license, and the required application fee.

112 – 04 – 01 – 05.   Photograph.

An unmounted passport photograph of the applicant must be attached in the space provided on the application before filing with the board. The photograph must have been taken within one year of the date of application.

112 – 04 – 01 – 06.   Examination requirements.

1. Those applicants for licensure who have obtained a passing score on the national board examinations shall be deemed to have met the examination requirement specified in North Dakota Century Code section 43 – 61 – 05.

2. The examination requirements for licensure must be successfully completed within four years from graduation. The board may grant an exception to this requirement for applicants who have concurrently pursued another graduate degree, and the applicant presents a verifiable, rational, and compelling explanation for not meeting the four-year time limit.

3. An applicant is permitted a maximum of five attempts to pass each part or component of the national board examination. If the applicant fails to pass each part or component of the national board examination after five attempts, the applicant is not eligible to apply for a license until one year has passed and must reapply as a new applicant.

112 – 04 – 01 – 07.   License issued.

When the board determines a candidate has successfully graduated from an approved school, passed the national board examination, and is a person of good moral character, the board shall issue the candidate a license to practice acupuncture.

112 – 04 – 01 – 08.   Location of practice — License displayed.

1. If a licensed acupuncturist moves from the acupuncturist's primary location, the office of the executive director must be notified of the change of location of the acupuncturist. A current certificate or duplicate certificate issued by the board must at all times be displayed prominently in each office location of the acupuncturist. In case of loss or destruction, a duplicate certificate may be issued by the board upon receipt of satisfactory evidence of the loss or destruction.

2. A licensed acupuncturist providing temporary services in offsite locations must carry a duplicate license wallet card and show the card upon request.

112 – 04 – 01 – 09.   License renewal.

1. Every acupuncturist who has been licensed by the board shall renew the license by remitting a renewal fee on or before December thirty-first of each even-numbered year and

completing the questionnaire provided by the board. For applicants who receive an initial license after July first in an even-numbered year, the license will be deemed to be automatically renewed on December thirty-first for an additional two years without payment of an additional renewal fee.

2. The applicant for renewal shall certify on the questionnaire that the continuing education requirements have been or will be met by December thirty-first. The applicant must keep records of completed continuing education. The board shall conduct random compliance audits of licensees. Failure to complete continuing education is considered unprofessional conduct.

3. A license renewal application received on or after January first of an odd-numbered year is a late renewal and requires a new completed application form, the renewal fee, plus a late fee set by the board. Proof of appropriate continuing education hours must be presented. A license that has not been renewed by December thirty-first in an even-numbered year is a lapsed license.

112 – 04 – 01 – 10.　Lapsed licenses.

Once a license has lapsed, the person who held the lapsed license may not practice acupuncture or use a title reserved under state law for individuals who are licensed by the board until a new license is issued. A person whose license has lapsed but who continues to practice acupuncture or use a restricted title violates state law and this chapter. Such a violation is grounds for denying an application by the former licensee for renewal of the lapsed license or for a new license.

112 – 04 – 01 – 11.　Fees.

The board charges the following nonrefundable fees:

1. Application. The fee for filing an application for an initial license is fifty dollars.

2. Initial license. The fee for an initial license is three hundred dollars. The licensing period is biennial, ending on December thirty-first every even-numbered year. The initial license fee shall be prorated quarterly based upon the time period remaining in the two-year cycle at application.

3. Temporary license. The temporary license fee for acupuncturists shall be one hundred dollars. The cost of the temporary license fee will be applied toward the initial license fee upon receipt of application for the initial license.

4. Renewal. Licenses renew on December thirty-first every even-numbered year. The renewal fee is two hundred dollars for active status and one hundred dollars for inactive status.

5. Change of status. To change from inactive to active status, the fee shall be prorated on a quarterly basis on the time period remaining in the two-year cycle.

6. Late filing. An additional late filing fee will be charged on renewal applications not received by December thirty-first every even-numbered year. The late filing fee for acupuncturists is seventy-five dollars.

7. Duplicate license. The duplicate license fee for an acupuncture license certificate is

twenty-five dollars. The duplicate license fee for an acupuncturist license wallet card is twenty dollars.

Chapter 112 – 04 – 02. Authority of Acupuncturists

112 – 04 – 02 – 01.   Rights and Privileges.

Unless otherwise limited by statute, licensed acupuncturists shall be entitled to the rights and privileges of health care practitioners in North Dakota in accordance with acupuncture and oriental medicine training. The practice of acupuncture in North Dakota Century Code section 43 – 61 – 01 includes aspects of oriental medicine, such as:

1. Using oriental medicine theory to assess and diagnose a patient;

2. Using oriental medicine theory to develop a plan to treat a patient; and

3. Prescribing and administering oriental medicine therapies as part of a patient treatment plan.

112 – 04 – 02 – 02.   Advertising.

Licensed acupuncturists will be privileged to advertise their practice in any legitimate manner set forth in the code of ethics adopted by the board under section 112 – 01 – 04 – 02, except as limited or prohibited by statute. Doctoral level licensed acupuncturists may use the prefix "doctor" or "Dr." in accordance with an accredited doctoral acupuncture degree but may not advertise any acupuncture title or designation except those established under North Dakota Century Code chapter 43 – 61 – 03.

112 – 04 – 02 – 03.   Authority to administer, prescribe, and dispense.

The practice of acupuncture includes the administration, prescription, dispensing, ordering, or performing of the following based on oriental medicine principles:

1. Food, nutritional supplements, herbs, and patent herbal remedies.

2. Health counseling, nutritional therapy, herbal therapy, oriental massage, exercises, and breathing techniques.

3. Acupuncture point stimulation by acupuncture needles, auriculotherapy, cupping, electricity, heat, dermal friction, gua sha, and touch.

112 – 04 – 02 – 04.   Needle acupuncture administration; acupuncture point stimulation.

1. A licensed acupuncturist shall administer needle acupuncture in accordance with acupuncture and oriental medicine training. Needles used in the practice of acupuncture shall only be prepackaged, single use, sterile acupuncture needles. These needles shall only be used on an individual patient in a single treatment session and disposed of according to federal standards for biohazard waste. Acupuncture points must be cleaned with alcohol or another approved clean needle technique (CNT) antiseptic prior to needle insertion.

2. A licensed acupuncturist must have a plan to manage patient adverse events, including allergy.

112 – 04 – 02 – 05.　Requirement to refer.

1. A licensed acupuncturist shall request a consultation or written diagnosis from a licensed physician for patients with potentially serious disorders. A referral to a licensed physician is required when a patient has signs or symptoms of:

a. Cardiac conditions including uncontrolled hypertension;

b. Acute, severe abdominal pain;

c. Acute, undiagnosed neurological changes;

d. Unexplained weight loss or gain in excess of fifteen percent of the body weight in less than a three-month period;

e. Suspected fracture or dislocation;

f. Suspected systemic infections;

g. Any serious undiagnosed hemorrhagic disorder; and

h. Acute respiratory distress without previous history.

2. A licensed acupuncturist shall refer a patient to a licensed physician in the event of:

a. Suspected pneumothorax; or

b. Broken acupuncture needle.

Chapter 112 – 04 – 03. Continuing Acupuncture Education

112 – 04 – 03 – 01.　Continuing education requirements.

1. All active licensees shall complete a minimum of thirty hours of approved continuing education credit during the biennial licensing cycle. Only hours earned at board-accepted continuing education programs will be allowed. One hour of credit is earned for every fifty minutes of actual class time.

a. CPR recertification is required each biennial cycle and is granted four continuing education units.

b. Two credits are required in either ethics or safety each biennial cycle.

2. An extension of time or other waiver to complete the hours required in subsection 1 shall be granted upon written application if the licensee failed to meet the requirements due to illness, military service, medical or religious missionary activity, or other extenuating circumstance.

112 – 04 – 03 – 02.　Exceptions.

The following licensed acupuncturists are not required to meet the continuing education requirements of this chapter:

1. Acupuncturists who are enrolled in full-time graduate acupuncture education programs (doctoral degrees, residencies, and fellowships).

2. Acupuncturists who hold a provisional temporary license, and acupuncturists who have not renewed their licenses for the first time since being granted a regular permanent license by

the board.

3. Acupuncturists who have retired from the active practice of acupuncture and oriental medicine. This exception is available only to retired acupuncturists who have completely and totally withdrawn from the practice of acupuncture and oriental medicine. Any acupuncturist seeking to be excused from completing continuing acupuncture education requirements under this subsection must submit an affidavit to the board (on the board's form) certifying that the acupuncturist will render no acupuncture services during the term of the next continuing education reporting period.

112 – 04 – 03 – 03. Board approval.

1. In order to receive board approval, a continuing education program must be accepted by the credentialing commission.

2. It is the responsibility of the licensee to verify the appropriate credit designation with the source of the program. All licensees must verify eligibility for continuing credit and the appropriate credit designation before taking any particular course.

112 – 04 – 03 – 04. Board audit.

Each biennium the board shall audit randomly selected acupuncturists to monitor compliance with the continuing education requirements. Any acupuncturist so audited will be required to furnish documentation of compliance, including the name of the continuing education provider, name of the program, hours of continuing education completed, dates of attendance, and verification of attendance. Any acupuncturist who fails to provide verification of compliance with the continuing education requirements will be subject to revocation of licensure. In order to facilitate the board's audits, every acupuncturist is required to maintain a record of all continuing education activities in which the acupuncturist has participated. Every acupuncturist shall maintain those records for a period of at least two years following the time when those containing education activities were reported to the board.

112 – 04 – 03 – 05. Inactive status.

On or before December thirty-first of each even-numbered year, licensees may elect to renew their licenses as inactive. The inactive status is at a reduced fee for those licensees who do not practice, consult, or provide any service relative to the acupuncture profession in the state. The inactive licensee does not have to provide proof of continuing education hours. Any inactive licensee may activate the license at any time by paying an additional fee and showing proof of thirty hours of continuing acupuncture education in the preceding twenty-four months.

Ohio

Ohio Revised Code Annotated

4762.01 Definitions

As used in this chapter:

(A) "Acupuncture" means a form of health care performed by the insertion and removal of specialized needles, with or without the use of supplemental techniques, to specific areas of the human body.

(B) "Chiropractor" means an individual licensed under Chapter 4734. of the Revised Code to engage in the practice of chiropractic.

(C) "General nonmedical nutritional information" means information on any of the following:

(1) Principles of good nutrition and food preparation;

(2) Foods to be included in the normal daily diet;

(3) Essential nutrients needed by the human body and recommended amounts of those nutrients;

(4) Foods and supplements that are good sources of essential nutrients;

(5) The actions of nutrients on the human body and the effects of nutrient deficiency and nutrient excess.

(D) "Herbal therapy" means the use of foods, herbs, vitamins, minerals, organ extracts, and homeopathy.

(E) "Homeopathy" means a noninvasive system of natural and alternative medicine that seeks to stimulate the human body's ability to heal itself through the use of small doses of highly diluted substances prepared from animal, vegetable, or mineral sources.

(F) "Moxibustion" means the use of an herbal heat source on one or more acupuncture points.

(G) "Oriental medicine" means a form of health care in which acupuncture is performed with or without the use of herbal therapy.

(H) "Physician" means an individual authorized under Chapter 4731. of the Revised Code to practice medicine and surgery, osteopathic medicine and surgery, or podiatric medicine and surgery.

(I) "Supplemental techniques" means the use of general nonmedical nutritional information, traditional and modern oriental therapeutics, heat therapy, moxibustion, acupressure and other forms of Chinese massage, and educational information regarding lifestyle modifications.

4762.01(1) Applicability of chapter to oriental medicine practitioners

On and after the effective date of this section, this chapter no longer applies to oriental medicine practitioners.

4762.02 License to practice; exemptions

(A) Except as provided in division (B), (C), or (D) of this section, no person shall do either of the following:

(1) Engage in the practice of oriental medicine unless the person holds a valid license to practice as an oriental medicine practitioner issued by the state medical board under this chapter;

(2) Engage in the practice of acupuncture unless the person holds a valid license to practice as an acupuncturist issued by the state medical board under this chapter.

(B) Division (A) of this section does not apply to a physician.

(C) Division (A) (1) of this section does not apply to the following:

(1) A person who engages in activities included in the practice of oriental medicine as part of a training program in oriental medicine, but only if both of the following conditions are met:

(a) The training program is operated by an educational institution that holds an effective certificate of authorization issued by the chancellor of higher education under section 1713.02 of the Revised Code or a school that holds an effective certificate of registration issued by the state board of career colleges and schools under section 3332.05 of the Revised Code.

(b) The person engages in the activities under the general supervision of an individual who holds a license to practice as an oriental medicine practitioner issued under this chapter and is not practicing within the supervisory period required by section 4762.10 of the Revised Code.

(2) To the extent that acupuncture is a component of oriental medicine, an individual who holds a license to practice as an acupuncturist issued under this chapter or a chiropractor who holds a certificate to practice acupuncture issued by the state chiropractic board under section 4734.283 of the Revised Code.

(D) Division (A) (2) of this section does not apply to the following:

(1) A person who performs acupuncture as part of a training program in acupuncture, but only if both of the following conditions are met:

(a) The training program is operated by an educational institution that holds an effective certificate of authorization issued by the chancellor of higher education under section 1713.02 of the Revised Code or a school that holds an effective certificate of registration issued by the state board of career colleges and schools under section 3332.05 of the Revised Code.

(b) The person performs the acupuncture under the general supervision of an acupuncturist who holds a license to practice as an acupuncturist issued under this chapter and is not practicing within the supervisory period required by section 4762.10 of the Revised Code.

(2) An individual who holds a license to practice as an oriental medicine practitioner issued under this chapter.

(3) A chiropractor who holds a certificate to practice acupuncture issued by the state chiropractic board under section 4734.283 of the Revised Code.

4762.03 Application; eligibility; review; fee

(A) An individual seeking a license to practice as an oriental medicine practitioner or license to practice as an acupuncturist shall file with the state medical board a written application on a form prescribed and supplied by the board.

(B) To be eligible for the license, an applicant shall meet all of the following conditions, as applicable:

(1) The applicant shall submit evidence satisfactory to the board that the applicant is at least eighteen years of age.

(2) In the case of an applicant seeking a license to practice as an oriental medicine practitioner, the applicant shall submit evidence satisfactory to the board of both of the following:

(a) That the applicant holds a current and active designation from the national certification commission for acupuncture and oriental medicine as either a diplomate in oriental medicine or diplomate of acupuncture and Chinese herbology;

(b) That the applicant has successfully completed, in the two-year period immediately preceding application for the license to practice, one course approved by the commission on federal food and drug administration dispensary and compounding guidelines and procedures.

(3) In the case of an applicant seeking a license to practice as an acupuncturist, the applicant shall submit evidence satisfactory to the board that the applicant holds a current and active designation from the national certification commission for acupuncture and oriental medicine as a diplomate in acupuncture.

(4) The applicant shall demonstrate to the board proficiency in spoken English by satisfying one of the following requirements:

(a) Passing the examination described in section 4731.142 of the Revised Code;

(b) Submitting evidence satisfactory to the board that the applicant was required to demonstrate proficiency in spoken English as a condition of obtaining designation from the national certification commission for acupuncture and oriental medicine as a diplomate in oriental medicine, diplomate of acupuncture and Chinese herbology, or diplomate in acupuncture;

(c) Submitting evidence satisfactory to the board that the applicant, in seeking a designation from the national certification commission for acupuncture and oriental medicine as a diplomate of oriental medicine, diplomate of acupuncture and Chinese herbology, or diplomate of acupuncture, has successfully completed in English the examination required for such a designation by the national certification commission for acupuncture and oriental medicine;

(d) In the case of an applicant seeking a license to practice as an oriental medicine practitioner, submitting evidence satisfactory to the board that the applicant has previously held a license to practice as an acupuncturist issued under section 4762.04 of the Revised Code.

(5) The applicant shall submit to the board any other information the board requires.

(6) The applicant shall pay to the board a fee of one hundred dollars, no part of which may be returned to the applicant.

(C) The board shall review all applications received under this section. The board shall determine whether an applicant meets the requirements to receive a license not later than sixty days after receiving a complete application.

4762.03(1)   Criminal records check

In addition to any other eligibility requirement set forth in this chapter, each applicant for a license to practice as an oriental medicine practitioner or license to practice as an acupuncturist shall comply with sections 4776.01 to 4776.04 of the Revised Code. The state medical board shall not grant to an applicant a license to practice unless the board, in its discretion, decides that the results of the criminal records check do not make the applicant ineligible for a license issued pursuant to section 4762.04 of the Revised Code.

4762.04   Registration and issuance of license

If the state medical board determines under section 4762.03 of the Revised Code that an applicant meets the requirements for a license to practice as an oriental medicine practitioner or license to practice as an acupuncturist, the secretary of the board shall register the applicant as an oriental medicine practitioner or acupuncturist, as appropriate, and issue to the applicant the appropriate license to practice. The license shall be valid for a two-year period unless revoked or suspended, shall expire on the date that is two years after the date of issuance, and may be renewed for additional two-year periods in accordance with section 4762.06 of the Revised Code.

4762.05   Duplicate licenses; fee

Upon application by the holder of a license to practice as an oriental medicine practitioner or license to practice as an acupuncturist, the state medical board shall issue a duplicate license to replace one that is missing or damaged, to reflect a name change, or for any other reasonable cause. The fee for a duplicate license is thirty-five dollars.

4762.06   License renewal

(A) A person seeking to renew a license to practice as an oriental medicine practitioner or license to practice as an acupuncturist shall, on or before the license's expiration date, apply to the state medical board for renewal. The board shall provide renewal notices to license holders at least one month prior to the expiration date.

Applications shall be submitted to the board in a manner prescribed by the board. Each application shall be accompanied by a biennial renewal fee of one hundred dollars.

The applicant shall report any criminal offense that constitutes grounds for refusing to issue a license under section 4762.13 of the Revised Code to which the applicant has pleaded guilty, of which the applicant has been found guilty, or for which the applicant has been found eligible for intervention in lieu of conviction, since last signing an application for a license to practice as an oriental medicine practitioner or license to practice as an acupuncturist.

(B) (1) To be eligible for renewal of a license to practice as an oriental medicine practitioner, an applicant shall certify to the board both of the following, as applicable:

(a) That the applicant has maintained a current and active designation from the national certification commission for acupuncture and oriental medicine as either a diplomate in oriental medicine or diplomate of acupuncture and Chinese herbology;

(b) That the applicant has successfully completed one six-hour course in herb and drug interaction approved by the national certification commission for acupuncture and oriental medicine in the four years immediately preceding the expiration date of the applicant's current and active designation from the commission as a diplomate in oriental medicine or diplomate of acupuncture and Chinese herbology.

(2) To be eligible for renewal of a license to practice as an acupuncturist, an applicant shall certify to the board that the acupuncturist has maintained a current and active designation from the national certification commission for acupuncture and oriental medicine as a diplomate in acupuncture.

(C) If an applicant submits a complete renewal application and qualifies for renewal pursuant to division (B) of this section, the board shall issue to the applicant a renewed license to practice.

(D) A license to practice that is not renewed on or before its expiration date is automatically suspended on its expiration date.

If a license has been suspended pursuant to this division for two years or less, the board shall reinstate the license upon an applicant's submission of a renewal application, the biennial renewal fee, and the applicable monetary penalty. The penalty for reinstatement is twenty-five dollars.

If a license has been suspended pursuant to this division for more than two years, it may be restored. Subject to section 4762.061 of the Revised Code, the board may restore the license upon an applicant's submission of a restoration application, the biennial renewal fee, and the applicable monetary penalty and compliance with sections 4776.01 to 4776.04 of the Revised Code. The board shall not restore a license unless the board, in its discretion, decides that the results of the criminal records check do not make the applicant ineligible for a certificate issued pursuant to section 4762.04 of the Revised Code. The penalty for restoration is fifty dollars.

4762.06(1) Restoration of license

(A) This section applies to both of the following:

(1) An applicant seeking restoration of a license issued under this chapter that has been in a suspended or inactive state for any cause for more than two years;

(2) An applicant seeking issuance of a license pursuant to this chapter who for more than two years has not been engaged in the practice of oriental medicine or acupuncture as either of the following:

(a) An active practitioner;

(b) A participant in a training program as described in section 4762.02 of the Revised Code.

(B) Before issuing a license to an applicant subject to this section or restoring a license to good standing for an applicant subject to this section, the state medical board may impose terms and conditions including any one or more of the following:

(1) Requiring the applicant to pass an oral or written examination, or both, to determine the applicant's present fitness to resume practice;

(2) Requiring the applicant to obtain additional training and to pass an examination upon completion of such training;

(3) Requiring an assessment of the applicant's physical skills for purposes of determining whether the applicant's coordination, fine motor skills, and dexterity are sufficient for performing evaluations and procedures in a manner that meets the minimal standards of care;

(4) Requiring an assessment of the applicant's skills in recognizing and understanding diseases and conditions;

(5) Requiring the applicant to undergo a comprehensive physical examination, which may include an assessment of physical abilities, evaluation of sensory capabilities, or screening for the presence of neurological disorders;

(6) Restricting or limiting the extent, scope, or type of practice of the applicant.

The board shall consider the moral background and the activities of the applicant during the period of suspension or inactivity. The board shall not issue or restore a license under this section unless the applicant complies with sections 4776.01 to 4776.04 of the Revised Code.

4762.08 Use of title

(A) A person who holds a license to practice as an oriental medicine practitioner issued under this chapter may use the following titles, initials, or abbreviations, or the equivalent of such titles, initials, or abbreviations, to identify the person as an oriental medicine practitioner: "Oriental Medicine Practitioner," "Licensed Oriental Medicine Practitioner," "L. O. M.," "Diplomate in Oriental Medicine (NCCAOM)," "Dipl.O.M. (NCCAOM)," "National Board Certified in Oriental Medicine (NCCAOM)," "Acupuncturist," "Licensed Acupuncturist,"

"L. Ac. and L.C.H.," "Diplomate of Acupuncture and Chinese Herbology (NCCAOM)," "Dipl. Ac. and Dipl. C.H. (NCCAOM)," or "National Board Certified in Acupuncture and Chinese Herbology (NCCAOM)." The person shall not use other titles, initials, or abbreviations in conjunction with the person's practice of oriental medicine, including the title "doctor."

(B) A person who holds a license to practice as an acupuncturist issued under this chapter may use the following titles, initials, or abbreviations, or the equivalent of such titles, initials, or abbreviations, to identify the person as an acupuncturist: "Acupuncturist," "Licensed Acupuncturist," "L. Ac.," "Diplomate in Acupuncture (NCCAOM)," "Dipl. Ac. (NCCAOM)," or "National Board Certified in Acupuncture (NCCAOM)." The person shall not use other titles, initials, or abbreviations in conjunction with the person's practice of acupuncture, including the title "doctor."

4762.09 Display of license and notice

An individual who holds a license to practice as an oriental medicine practitioner or license to practice as an acupuncturist issued under this chapter shall conspicuously display at the individual's primary place of business both of the following:

(A) The individual's license, as evidence that the individual is authorized to practice in this state;

(B) A notice specifying that the practice of oriental medicine or acupuncture, as applicable, under the license is regulated by the state medical board and the address and telephone number of the board's office.

4762.10 Supervisory period; exercise of powers and duties

The following, as applicable, apply to an individual who holds a license to practice as an oriental medicine practitioner or license to practice as an acupuncturist:

(A) On receipt of an initial license to practice, the practice of the oriental medicine practitioner or acupuncturist is subject to a supervisory period. The supervisory period shall begin on the date the initial license is granted and end one year thereafter, except that if the oriental medicine practitioner or acupuncturist is subject during that year to disciplinary action taken by the state medical board pursuant to section 4762.13 of the Revised Code, the supervision shall continue until the practitioner or acupuncturist has not been subject to any disciplinary action for one year.

(B) During the supervisory period, both of the following apply to an oriental medicine practitioner's or acupuncturist's practice in addition to the applicable requirements of divisions (D) and (E) of this section:

(1) An oriental medicine practitioner shall perform oriental medicine or acupuncture for a patient only if the patient has received a written referral or prescription for oriental medicine or acupuncture from a physician or for acupuncture from a chiropractor. An acupuncturist shall perform acupuncture for a patient only if the patient has received a written referral or prescription

for acupuncture from a physician or chiropractor. As specified in the referral or prescription, the oriental medicine practitioner or acupuncturist shall provide reports to the physician or chiropractor on the patient's condition or progress in treatment and comply with the conditions or restrictions on the practitioner's or acupuncturist's course of treatment.

(2) The oriental medicine practitioner or acupuncturist shall perform oriental medicine or acupuncture under the general supervision of the patient's referring or prescribing physician or chiropractor, except that an oriental medicine practitioner using herbal therapy in the treatment of a patient shall not provide herbal therapy under the general supervision of a chiropractor. General supervision does not require that the oriental medicine practitioner or acupuncturist and supervising physician or chiropractor practice in the same office.

(C) After the supervisory period has ended, both of the following apply to an oriental medicine practitioner's or acupuncturist's practice in addition to the applicable requirements of divisions (D) and (E) of this section:

(1) Before treating a patient for a particular condition, an oriental medicine practitioner or acupuncturist shall confirm whether the patient has undergone within the past six months a diagnostic examination that was related to the condition for which the patient is seeking oriental medicine or acupuncture and was performed by a physician or chiropractor acting within the physician's or chiropractor's scope of practice. Confirmation that the diagnostic examination was performed may be made by obtaining from the patient a signed form stating that the patient has undergone the examination.

(2) If the patient does not provide the signed form specified in division (C) (1) of this section or an oriental medicine practitioner or acupuncturist otherwise determines that the patient has not undergone the diagnostic examination specified in that division, the practitioner or acupuncturist shall provide to the patient a written recommendation to undergo a diagnostic examination by a physician or chiropractor.

(D) In an individual's practice of oriental medicine or acupuncture pursuant to a license to practice issued under this chapter, all of the following apply:

(1) Prior to treating a patient, the individual shall advise the patient that oriental medicine or acupuncture, as applicable, is not a substitute for conventional medical diagnosis and treatment.

(2) On initially meeting a patient in person, the individual shall provide in writing the individual's name, business address, and business telephone number, and information on oriental medicine or acupuncture, as applicable, including the techniques that are used.

(3) While treating a patient, the individual shall not make a diagnosis. If a patient's condition is not improving or a patient requires emergency medical treatment, the individual shall consult promptly with a physician.

(4) The individual shall maintain records for each patient treated. The records shall be confidential and shall be retained for not less than three years following termination of treatment.

The individual shall include in a patient's records the written referral or prescription pursuant to which the patient is treated during a supervisory period and any written referral or prescription for oriental medicine or acupuncture received for a patient being treated after the supervisory period.

(E) In an individual's practice of oriental medicine by using herbal therapy in the treatment of a patient, all of the following apply:

(1) The oriental medicine practitioner shall provide to the patient counseling and treatment instructions. The treatment instructions shall do all of the following:

(a) Explain the need for herbal therapy;

(b) Instruct the patient how to take the herbal therapy;

(c) Explain possible contraindications to the herbal therapy and provide sources of care in case of an adverse reaction;

(d) Instruct the patient to inform the patient's other health care providers, including the patient's pharmacist, of the herbal therapy that has been provided to the patient.

(2) The oriental medicine practitioner shall document all of the following in the patient's record:

(a) The type, amount, and strength of herbal therapy recommended for the patient's use;

(b) The counseling and treatment instructions provided to the patient under division (E) (1) of this section;

(c) Any adverse reaction reported by the patient in conjunction with the use of herbal therapy.

(3) The oriental medicine practitioner shall report to the state medical board any adverse reactions reported by the patient under division (E) (2) (c) of this section.

4762.11   Powers and duties of supervising physician or chiropractor

All of the following apply to a supervising physician or chiropractor, as applicable, during an oriental medicine practitioner's or acupuncturist's supervisory period required by section 4762.10 of the Revised Code:

(A) Before a physician makes the referral or issues a prescription for oriental medicine or acupuncture, the physician shall perform a medical diagnostic examination of the patient or review the results of a medical diagnostic examination recently performed by another physician. Before a chiropractor makes a referral or issues a prescription for oriental medicine or acupuncture, the chiropractor shall perform a chiropractic diagnostic examination of the patient or review the results of a chiropractic diagnostic examination recently performed by another chiropractor.

(B) The physician or chiropractor shall make the referral or prescription in writing and specify in the referral or prescription all of the following:

(1) The physician's or chiropractor's diagnosis of the ailment or condition that is to be

treated by oriental medicine or acupuncture;

(2) A time by which or the intervals at which the oriental medicine practitioner or acupuncturist must provide reports to the physician or chiropractor regarding the patient's condition or progress in treatment;

(3) The conditions or restrictions placed in accordance with division (C) of this section on the oriental medicine practitioner's or acupuncturist's course of treatment.

(C) In the case of a physician, the physician shall place conditions or restrictions on the oriental medicine practitioner's or acupuncturist's course of treatment in compliance with accepted or prevailing standards of medical care, or, in the case of a chiropractor, the chiropractor shall place conditions or restrictions on the practitioner's or acupuncturist's course of treatment in compliance with accepted or prevailing standards of chiropractic care.

(D) The physician or chiropractor shall be personally available for consultation with the oriental medicine practitioner or acupuncturist. If the physician or chiropractor is not on the premises at which oriental medicine or acupuncture is performed, the physician or chiropractor shall be readily available to the practitioner or acupuncturist through some means of telecommunication and be in a location that under normal circumstances is not more than sixty minutes travel time away from the location where the practitioner or acupuncturist is practicing.

(E) A chiropractor shall not supervise an oriental medicine practitioner in the practitioner's use of herbal therapy in the treatment of a patient.

4762.12　Reimbursement of supervising physician or chiropractor

In the case of a patient with a claim under Chapter 4121. or 4123. of the Revised Code, a supervising physician or chiropractor is eligible to be reimbursed for referring the patient to an oriental medicine practitioner or acupuncturist or for prescribing oriental medicine or acupuncture for the patient only if the physician has attained knowledge in the treatment of patients with oriental medicine or acupuncture, or the chiropractor has attained knowledge in the treatment of patients with acupuncture, as demonstrated by successful completion of a relevant course of study administered by a college of medicine, osteopathic medicine, podiatric medicine, or chiropractic acceptable to the bureau of workers' compensation or administered by another entity acceptable to the bureau.

4762.13　Discipline

(A) The state medical board, by an affirmative vote of not fewer than six members, may revoke or may refuse to grant a license to practice as an oriental medicine practitioner or license to practice as an acupuncturist to a person found by the board to have committed fraud, misrepresentation, or deception in applying for or securing the license.

(B) The board, by an affirmative vote of not fewer than six members, shall, except as provided in division (C) of this section, and to the extent permitted by law, limit, revoke, or suspend an individual's license to practice, refuse to issue a license to an applicant, refuse to renew a license, refuse to reinstate a license, or reprimand or place on probation the holder of a license for any of the following reasons:

(1) Permitting the holder's name or license to be used by another person;

(2) Failure to comply with the requirements of this chapter, Chapter 4731. of the Revised Code, or any rules adopted by the board;

(3) Violating or attempting to violate, directly or indirectly, or assisting in or abetting the violation of, or conspiring to violate, any provision of this chapter, Chapter 4731. of the Revised Code, or the rules adopted by the board;

(4) A departure from, or failure to conform to, minimal standards of care of similar practitioners under the same or similar circumstances whether or not actual injury to the patient is established;

(5) Inability to practice according to acceptable and prevailing standards of care by reason of mental illness or physical illness, including physical deterioration that adversely affects cognitive, motor, or perceptive skills;

(6) Impairment of ability to practice according to acceptable and prevailing standards of care because of habitual or excessive use or abuse of drugs, alcohol, or other substances that impair ability to practice;

(7) Willfully betraying a professional confidence;

(8) Making a false, fraudulent, deceptive, or misleading statement in soliciting or advertising for patients or in securing or attempting to secure a license to practice as an oriental medicine practitioner or license to practice as an acupuncturist.

As used in this division, "false, fraudulent, deceptive, or misleading statement" means a statement that includes a misrepresentation of fact, is likely to mislead or deceive because of a failure to disclose material facts, is intended or is likely to create false or unjustified expectations of favorable results, or includes representations or implications that in reasonable probability will cause an ordinarily prudent person to misunderstand or be deceived.

(9) Representing, with the purpose of obtaining compensation or other advantage personally or for any other person, that an incurable disease or injury, or other incurable condition, can be permanently cured;

(10) The obtaining of, or attempting to obtain, money or a thing of value by fraudulent misrepresentations in the course of practice;

(11) A plea of guilty to, a judicial finding of guilt of, or a judicial finding of eligibility for intervention in lieu of conviction for, a felony;

(12) Commission of an act that constitutes a felony in this state, regardless of the jurisdiction in which the act was committed;

(13) A plea of guilty to, a judicial finding of guilt of, or a judicial finding of eligibility for intervention in lieu of conviction for, a misdemeanor committed in the course of practice;

(14) A plea of guilty to, a judicial finding of guilt of, or a judicial finding of eligibility for intervention in lieu of conviction for, a misdemeanor involving moral turpitude;

(15) Commission of an act in the course of practice that constitutes a misdemeanor in this state, regardless of the jurisdiction in which the act was committed;

(16) Commission of an act involving moral turpitude that constitutes a misdemeanor in this state, regardless of the jurisdiction in which the act was committed;

(17) A plea of guilty to, a judicial finding of guilt of, or a judicial finding of eligibility for intervention in lieu of conviction for violating any state or federal law regulating the possession, distribution, or use of any drug, including trafficking in drugs;

(18) Any of the following actions taken by the state agency responsible for regulating the practice of oriental medicine or acupuncture in another jurisdiction, for any reason other than the nonpayment of fees: the limitation, revocation, or suspension of an individual's license to practice; acceptance of an individual's license surrender; denial of a license; refusal to renew or reinstate a license; imposition of probation; or issuance of an order of censure or other reprimand;

(19) Violation of the conditions placed by the board on a license to practice as an oriental medicine practitioner or license to practice as an acupuncturist;

(20) Failure to use universal blood and body fluid precautions established by rules adopted under section 4731.051 of the Revised Code;

(21) Failure to cooperate in an investigation conducted by the board under section 4762.14 of the Revised Code, including failure to comply with a subpoena or order issued by the board or failure to answer truthfully a question presented by the board at a deposition or in written interrogatories, except that failure to cooperate with an investigation shall not constitute grounds for discipline under this section if a court of competent jurisdiction has issued an order that either quashes a subpoena or permits the individual to withhold the testimony or evidence in issue;

(22) Failure to comply with the standards of the national certification commission for acupuncture and oriental medicine regarding professional ethics, commitment to patients, commitment to the profession, and commitment to the public;

(23) Failure to have adequate professional liability insurance coverage in accordance with section 4762.22 of the Revised Code;

(24) Failure to maintain a current and active designation as a diplomate in oriental medicine, diplomate of acupuncture and Chinese herbology, or diplomate in acupuncture, as applicable, from the national certification commission for acupuncture and oriental medicine, including revocation by the commission of the individual's designation, failure by the individual to meet the commission's requirements for redesignation, or failure to notify the board that the appropriate designation has not been maintained.

(C) The board shall not refuse to issue a certificate to an applicant because of a plea of guilty to, a judicial finding of guilt of, or a judicial finding of eligibility for intervention in lieu of conviction for an offense unless the refusal is in accordance with section 9.79 of the Revised Code.

(D) Disciplinary actions taken by the board under divisions (A) and (B) of this section shall be taken pursuant to an adjudication under Chapter 119. of the Revised Code, except that in lieu of an adjudication, the board may enter into a consent agreement with an oriental medicine practitioner or acupuncturist or applicant to resolve an allegation of a violation of this chapter or any rule adopted under it. A consent agreement, when ratified by an affirmative vote of not fewer than six members of the board, shall constitute the findings and order of the board with respect to the matter addressed in the agreement. If the board refuses to ratify a consent agreement, the admissions and findings contained in the consent agreement shall be of no force or effect.

(E) For purposes of divisions (B) (12), (15), and (16) of this section, the commission of the act may be established by a finding by the board, pursuant to an adjudication under Chapter 119. of the Revised Code, that the applicant or license holder committed the act in question. The board shall have no jurisdiction under these divisions in cases where the trial court renders a final judgment in the license holder's favor and that judgment is based upon an adjudication on the merits. The board shall have jurisdiction under these divisions in cases where the trial court issues an order of dismissal upon technical or procedural grounds.

(F) The sealing of conviction records by any court shall have no effect upon a prior board order entered under the provisions of this section or upon the board's jurisdiction to take action under the provisions of this section if, based upon a plea of guilty, a judicial finding of guilt, or a judicial finding of eligibility for intervention in lieu of conviction, the board issued a notice of opportunity for a hearing or entered into a consent agreement prior to the court's order to seal the records. The board shall not be required to seal, destroy, redact, or otherwise modify its records to reflect the court's sealing of conviction records.

(G) For purposes of this division, any individual who holds a license to practice issued under this chapter, or applies for a license to practice, shall be deemed to have given consent to submit to a mental or physical examination when directed to do so in writing by the board and to have waived all objections to the admissibility of testimony or examination reports that constitute a privileged communication.

(1) In enforcing division (B) (5) of this section, the board, upon a showing of a possible violation, may compel any individual who holds a license to practice issued under this chapter or who has applied for a license pursuant to this chapter to submit to a mental examination, physical examination, including an HIV test, or both a mental and physical examination. The expense of the examination is the responsibility of the individual compelled to be examined. Failure to submit to a mental or physical examination or consent to an HIV test ordered by the board constitutes an admission of the allegations against the individual unless the

failure is due to circumstances beyond the individual's control, and a default and final order may be entered without the taking of testimony or presentation of evidence. If the board finds an oriental medicine practitioner or acupuncturist unable to practice because of the reasons set forth in division (B) (5) of this section, the board shall require the individual to submit to care, counseling, or treatment by physicians approved or designated by the board, as a condition for an initial, continued, reinstated, or renewed license to practice. An individual affected by this division shall be afforded an opportunity to demonstrate to the board the ability to resume practicing in compliance with acceptable and prevailing standards of care.

(2) For purposes of division (B) (6) of this section, if the board has reason to believe that any individual who holds a license to practice issued under this chapter or any applicant for a license suffers such impairment, the board may compel the individual to submit to a mental or physical examination, or both. The expense of the examination is the responsibility of the individual compelled to be examined. Any mental or physical examination required under this division shall be undertaken by a treatment provider or physician qualified to conduct such examination and chosen by the board.

Failure to submit to a mental or physical examination ordered by the board constitutes an admission of the allegations against the individual unless the failure is due to circumstances beyond the individual's control, and a default and final order may be entered without the taking of testimony or presentation of evidence. If the board determines that the individual's ability to practice is impaired, the board shall suspend the individual's license or deny the individual's application and shall require the individual, as a condition for an initial, continued, reinstated, or renewed license, to submit to treatment.

Before being eligible to apply for reinstatement of a license suspended under this division, the oriental medicine practitioner or acupuncturist shall demonstrate to the board the ability to resume practice in compliance with acceptable and prevailing standards of care. The demonstration shall include the following:

(a) Certification from a treatment provider approved under section 4731.25 of the Revised Code that the individual has successfully completed any required inpatient treatment;

(b) Evidence of continuing full compliance with an aftercare contract or consent agreement;

(c) Two written reports indicating that the individual's ability to practice has been assessed and that the individual has been found capable of practicing according to acceptable and prevailing standards of care. The reports shall be made by individuals or providers approved by the board for making such assessments and shall describe the basis for their determination.

The board may reinstate a license suspended under this division after such demonstration and after the individual has entered into a written consent agreement.

When the impaired individual resumes practice, the board shall require continued monitoring of the individual. The monitoring shall include monitoring of compliance with the written consent agreement entered into before reinstatement or with conditions imposed by board order after a hearing, and, upon termination of the consent agreement, submission to the board for at least two years of annual written progress reports made under penalty of falsification stating whether the individual has maintained sobriety.

(H) If the secretary and supervising member determine both of the following, they may recommend that the board suspend an individual's license to practice without a prior hearing:

(1) That there is clear and convincing evidence that an oriental medicine practitioner or acupuncturist has violated division (B) of this section;

(2) That the individual's continued practice presents a danger of immediate and serious harm to the public.

Written allegations shall be prepared for consideration by the board. The board, upon review of the allegations and by an affirmative vote of not fewer than six of its members, excluding the secretary and supervising member, may suspend a license without a prior hearing. A telephone conference call may be utilized for reviewing the allegations and taking the vote on the summary suspension.

The board shall issue a written order of suspension by certified mail or in person in accordance with section 119.07 of the Revised Code. The order shall not be subject to suspension by the court during pendency of any appeal filed under section 119.12 of the Revised Code. If the oriental medicine practitioner or acupuncturist requests an adjudicatory hearing by the board, the date set for the hearing shall be within fifteen days, but not earlier than seven days, after the hearing is requested, unless otherwise agreed to by both the board and the license holder.

A summary suspension imposed under this division shall remain in effect, unless reversed on appeal, until a final adjudicative order issued by the board pursuant to this section and Chapter 119. of the Revised Code becomes effective. The board shall issue its final adjudicative order within sixty days after completion of its hearing. Failure to issue the order within sixty days shall result in dissolution of the summary suspension order, but shall not invalidate any subsequent, final adjudicative order.

(I) If the board takes action under division (B) (11), (13), or (14) of this section, and the judicial finding of guilt, guilty plea, or judicial finding of eligibility for intervention in lieu of conviction is overturned on appeal, upon exhaustion of the criminal appeal, a petition for reconsideration of the order may be filed with the board along with appropriate court documents. Upon receipt of a petition and supporting court documents, the board shall reinstate the license. The board may then hold an adjudication under Chapter 119. of the Revised Code to determine whether the individual committed the act in question. Notice of opportunity for hearing shall be given in accordance with Chapter 119. of the Revised Code. If the board finds, pursuant to an adjudication held under this division, that the individual committed the act, or if no hearing is requested, it may order any of the sanctions specified in division (B) of this section.

(J) The license to practice of an oriental medicine practitioner or acupuncturist and the practitioner's or acupuncturist's practice in this state are automatically suspended as of the date the practitioner or acupuncturist pleads guilty to, is found by a judge or jury to be guilty of, or is subject to a judicial finding of eligibility for intervention in lieu of conviction in this state or treatment or intervention in lieu of conviction in another jurisdiction for any of the following criminal offenses in this state or a substantially equivalent criminal offense in another jurisdiction: aggravated murder, murder, voluntary manslaughter, felonious assault, kidnapping, rape, sexual battery, gross sexual imposition, aggravated arson, aggravated robbery, or aggravated burglary. Continued practice after the suspension shall be considered practicing without a license.

The board shall notify the individual subject to the suspension by certified mail or in person in accordance with section 119.07 of the Revised Code. If an individual whose license is suspended under this division fails to make a timely request for an adjudication under Chapter 119. of the Revised Code, the board shall enter a final order permanently revoking the individual's license.

(K) In any instance in which the board is required by Chapter 119. of the Revised Code to give notice of opportunity for hearing and the individual subject to the notice does not timely request a hearing in accordance with section 119.07 of the Revised Code, the board is not required to hold a hearing, but may adopt, by an affirmative vote of not fewer than six of its members, a final order that contains the board's findings. In the final order, the board may order any of the sanctions identified under division (A) or (B) of this section.

(L) Any action taken by the board under division (B) of this section resulting in a suspension shall be accompanied by a written statement of the conditions under which the license may be reinstated. The board shall adopt rules in accordance with Chapter 119. of the Revised Code governing conditions to be imposed for reinstatement. Reinstatement of a license suspended pursuant to division (B) of this section requires an affirmative vote of not fewer than six members of the board.

(M) When the board refuses to grant or issue a license to an applicant, revokes an individual's license, refuses to renew an individual's license, or refuses to reinstate an individual's license, the board may specify that its action is permanent. An individual subject to a permanent action taken by the board is forever thereafter ineligible to hold a license to practice as an oriental medicine practitioner or license to practice as an acupuncturist and the board shall not accept an application for reinstatement of the license or for issuance of a new license.

(N) Notwithstanding any other provision of the Revised Code, all of the following apply:

(1) The surrender of a license to practice as an oriental medicine practitioner or license to practice as an acupuncturist issued under this chapter is not effective unless or until accepted by the board. Reinstatement of a license surrendered to the board requires an affirmative vote of not fewer than six members of the board.

(2) An application made under this chapter for a license may not be withdrawn without approval of the board.

(3) Failure by an individual to renew a license in accordance with section 4762.06 of the Revised Code shall not remove or limit the board's jurisdiction to take disciplinary action under this section against the individual.

4762.13(1) Suspension of license for default on child support

On receipt of a notice pursuant to section 3123.43 of the Revised Code, the state medical board shall comply with sections 3123.41 to 3123.50 of the Revised Code and any applicable rules adopted under section 3123.63 of the Revised Code with respect to a license to practice as an oriental medicine practitioner or license to practice as an acupuncturist issued pursuant to this chapter.

4762.13(2) Mental illness or incompetence; suspension of license

If the state medical board has reason to believe that any person who has been granted under this chapter a license to practice as an oriental medicine practitioner or license to practice as an acupuncturist is mentally ill or mentally incompetent, it may file in the probate court of the county in which the person has a legal residence an affidavit in the form prescribed in section 5122.11 of the Revised Code and signed by the board secretary or a member of the board secretary's staff, whereupon the same proceedings shall be had as provided in Chapter 5122. of the Revised Code. The attorney general may represent the board in any proceeding commenced under this section.

If any person who has been granted a license is adjudged by a probate court to be mentally ill or mentally incompetent, the person's license shall be automatically suspended until the person has filed with the state medical board a certified copy of an adjudication by a probate court of the person's subsequent restoration to competency or has submitted to the board proof, satisfactory to the board, that the person has been discharged as having a restoration to competency in the manner and form provided in section 5122.38 of the Revised Code. The judge of the probate court shall forthwith notify the state medical board of an adjudication of mental illness or mental incompetence, and shall note any suspension of a license in the margin of the court's record of such license.

4762.13(3) Civil penalties

(A) (1) If an oriental medicine practitioner or acupuncturist violates any section of this chapter or any rule adopted under this chapter, the state medical board may, pursuant to an adjudication under Chapter 119. of the Revised Code and an affirmative vote of not fewer than six of its members, impose a civil penalty. The amount of the civil penalty shall be determined by the board in accordance with the guidelines adopted under division (A) (2) of this section. The civil penalty may be in addition to any other action the board may take under section 4762.13 of the Revised Code.

(2) The board shall adopt and may amend guidelines regarding the amounts of civil penalties to be imposed under this section. Adoption or amendment of the guidelines requires the approval of not fewer than six board members.

Under the guidelines, no civil penalty amount shall exceed twenty thousand dollars.

(B) Amounts received from payment of civil penalties imposed under this section shall be deposited by the board in accordance with section 4731.24 of the Revised Code. Amounts received from payment of civil penalties imposed for violations of division (B) (6) of section 4762.13 of the Revised Code shall be used by the board solely for investigations, enforcement, and compliance monitoring.

4762.14 Investigations of alleged violations

(A) The state medical board shall investigate evidence that appears to show that any person has violated this chapter or the rules adopted under it. Any person may report to the board in a signed writing any information the person has that appears to show a violation of any provision of this chapter or the rules adopted under it. In the absence of bad faith, a person who reports such information or testifies before the board in an adjudication conducted under Chapter 119. of the Revised Code shall not be liable for civil damages as a result of reporting the information or providing testimony. Each complaint or allegation of a violation received by the board shall be assigned a case number and be recorded by the board.

(B) Investigations of alleged violations of this chapter or rules adopted under it shall be supervised by the supervising member elected by the board in accordance with section 4731.02 of the Revised Code and by the secretary as provided in section 4762.17 of the Revised Code. The board's president may designate another member of the board to supervise the investigation in place of the supervising member. A member of the board who supervises the investigation of a case shall not participate in further adjudication of the case.

(C) In investigating a possible violation of this chapter or the rules adopted under it, the board may administer oaths, order the taking of depositions, issue subpoenas, and compel the attendance of witnesses and production of books, accounts, papers, records, documents, and testimony, except that a subpoena for patient record information shall not be issued without consultation with the attorney general's office and approval of the secretary and supervising member of the board. Before issuance of a subpoena for patient record information, the secretary and supervising member shall determine whether there is probable cause to believe that the complaint filed alleges a violation of this chapter or the rules adopted under it and that the records sought are relevant to the alleged violation and material to the investigation. The subpoena may apply only to records that cover a reasonable period of time surrounding the alleged violation.

On failure to comply with any subpoena issued by the board and after reasonable notice to the person being subpoenaed, the board may move for an order compelling the production of persons or records pursuant to the Rules of Civil Procedure.

A subpoena issued by the board may be served by a sheriff, the sheriff's deputy, or a board employee designated by the board. Service of a subpoena issued by the board may be made by delivering a copy of the subpoena to the person named therein, reading it to the person, or leaving it at the person's usual place of residence. When the person being served is an oriental medicine practitioner or acupuncturist, service of the subpoena may be made by certified mail, restricted delivery, return receipt requested, and the subpoena shall be deemed served on the date delivery is made or the date the person refuses to accept delivery.

A sheriff's deputy who serves a subpoena shall receive the same fees as a sheriff. Each witness who appears before the board in obedience to a subpoena shall receive the fees and mileage provided for under section 119.094 of the Revised Code.

(D) All hearings and investigations of the board shall be considered civil actions for the purposes of section 2305.252 of the Revised Code.

(E) Information received by the board pursuant to an investigation is confidential and not subject to discovery in any civil action.

The board shall conduct all investigations and proceedings in a manner that protects the confidentiality of patients and persons who file complaints with the board. The board shall not make public the names or any other identifying information about patients or complainants unless proper consent is given.

The board may share any information it receives pursuant to an investigation, including patient records and patient record information, with law enforcement agencies, other licensing boards, and other governmental agencies that are prosecuting, adjudicating, or investigating alleged violations of statutes or administrative rules. An agency or board that receives the information shall comply with the same requirements regarding confidentiality as those with which the state medical board must comply, notwithstanding any conflicting provision of the Revised Code or procedure of the agency or board that applies when it is dealing with other information in its possession. In a judicial proceeding, the information may be admitted into evidence only in accordance with the Rules of Evidence, but the court shall require that appropriate measures are taken to ensure that confidentiality is maintained with respect to any part of the information that contains names or other identifying information about patients or complainants whose confidentiality was protected by the state medical board when the information was in the board's possession. Measures to ensure confidentiality that may be taken by the court include sealing its records or deleting specific information from its records.

(F) The state medical board shall develop requirements for and provide appropriate initial training and continuing education for investigators employed by the board to carry out its duties under this chapter. The training and continuing education may include enrollment in courses operated or approved by the Ohio peace officer training commission that the board considers appropriate under conditions set forth in section 109.79 of the Revised Code.

(G) On a quarterly basis, the board shall prepare a report that documents the disposition of all cases during the preceding three months. The report shall contain the following information for each case with which the board has completed its activities:

(1) The case number assigned to the complaint or alleged violation;

(2) The type of license, if any, held by the individual against whom the complaint is directed;

(3) A description of the allegations contained in the complaint;

(4) The disposition of the case.

The report shall state how many cases are still pending, and shall be prepared in a manner that protects the identity of each person involved in each case. The report is a public record for purposes of section 149.43 of the Revised Code.

4762.15 Prosecutor to notify state medical board of conviction of acupuncturist or oriental medicine practitioner

(A) As used in this section, "prosecutor" has the same meaning as in section 2935.01 of the Revised Code.

(B) Whenever any person holding a valid license to practice as an oriental medicine practitioner or valid license to practice as an acupuncturist issued pursuant to this chapter pleads guilty to, is subject to a judicial finding of guilt of, or is subject to a judicial finding of eligibility for intervention in lieu of conviction for a violation of Chapter 2907., 2925., or 3719. of the Revised Code or of any substantively comparable ordinance of a municipal corporation in connection with the person's practice, the prosecutor in the case, on forms prescribed and provided by the state medical board, shall promptly notify the board of the conviction. Within thirty days of receipt of that information, the board shall initiate action in accordance with Chapter 119. of the Revised Code to determine whether to suspend or revoke the license under section 4762.13 of the Revised Code.

(C) The prosecutor in any case against any person holding a valid license issued pursuant to this chapter, on forms prescribed and provided by the state medical board, shall notify the board of any of the following:

(1) A plea of guilty to, a finding of guilt by a jury or court of, or judicial finding of eligibility for intervention in lieu of conviction for a felony, or a case in which the trial court issues an order of dismissal upon technical or procedural grounds of a felony charge;

(2) A plea of guilty to, a finding of guilt by a jury or court of, or judicial finding of eligibility for intervention in lieu of conviction for a misdemeanor committed in the course of practice, or a case in which the trial court issues an order of dismissal upon technical or procedural grounds of a charge of a misdemeanor, if the alleged act was committed in the course of practice;

（3）A plea of guilty to, a finding of guilt by a jury or court of, or judicial finding of eligibility for intervention in lieu of conviction for a misdemeanor involving moral turpitude, or a case in which the trial court issues an order of dismissal upon technical or procedural grounds of a charge of a misdemeanor involving moral turpitude.

The report shall include the name and address of the license holder, the nature of the offense for which the action was taken, and the certified court documents recording the action.

4762.16 Disciplinary action by health care facility; reports to state medical board or monitoring organization; malpractice suits

（A）Within sixty days after the imposition of any formal disciplinary action taken by any health care facility, including a hospital, health care facility operated by a health insuring corporation, ambulatory surgical center, or similar facility, against any individual holding a valid license to practice as an oriental medicine practitioner or valid license to practice as an acupuncturist, the chief administrator or executive officer of the facility shall report to the state medical board the name of the individual, the action taken by the facility, and a summary of the underlying facts leading to the action taken. Upon request, the board shall be provided certified copies of the patient records that were the basis for the facility's action. Prior to release to the board, the summary shall be approved by the peer review committee that reviewed the case or by the governing board of the facility.

The filing of a report with the board or decision not to file a report, investigation by the board, or any disciplinary action taken by the board, does not preclude a health care facility from taking disciplinary action against an oriental medicine practitioner or acupuncturist.

In the absence of fraud or bad faith, no individual or entity that provides patient records to the board shall be liable in damages to any person as a result of providing the records.

（B）（1）Except as provided in division（B）（2）of this section, an oriental medicine practitioner or acupuncturist, professional association or society of oriental medicine practitioners or acupuncturists, physician, or professional association or society of physicians that believes a violation of any provision of this chapter, Chapter 4731. of the Revised Code, or rule of the board has occurred shall report to the board the information upon which the belief is based.

（2）An oriental medicine practitioner or acupuncturist, professional association or society of oriental medicine practitioners or acupuncturists, physician, or professional association or society of physicians that believes a violation of division（B）（6）of section 4762.13 of the Revised Code has occurred shall report the information upon which the belief is based to the monitoring organization conducting the program established by the board under section 4731.251 of the Revised Code. If any such report is made to the board, it shall be referred to the monitoring organization unless the board is aware that the individual who is the subject of the report does not meet the program eligibility requirements of section 4731.252 of the Revised Code.

(C) Any professional association or society composed primarily of oriental medicine practitioners or acupuncturists that suspends or revokes an individual's membership for violations of professional ethics, or for reasons of professional incompetence or professional malpractice, within sixty days after a final decision, shall report to the board, on forms prescribed and provided by the board, the name of the individual, the action taken by the professional organization, and a summary of the underlying facts leading to the action taken.

The filing of a report with the board or decision not to file a report, investigation by the board, or any disciplinary action taken by the board, does not preclude a professional organization from taking disciplinary action against an individual.

(D) Any insurer providing professional liability insurance to any person holding a valid license to practice as an oriental medicine practitioner or valid license to practice as an acupuncturist or any other entity that seeks to indemnify the professional liability of an oriental medicine practitioner or acupuncturist shall notify the board within thirty days after the final disposition of any written claim for damages where such disposition results in a payment exceeding twenty-five thousand dollars. The notice shall contain the following information:

(1) The name and address of the person submitting the notification;

(2) The name and address of the insured who is the subject of the claim;

(3) The name of the person filing the written claim;

(4) The date of final disposition;

(5) If applicable, the identity of the court in which the final disposition of the claim took place.

(E) The board may investigate possible violations of this chapter or the rules adopted under it that are brought to its attention as a result of the reporting requirements of this section, except that the board shall conduct an investigation if a possible violation involves repeated malpractice. As used in this division, "repeated malpractice" means three or more claims for malpractice within the previous five-year period, each resulting in a judgment or settlement in excess of twenty-five thousand dollars in favor of the claimant, and each involving negligent conduct by the oriental medicine practitioner or acupuncturist.

(F) All summaries, reports, and records received and maintained by the board pursuant to this section shall be held in confidence and shall not be subject to discovery or introduction in evidence in any federal or state civil action involving an oriental medicine practitioner, acupuncturist, supervising physician, or health care facility arising out of matters that are the subject of the reporting required by this section. The board may use the information obtained only as the basis for an investigation, as evidence in a disciplinary hearing against an oriental medicine practitioner, acupuncturist, or supervising physician, or in any subsequent trial or appeal of a board action or order.

The board may disclose the summaries and reports it receives under this section only to health care facility committees within or outside this state that are involved in credentialing or recredentialing an oriental medicine practitioner, acupuncturist, or supervising physician or reviewing their privilege to practice within a particular facility. The board shall indicate whether or not the information has been verified. Information transmitted by the board shall be subject to the same confidentiality provisions as when maintained by the board.

(G) Except for reports filed by an individual pursuant to division (B) of this section, the board shall send a copy of any reports or summaries it receives pursuant to this section to the acupuncturist. The oriental medicine practitioner or acupuncturist shall have the right to file a statement with the board concerning the correctness or relevance of the information. The statement shall at all times accompany that part of the record in contention.

(H) An individual or entity that reports to the board, reports to the monitoring organization described in section 4731.251 of the Revised Code, or refers an impaired oriental medicine practitioner or impaired acupuncturist to a treatment provider approved by the board under section 4731.25 of the Revised Code shall not be subject to suit for civil damages as a result of the report, referral, or provision of the information.

(I) In the absence of fraud or bad faith, a professional association or society of oriental medicine practitioners or acupuncturists that sponsors a committee or program to provide peer assistance to an oriental medicine practitioner or acupuncturist with substance abuse problems, a representative or agent of such a committee or program, a representative or agent of the monitoring organization described in section 4731.251 of the Revised Code, and a member of the state medical board shall not be held liable in damages to any person by reason of actions taken to refer an oriental medicine practitioner or acupuncturist to a treatment provider approved under section 4731.25 of the Revised Code for examination or treatment.

4762.17　Enforcement of laws

The secretary of the state medical board shall enforce the laws relating to the practice of oriental medicine and acupuncture. If the secretary has knowledge or notice of a violation of this chapter or the rules adopted under it, the secretary shall investigate the matter, and, upon probable cause appearing, file a complaint and prosecute the offender. When requested by the secretary, the prosecuting attorney of the proper county shall take charge of and conduct the prosecution.

4762.18　Injunctive relief

(A) Subject to division (E) of this section, the attorney general, the prosecuting attorney of any county in which the offense was committed or the offender resides, the state medical board, or any other person having knowledge of a person engaged either directly or by complicity in the practice of oriental medicine or acupuncture without having first obtained a license to do so pursuant to this chapter, may, in accord with provisions of the Revised Code governing injunctions, maintain an action in the name of the state to enjoin any person from engaging either directly or by complicity in the unlawful practice of oriental medicine or acupuncture by applying for an injunction in any court of competent jurisdiction.

(B) Prior to application for an injunction under division (A) of this section, the secretary of the state medical board shall notify the person allegedly engaged either directly or by complicity in the unlawful practice of oriental medicine or acupuncture by registered mail that the secretary has received information indicating that this person is so engaged. The person shall answer the secretary within thirty days showing that the person is either properly licensed for the stated activity or that the person is not in violation of this chapter. If the answer is not forthcoming within thirty days after notice by the secretary, the secretary shall request that the attorney general, the prosecuting attorney of the county in which the offense was committed or the offender resides, or the state medical board proceed as authorized in this section.

(C) Upon the filing of a verified petition in court, the court shall conduct a hearing on the petition and shall give the same preference to this proceeding as is given all proceedings under Chapter 119. of the Revised Code, irrespective of the position of the proceeding on the calendar of the court.

(D) Injunction proceedings as authorized by this section shall be in addition to, and not in lieu of, all penalties and other remedies provided in this chapter.

(E) An injunction proceeding permitted by division (A) of this section may not be maintained against a person described in division (B) of section 4762.02 of the Revised Code or a chiropractor who holds a valid certificate to practice acupuncture issued under section 4734.283 of the Revised Code.

4762.19 Rules

The state medical board may adopt any rules necessary to govern the practice of oriental medicine, the practice of acupuncture, the supervisory relationship between oriental medicine practitioners or acupuncturists and supervising physicians, the use of herbal therapy by oriental medicine practitioners, and the administration and enforcement of this chapter. Rules adopted under this section shall be adopted in accordance with Chapter 119. of the Revised Code.

4762.20 Fees

The state medical board, subject to the approval of the controlling board, may establish fees in excess of the amounts specified in this chapter, except that the fees may not exceed the specified amounts by more than fifty per cent.

All fees, penalties, and other funds received by the board under this chapter shall be deposited in accordance with section 4731.24 of the Revised Code.

4762.21 Immunities of state medical board

In the absence of fraud or bad faith, the state medical board, a current or former board member, an agent of the board, a person formally requested by the board to be the board's representative, or an employee of the board shall not be held liable in damages to any person as the result of any act, omission, proceeding, conduct, or decision related to official duties undertaken or performed pursuant to this chapter. If any such person asks to be defended by the state against any claim or action arising out of any act, omission, proceeding, conduct, or decision related to the person's official duties, and if the request is made in writing at a reasonable time before trial and the person requesting defense cooperates in good faith in the defense of the claim or action, the state shall provide and pay for the person's defense and shall pay any resulting judgment, compromise, or settlement. At no time shall the state pay any part of a claim or judgment that is for punitive or exemplary damages.

4762.22　Professional liability insurance

An individual who holds a license to practice as an oriental medicine practitioner or license to practice as an acupuncturist issued under this chapter shall have professional liability insurance coverage in an amount that is not less than five hundred thousand dollars.

4762.23　Compliance with RC 4776.20

The state medical board shall comply with section 4776.20 of the Revised Code.

4762.99　Penalties

(A) Whoever violates section 4762.02 of the Revised Code is guilty of a misdemeanor of the first degree on a first offense; on each subsequent offense, the person is guilty of a felony of the fourth degree.

(B) Whoever violates division (A), (B), (C), or (D) of section 4762.16 of the Revised Code is guilty of a minor misdemeanor on a first offense; on each subsequent offense the person is guilty of a misdemeanor of the fourth degree, except that an individual guilty of a subsequent offense shall not be subject to imprisonment, but to a fine alone of up to one thousand dollars for each offense.

Ohio Administrative Code Annotated

4734 - 10 - 01　Maintaining a certificate to practice acupuncture

(A) Each chiropractic physician issued a certificate to practice acupuncture by the board shall maintain a current license to practice chiropractic in the state of Ohio.

(B) If at any time a chiropractic physician's license to practice chiropractic in Ohio is suspended, revoked, placed inactive, or forfeited, the certificate to practice acupuncture issued by the state chiropractic board shall likewise be suspended, revoked, placed inactive, or forfeited without further administrative action.

(C) At no time shall a chiropractic physician hold an active certificate to practice acupuncture without simultaneously holding a valid, current license to practice chiropractic in the state of Ohio.

4734 – 10 – 02　Acupuncture course of study approval

(A) It shall be the objective of each board-approved acupuncture educational provider to prepare each chiropractic physician to demonstrate professional competence to become an acupuncture provider.

(B) Each educational provider that seeks board approval of an acupuncture course of study shall file a request for approval with the board. The request shall include:

(1) Evidence that the program meets the requirements outlined in section 4734.211 of the Revised Code;

(2) An outline for the entire course of study;

(3) Accreditation held by the educational provider, to include programs that are accredited;

(4) Evidence that the course of study will prepare students to become a competent acupuncture provider;

(5) A vitae of each instructor, to include the instructors' faculty status with the educational provider seeking approval;

(6) Evidence that the course of study is accepted by the national board of chiropractic examiners to allow students to sit for the acupuncture examination;

(7) Other information as deemed appropriate by the board.

(C) The board may review the request and supporting documentation and/or appoint a committee to review the materials.

(D) Board-approved acupuncture educational providers may accept transfer hours towards the required three hundred hours of acupuncture education for those chiropractic physicians who have previously earned acupuncture education. The educational provider shall ensure that any accepted transferred hours are appropriate and acceptable to utilize towards the three hundred hour course requirement as outlined in section 4734.211 of the Revised Code. The board-approved acupuncture educational provider shall reflect all transferred coursework on the chiropractic physician's final transcript.

(E) The educational institution shall ensure appropriate attendance and monitoring procedures for the course of study.

(F) The board may withdraw approval of an acupuncture course of study at any time if such program is not in compliance with the provisions of this rule. If, in the opinion of the board, there is evidence that an entity having status of board-approved acupuncture educational provider is not in compliance with this rule, the board shall issue a warning letter to the program stating that board-approved status may be withdrawn and the reasons for the action. Such letter shall be sent at least thirty days prior to such contemplated action by the board. Reinstatement of board-approved status may be granted by the board if the educational provider furnishes proof of compliance with this rule.

4734 - 10 - 03 Application for acupuncture certificate

（A）Each applicant for a certificate to practice acupuncture shall apply in the manner prescribed by the board and submit a one hundred dollar non-refundable application fee. The application and fee shall be valid for one year from the initial application date. The applicant shall submit satisfactory evidence of his or her qualifications to receive a certificate to practice acupuncture in the state of Ohio as prescribed by section 4734.282 of the Revised Code. All required credentials must be sent directly from the issuing entity.

（B）The board may refuse or deny an applicant for a certificate to practice acupuncture in this state if the applicant does not meet the licensure requirements as outlined in section 4734.282 of the Revised Code or has committed any act which indicates that the applicant does not possess the character and fitness to practice acupuncture, including any act that would be grounds for disciplinary action as outlined in section 4734.31 of the Revised Code. The burden of proof is on the applicant to prove by clear and convincing evidence to the board that he or she meets the conditions for receipt of a certificate to practice acupuncture.

（C）Any applicant that the board proposes to refuse or deny a certificate to practice acupuncture shall be entitled to a hearing on the question of such proposed refusal or denial.

4734 - 10 - 04 Acupuncture certificate renewal requirements — Repealed

4734 - 10 - 05 Acupuncture referral — Repealed

4734 - 10 - 06 Inactive acupuncture certificate; restoration of acupuncture certificate

（A）A licensee holding an inactive acupuncture certificate may apply to have the certificate restored in the manner prescribed by the board and shall complete an application and supply all information necessary to process the application. An acupuncture certificate shall not be restored unless the licensee's chiropractic license is current.

（1）If an application for restoration is received before the first day of the second year of the CE period, the applicant shall submit a non-refundable payment of one hundred dollars and evidence of twelve hours of acupuncture CE earned in accordance with the provisions of rule 4734 - 7 - 01 of the Administrative Code within the twenty-four months immediately preceding the date of the application.

（2）If an application for restoration is received on or after the first day of the second year of the CE period, the applicant shall submit a non-refundable payment of fifty dollars and evidence of six hours of acupuncture CE earned in accordance with the provisions of rule 4734 - 7 - 01 of the Administrative Code within the twenty-four months immediately preceding the date of the application.

（B）The board shall consider the length of inactivity and the moral character and activities of the applicant during the inactive certificate period and may impose any of the terms and conditions for restoration outlined in division（B）of section 4734.286 of the Revised Code.

（C）The board may refuse or deny an applicant for restoration of his or her inactive certificate if the applicant does not meet the requirements as outlined in this chapter or section 4734.286 of the Revised Code or has committed any act which indicates that the applicant does not possess the character and fitness to practice acupuncture, including any act that would be grounds for disciplinary action as outlined in section 4734.31 of the Revised Code. The burden of proof is on the applicant to prove by clear and convincing evidence to the board that he or she meets the conditions for certificate restoration.

Kansas

Kansas Statutes Annotated

65 – 7601. Citation of act

K.S.A. 65 – 7601 through 65 – 7624, and amendments thereto, shall be known and may be cited as the acupuncture practice act.

65 – 7602. Definitions

As used in the acupuncture practice act:

(a) "ACAOM" means the national accrediting agency recognized by the U. S. department of education that provides accreditation for educational programs for acupuncture and oriental medicine. For purposes of the acupuncture practice act, the term ACAOM shall also include any entity deemed by the board to be the equivalent of ACAOM.

(b) "Act" means the acupuncture practice act.

(c) "Acupuncture" means the use of needles inserted into the human body by piercing of the skin and related modalities for the assessment, evaluation, prevention, treatment or correction of any abnormal physiology or pain by means of controlling and regulating the flow and balance of energy in the body and stimulating the body to restore itself to its proper functioning and state of health.

(d) "Board" means the state board of healing arts.

(e) "Council" means the acupuncture advisory council established by K.S.A. 65 – 7613, and amendments thereto.

(f) "Licensed acupuncturist" means any person licensed to practice acupuncture under the acupuncture practice act.

(g) "NCCAOM" means the national certification commission for acupuncture and oriental medicine. NCCAOM is a national organization that validates entry-level competency in the practice of acupuncture and oriental medicine through the administration of professional certification examinations. For purposes of the acupuncture practice act, the term NCCAOM shall also include any entity deemed by the board to be the equivalent of the NCCAOM.

(h) "Physician" means a person licensed to practice medicine and surgery or osteopathy in Kansas.

(i) "Practice of acupuncture" includes, but is not limited to:

(1) Techniques sometimes called "dry needling," "trigger point therapy," "intramuscular therapy," "auricular detox treatment" and similar terms;

(2) mechanical, thermal, pressure, suction, friction, electrical, magnetic, light, sound, vibration, manual and electromagnetic treatment;

(3) the use, application or recommendation of therapeutic exercises, breathing techniques, meditation and dietary and nutritional counselings; and

(4) the use and recommendation of herbal products and nutritional supplements, according to the acupuncturist's level of training and certification by the NCCAOM or its equivalent.

(j) "Practice of acupuncture" does not include:

(1) Prescribing, dispensing or administering of any controlled substances as defined in K.S.A. 65 – 4101 et seq., and amendments thereto, or any prescription-only drugs;

(2) the practice of medicine and surgery, including obstetrics and the use of lasers or ionizing radiation;

(3) the practice of osteopathic medicine and surgery or osteopathic manipulative treatment;

(4) the practice of chiropractic;

(5) the practice of dentistry; or

(6) the practice of podiatry.

65 – 7603.　License prerequisite to practice acupuncture; representation as acupuncturist; penalties

(a) On and after July 1, 2017, except as otherwise provided in this act, no person shall practice acupuncture unless such person possesses a current and valid acupuncture license issued under this act.

(b) (1) No person shall depict oneself orally or in writing, expressly or by implication, as a holder of a license who does not hold a current license under this act.

(2) Only persons licensed under this act shall be entitled to use the title "licensed acupuncturist" or the designated letters "L. Ac."

(3) Nothing in this section shall be construed to prohibit an acupuncturist licensed under this act from listing or using in conjunction with their name any letters, words, abbreviations or other insignia to denote any educational degrees, certifications or credentials which such licensed acupuncturist has earned.

(4) Violation of this section shall constitute a class B misdemeanor.

65 – 7604.　Acupuncture needles; requirements

Needles used in the practice of acupuncture shall only be prepackaged, single-use and sterile. These needles shall only be used on an individual patient in a single treatment session.

65 – 7605.　Persons not required to hold acupuncturist license

(a) The following shall be exempt from the requirements for an acupuncture license pursuant to this act:

(1) Any person licensed in this state to practice medicine and surgery, osteopathy, dentistry or podiatry, a licensed chiropractor or a licensed naturopathic doctor, if the person confines the person's acts or practice to the scope of practice authorized by their health professional licensing laws and does not represent to the public that the person is licensed under this act;

(2) any herbalist or herbal retailer who does not hold oneself out to be a licensed acupuncturist;

(3) any health care provider in the United States armed forces, federal facilities and other military service when acting in the line of duty in this state;

(4) any student, trainee or visiting teacher of acupuncture, oriental medicine or herbology who is designated as a student, trainee or visiting teacher while participating in a course of study or training under the supervision of a licensed acupuncturist licensed under this act in a program that the council has approved. This includes continuing education programs and any acupuncture or herbology programs that are a recognized route by the NCCAOM, or its equivalent, to certification;

(5) any person rendering assistance in the case of an emergency or disaster relief;

(6) any person practicing self-care or any family member providing gratuitous care, so long as such person or family member does not represent or hold oneself out to the public to be an acupuncturist;

(7) any person who massages, so long as such person does not practice acupuncture or hold oneself out to be a licensed acupuncturist;

(8) any person whose professional services are performed pursuant to delegation by and under the supervision of a practitioner licensed under this act;

(9) any team acupuncturist or herbology practitioner, who is traveling with and treating those associated with an out-of-state or national team that is temporarily in the state for training or competition purposes; and

(10) any person licensed as a physical therapist when performing dry needling, trigger point therapy or services specifically authorized in accordance with the provisions of the physical therapy practice act.

(b) This section shall take effect on and after July 1, 2017.

65 – 7606.　License to practice acupuncture by examination; prerequisites

An applicant for licensure as an acupuncturist shall file an application, on forms provided by the board, showing to the satisfaction of the board that the applicant:

(a) Is at least 21 years of age;

(b) has successfully completed secondary schooling or its equivalent;

(c) has satisfactorily completed a course of study involving acupuncture from an accredited school of acupuncture which the board shall determine to have educational standards substantially equivalent to the minimum educational standards for acupuncture colleges as established by the ACAOM or NCCAOM;

(d) has satisfactorily passed a license examination approved by the board;

(e) has the reasonable ability to communicate in English; and

(f) has paid all fees required for licensure pursuant to K.S.A. 65 – 7611, and amendments thereto.

65 – 7607. License to practice acupuncture by endorsement; prerequisite

(a) The board, without examination, may issue a license to a person who has been in the active practice of acupuncture in some other state, territory, the District of Columbia or other country upon certification by the proper licensing authority of that state, territory, District of Columbia or other country certifying that the applicant is duly licensed, that the applicant's license has never been limited, suspended or revoked, that the licensee has never been censured or received other disciplinary actions and that, so far as the records of such authority are concerned, the applicant is entitled to such licensing authority's endorsement. The applicant shall also present proof satisfactory to the board:

(1) That the state, territory, District of Columbia or country in which the applicant last practiced has and maintains standards at least equal to those maintained in Kansas;

(2) that the applicant's original license was based upon an examination at least equal in quality to the examination required in this state and that the passing grade required to obtain such original license was comparable to that required in this state;

(3) the date of the applicant's original license and all endorsed licenses and the date and place from which any license was attained;

(4) the applicant has been actively engaged in practice under such license or licenses since issued. The board may adopt rules and regulations establishing qualitative and quantitative practice activities which qualify as active practice;

(5) that the applicant has a reasonable ability to communicate in English; and

(6) that the applicant has paid all the application fees as prescribed by K.S.A. 65 – 7611, and amendments thereto.

(b) An applicant for a license by endorsement shall not be licensed unless, as determined by the board, the applicant's individual qualifications are substantially equivalent to the Kansas requirements for licensure under the acupuncture practice act.

65 – 7608. Waiver of certain license prerequisites

The board shall waive the education and examination requirements for an applicant who submits an application on or before January 1, 2018, and who, on or before July 1, 2017:

(a) Is 21 years of age or older;

(b) has successfully completed secondary schooling or its equivalent;

(c) (1) (A) has completed a minimum of 1,350 hours of study, excluding online study in the field of acupuncture; and

(B) has been engaged in the practice of acupuncture with a minimum of 1,500 patient visits during a period of at least three of the five years immediately preceding July 1, 2017, as evidenced by two affidavits from office partners, clinic supervisors or other individuals approved by the board, who have personal knowledge of the years of practice and number of patients visiting the applicant for acupuncture. The board may adopt rules and regulations for further verification of the applicant's practice of acupuncture; or

(2) has satisfactorily passed a license examination approved by the board;

(d) has a reasonable ability to communicate in English; and

(e) has paid all fees required for licensure as prescribed by K. S. A. 65 - 7611, and amendments thereto.

65 - 7609.   Renewal date of license; requirements to maintain license; notice of renewal and cancellation; cancellation of license; reinstatement of license; designation of license

(a) The license shall be canceled on March 31 of each year unless renewed in the manner prescribed by the board. In each case in which a license is renewed for a period of time of less than 12 months, the board may prorate the amount of the fee established under K. S. A. 65 - 7611, and amendments thereto. The request for renewal shall be on a form provided by the board and shall be accompanied by the prescribed fee, which shall be paid not later than the renewal date of the license.

(b) There is hereby created a designation of an active license. The board is authorized to issue an active license to any licensee who makes written application for such license on a form provided by the board and remits the fee established pursuant to K. S. A. 65 - 7611, and amendments thereto. The board shall require every active licensee to submit evidence of satisfactory completion of a program of continuing education required by the board. The requirements for continuing education for licensed acupuncturists shall be established by rules and regulations adopted by the board.

(c) The board, prior to renewal of a license, shall require an active licensee to submit to the board evidence satisfactory to the board that the licensee is maintaining a policy of professional liability insurance. The board shall fix by rules and regulations the minimum level of coverage for such professional liability insurance.

(d) At least 30 days before the renewal date of a licensee's license, the board shall notify the licensee of the renewal date by mail addressed to the licensee's last known mailing address. If the licensee fails to submit the renewal application and pay the renewal fee by the renewal date of the license, the licensee shall be given notice that the licensee has failed to submit the renewal application and pay the renewal fee by the renewal date of the license, that the license will be deemed canceled if not renewed within 30 days following the renewal date, that upon receipt of the renewal application and renewal fee and an additional late fee established by rules and regulations not to exceed $500 within the 30 - day period, the license will not be canceled and that, if both fees are not received within the 30 - day period, the license shall be deemed canceled by operation of law and without further proceedings.

(e) Any license canceled for failure to renew may be reinstated within two years of cancellation upon recommendation of the board and upon payment of the renewal fees then due and upon proof of compliance with the continuing education requirements established by the board by rules and regulations. Any person who has not been in the active practice of acupuncture for which reinstatement is sought or who has not been engaged in a formal educational program during the two years preceding the application for reinstatement may be required to complete such additional testing, training or education as the board may deem necessary to establish the licensee's present ability to practice with reasonable skill and safety.

(f) There is hereby created a designation of an exempt license. The board is authorized to issue an exempt license to any licensee who makes written application for such license on a form provided by the board and remits the fee established pursuant to K. S. A. 65 - 7611, and amendments thereto. The board may issue an exempt license to a person who is not regularly engaged in the practice of acupuncture in Kansas and who does not hold oneself out to the public as being professionally engaged in such practice. An exempt license shall entitle the holder to all privileges attendant to the practice of acupuncture for which such license is issued. Each exempt license may be renewed subject to the provisions of this section. Each exempt licensee shall be subject to all provisions of the acupuncture practice act, except as otherwise provided in this subsection. The holder of an exempt license may be required to submit evidence of satisfactory completion of a program of continuing education required by this section. The requirements for continuing education for exempt licensees shall be established by rules and regulations adopted by the board. Each exempt licensee may apply for an active license to regularly engage in the practice of acupuncture upon filing a written application with the board. The request shall be on a form provided by the board and shall be accompanied by the license fee established pursuant to K.S.A. 65 - 7611, and amendments thereto. For the licensee whose license has been exempt for less than two years, the board shall adopt rules and regulations establishing appropriate continuing education requirements for exempt licensees to become licensed to regularly practice acupuncture within Kansas. Any licensee whose license has been exempt for more than two years and who has not been in the active practice of acupuncture since the license has been exempt may be required to complete such additional testing, training or education as the board may deem necessary to establish the licensee's present ability to practice with reasonable skill and safety. Nothing in this subsection shall be construed to prohibit a person holding an exempt license from serving as a paid employee of: (1) A local health department as defined by K.S.A. 65 - 241, and amendments thereto; or (2) an indigent health care clinic as defined by K.S.A. 75 - 6102, and amendments thereto.

(g) There is hereby created the designation of inactive license. The board is authorized to issue an inactive license to any licensee who makes written application for such license on a form provided by the board and remits the fee established pursuant to K.S.A. 65 - 7611, and amendments thereto. The board may issue an inactive license only to a person who is not regularly engaged in the practice of acupuncture in Kansas and who does not hold oneself out to the public as being professionally engaged in such practice. An inactive license shall not entitle the holder to practice acupuncture in this state. Each inactive license may be renewed subject to the provisions of this section. Each inactive licensee shall be subject to all provisions of the acupuncture practice act, except as otherwise provided in this subsection. The holder of an inactive license shall not be required to submit evidence of satisfactory completion of a program of continuing education required by subsection (b). Each inactive licensee may apply for an active license upon filing a written application with the board. The request shall be on a form provided by the board and shall be accompanied by the license fee established pursuant to K.S.A. 65 - 7611, and amendments thereto. For those licensees whose licenses have been inactive for less than two years, the board shall adopt rules and regulations establishing appropriate continuing education requirements for inactive licensees to become licensed to regularly practice acupuncture within Kansas. Any licensee whose license has been inactive for more than two years and who has not been in the active practice of acupuncture or engaged in a formal education program since the license has been inactive may be required to complete such additional testing, training or education as the board may deem necessary to establish the licensee's present ability to practice with reasonable skill and safety.

(h) This section shall take effect on and after July 1, 2017.

65 - 7610. Reinstatement of revoked license; requirements; procedure

A person whose license has been revoked may apply for reinstatement after the expiration of three years from the effective date of the revocation. Application for reinstatement shall be on a form provided by the board and shall be accompanied by the fee established by the board in accordance with K.S.A. 65 - 7611, and amendments thereto. The burden of proof by clear and convincing evidence shall be on the applicant to show sufficient rehabilitation to justify reinstatement. If the board determines that a license should not be reinstated, the person shall not be eligible to reapply for reinstatement for three years from the effective date of the denial. All proceedings conducted on an application for reinstatement shall be in accordance with the Kansas administrative procedure act and shall be reviewable in accordance with the Kansas judicial review act. The board, on its own motion, may stay the effectiveness of an order of revocation of license.

65 - 7611. Fees; collection by state board of healing arts

The board shall charge and collect in advance nonrefundable fees for acupuncturists as established by the board by rules and regulations, not to exceed:

Initial application for licensure	$700
Annual renewal for active license — paper	$300
Annual renewal for active license — online	$250
Annual renewal for inactive license — paper	$200
Annual renewal for inactive license — online	$150
Annual renewal for exempt license — paper	$200
Annual renewal for exempt license — online	$150
Late renewal fee	$100
Conversion from inactive to active license	$300
Conversion from exempt to active license	$300
Application for reinstatement of revoked license	$1,000
Certified copy of license	$25
Written verification of license	$25

65 - 7612. Fees, disposition of

The board shall remit all moneys received by or for the board from fees, charges or penalties to the state treasurer in accordance with the provisions of K.S.A. 75 - 4215, and amendments thereto. Upon receipt of each such remittance, the state treasurer shall deposit the entire amount in the state treasury. Ten percent of such amount shall be credited to the state general fund and the balance shall be credited to the healing arts fee fund. All expenditures from the healing arts fee fund shall be made in accordance with appropriation acts upon warrants of the director of accounts and reports issued pursuant to vouchers approved by the president of the board or by a person or persons designated by the president.

65 - 7613. Acupuncture advisory council; appointments and terms of members; meetings; reimbursement

(a) There is hereby established the acupuncture advisory council to assist the state board of healing arts in carrying out the provisions of this act. The council shall consist of five members, all citizens and residents of the state of Kansas, appointed as follows:

（1）The board shall appoint one member who is a physician licensed to practice medicine and surgery or osteopathy. The member appointed by the board shall serve at the pleasure of the board. The governor shall appoint three acupuncturists who have at least three years' experience in acupuncture preceding appointment and are actively engaged, in this state, in the practice of acupuncture or the teaching of acupuncture. At least two of the governor's appointments shall be made from a list of four nominees submitted by the Kansas association of oriental medicine. The governor shall appoint one member from the public sector who is not engaged, directly or indirectly, in the provision of health services. Insofar as possible, persons appointed by the governor to the council shall be from different geographic areas.

（2）The members appointed by the governor shall be appointed for terms of four years and until a successor is appointed. If a vacancy occurs on the council, the appointing authority of the position which has become vacant shall appoint a person of like qualifications to fill the vacant position for the unexpired term.

（b）The council shall meet at least once each year at a time of its choosing at the board's main office and at such other times as may be necessary on the chairperson's call or on the request of a majority of the council's members.

（c）A majority of the council constitutes a quorum. No action may be taken by the council except by affirmative vote of the majority of the members present and voting.

（d）Members of the council attending meetings of the council, or a subcommittee of the council, shall be paid amounts provided in K.S.A. 75 – 3223 （e）, and amendments thereto, from the healing arts fee fund.

65 – 7614. Same; duties

The acupuncture advisory council shall advise the board regarding：

（a）Examination, licensing and other fees；

（b）rules and regulations to be adopted to carry out the provisions of this act；

（c）the number of yearly continuing education hours required to maintain active licensure；

（d）changes and new requirements taking place in the areas of acupuncture；and

（e）such other duties and responsibilities as the board may assign.

65 – 7615. Rules and regulations

The board shall promulgate all necessary rules and regulations which may be necessary to administer the provisions of this act and to supplement the provisions herein.

65 – 7616. Disciplinary action against licensee；grounds for discipline；procedure；confidentiality of certain investigatory records

（a）A licensee's license may be revoked, suspended, limited or placed on probation, or the licensee may be publicly censured, or an application for a license or for reinstatement of a license may be denied upon a finding of the existence of any of the following grounds：

（1）The licensee has committed an act of unprofessional conduct as defined by rules and regulations adopted by the board;

(2) the licensee has committed fraud or misrepresentation in applying for or securing an original, renewal or reinstated license;

(3) the licensee has committed an act of professional incompetency as defined by rules and regulations adopted by the board;

(4) the licensee has been convicted of a felony;

(5) the licensee has violated any provision of the acupuncture practice act;

(6) the licensee has violated any lawful order or rule and regulation of the board;

(7) the licensee has been found to be mentally ill, disabled, not guilty by reason of insanity, not guilty because the licensee suffers from a mental disease or defect or incompetent to stand trial by a court of competent jurisdiction;

(8) the licensee has failed to report to the board any adverse action taken against the licensee by another state or licensing jurisdiction, a peer review body, a health care facility, a professional association or society, a governmental agency, a law enforcement agency or a court for acts or conduct similar to acts or conduct which would constitute grounds for disciplinary action under this section;

(9) the licensee has surrendered a license or authorization to practice as an acupuncturist in another state or jurisdiction, has agreed to a limitation or restriction of privileges at any medical care facility or has surrendered the licensee's membership on any professional staff or in any professional association or society while under investigation for acts or conduct similar to acts or conduct which would constitute grounds for disciplinary action under this section;

(10) the licensee has failed to report to the board the surrender of the licensee's license or authorization to practice as an acupuncturist in another state or jurisdiction or the surrender of the licensee's membership on any professional staff or in any professional association or society while under investigation for acts or conduct similar to acts or conduct which would constitute grounds for disciplinary action under this section;

(11) the licensee has an adverse judgment, award or settlement rendered against the licensee resulting from a medical liability claim related to acts or conduct similar to acts or conduct which would constitute grounds for disciplinary action under this section;

(12) the licensee has failed to report to the board any adverse judgment, settlement or award against the licensee resulting from a medical malpractice liability claim related to acts or conduct similar to acts or conduct which would constitute grounds for disciplinary action under this section; or

(13) the licensee's ability to practice with reasonable skill and safety to patients is impaired by reason of physical or mental illness, or use of alcohol, drugs or controlled substances. When reasonable suspicion of impairment exists, the board may take action in accordance with K.S.A. 65 – 2842, and amendments thereto. All information, reports, findings and other records relating

to impairment shall be confidential and not subject to discovery by or release to any person or entity outside of a board proceeding. This provision regarding confidentiality shall expire on July 1, 2022, unless the legislature reviews and reenacts such provision pursuant to K.S.A. 45 - 229, and amendments thereto, prior to July 1, 2022.

(b) The denial, refusal to renew, suspension, limitation, probation or revocation of a license or other sanction may be ordered by the board upon a finding of a violation of the acupuncture practice act. All administrative proceedings conducted pursuant to this act shall be in accordance with the Kansas administrative procedure act and shall be reviewable in accordance with the Kansas judicial review act.

(c) This section shall take effect on and after July 1, 2017.

65 - 7617. Same; jurisdiction; procedure; stipulations; emergency proceedings

(a) The board shall have jurisdiction of proceedings to take disciplinary action against any licensee practicing under the acupuncture practice act. Any such action shall be taken in accordance with the Kansas administrative procedure act.

(b) Either before or after formal charges have been filed, the board and the licensee may enter into a stipulation which shall be binding upon the board and the licensee entering into such stipulation, and the board may enter its findings of fact and enforcement order based upon such stipulation without the necessity of filing any formal charges or holding hearings in the case. An enforcement order based upon a stipulation may order any disciplinary action against the licensee entering into such stipulation.

(c) The board may temporarily suspend or temporarily limit the license of any licensee in accordance with the emergency adjudicative proceedings provisions under the Kansas administrative procedure act if the board determines that there is cause to believe that grounds exist for disciplinary action against the licensee and that the licensee's continuation of practice would constitute an imminent danger to public health and safety.

(d) Judicial review and civil enforcement of any agency action under this act shall be in accordance with the Kansas judicial review act.

65 - 7618. Non-disciplinary resolutions; procedure

The board or a committee of the board may implement non-disciplinary resolutions concerning a licensed acupuncturist consistent with the provisions of K.S.A. 65 - 2838a, and amendments thereto.

65 - 7619. Administrative fines

The state board of healing arts, in addition to any other penalty prescribed under the acupuncture practice act, may assess a civil fine, after proper notice and an opportunity to be heard, against a licensee for a violation of the acupuncture practice act in an amount not to exceed $2,000 for a first violation, $5,000 for a second violation and $10,000 for a third violation and any subsequent violation. All fines assessed and collected under this section shall be remitted to the state treasurer in accordance with the provisions of K.S.A. 75 – 4218[1], and amendments thereto. Upon receipt of each such remittance, the state treasurer shall deposit the entire amount in the state treasury to the credit of the state general fund. Fines collected under this section shall be considered administrative fines pursuant to 11 U.S.C. § 523.

65 – 7620. Confidentiality of complaints and related reports, records or information; exceptions

(a) Any complaint or report, record or other information relating to a complaint which is received, obtained or maintained by the board shall be confidential and shall not be disclosed by the board or its employees in a manner which identifies or enables identification of the person who is the subject or source of the information, except the information may be disclosed:

(1) In any proceeding conducted by the board under the law or in an appeal of an order of the board entered in a proceeding, or to any party to a proceeding or appeal or the party's attorney;

(2) to the person who is the subject of the information or to any person or entity when requested by the person who is the subject of the information, but the board may require disclosure in such a manner that will prevent identification of any other person who is the subject or source of the information; or

(3) to a state or federal licensing, regulatory or enforcement agency with jurisdiction over the subject of the information or to an agency with jurisdiction over acts or conduct similar to acts or conduct which would constitute grounds for action under this act.

(b) Any confidential complaint or report, record or other information disclosed by the board as authorized by this section shall not be re-disclosed by the receiving agency except as otherwise authorized by law.

(c) This section regarding confidentiality shall expire on July 1, 2022, unless the legislature reviews and reenacts such provision pursuant to K.S.A. 45 – 229, and amendments thereto, prior to July 1, 2022.

65 – 7621. Reporting alleged incidents of malpractice; civil immunity; when

(a) No person reporting to the state board of healing arts in good faith any information such person may have relating to alleged incidents of malpractice, or the qualifications, fitness or character of, or disciplinary action taken against a person licensed, registered or certified by the board shall be subject to a civil action for damages as a result of reporting such information.

(b) Any state, regional or local association composed of persons licensed to practice acupuncture and the individual members of any committee thereof, which in good faith investigates or communicates information pertaining to the alleged incidents of malpractice, or the qualifications, fitness or character of, or disciplinary action taken against any licensee, registrant or certificate holder to the state board of healing arts or to any committee or agent thereof, shall be immune from liability in any civil action that is based upon such investigation or transmittal of information if the investigation and communication was made in good faith and did not represent as true any matter not reasonably believed to be true.

65 – 7622. Acupuncturist-patient privilege

(a) The confidential relations and communications between a licensed acupuncturist and the acupuncturist's patient are placed on the same basis as those established between a physician and a physician's patient in K.S.A. 60 – 427, and amendments thereto.

(b) This section shall take effect on and after July 1, 2017.

65 – 7623. Injunction against violation of act

(a) When it appears that any person is violating any provision of this act, the board may bring an action in the name of the state in a court of competent jurisdiction for an injunction against such violation without regard as to whether proceedings have been or may be instituted before the board or whether criminal proceedings have been or may be instituted.

(b) This section shall take effect on and after July 1, 2017.

65 – 7624. Severability of act

If any provision of the acupuncture practice act or application thereof to any person or circumstance is held invalid, such invalidity shall not affect other provisions or applications of the acupuncture practice act which can be given effect without the invalid provision or application, and to this end the provisions of the acupuncture practice act are declared to be severable.

Kansas Administrative Regulations

100 – 76 – 1. Fees.

(a) The following fees shall be collected by the board:

(1) Application for license	$165.00
(2) Annual renewal of active license:	
(A) Paper renewal	$150.00
(B) On-line renewal	$125.00
(3) Annual renewal of inactive license:	
(A) Paper renewal	$125.00
(B) On-line renewal	$100.00
(4) Annual renewal of exempt license:	
(A) Paper renewal	$125.00

续　表

(B) On-line renewal	$100.00
(5) Conversion from inactive to active license	$75.00
(6) Conversion from exempt to active license	$75.00
(7) Late renewal:	
(A) Paper renewal	$50.00
(B) On-line renewal	$25.00
(8) Application for reinstatement of canceled license	$165.00
(9) Application for reinstatement of revoked license	$500.00
(10) Certified copy of license	$20.00
(11) Written verification of license	$20.00

(b) If a licensed acupuncturist's initial licensure period is six months or less before the first annual renewal period, the first annual renewal fee shall be prorated at $10.00 per month for any full or partial month.

100 – 76 – 2.　Licensure by examination.

Each applicant for licensure by examination shall provide the following or the substantial equivalent of the following as determined by the board:

(a) Documentation of successful completion of the certification examination offered by the NCCAOM or an entity with standards equivalent to the standards of NCCAOM at the time the applicant completed the examination as determined by the board. The certification examination shall include the following components:

(1) Foundations of oriental medicine;

(2) acupuncture with point location; and

(3) biomedicine, except that the biomedicine component of the examination shall not be required for any applicant who completed the NCCAOM certification, or its equivalent, before 2005; and

(b) a copy of a clean needle technique (CNT) certificate from the council of colleges of acupuncture and oriental medicine (CCAOM) or NCCAOM.

100 – 76 – 3.　Waiver of examination and education.

(a) Pursuant to K.S.A. 2017 Supp. 65 – 7608 and amendments thereto, certain license prerequisites for education and examination shall be waived by the board for each applicant who submits an application on or before January 1, 2018 and provides the following:

(1) Proof that the applicant has completed at least 1,350 hours of curriculum-based study,

an approved apprenticeship, or a tutorial program, or a combination of these, excluding on-line study, in the field of acupuncture. Proof of hours may be shown by successful completion of a curriculum-based program, an approved apprenticeship, or a tutorial program, or a combination of these, that meets the standards of the NCCAOM or any entity determined by the board to be the equivalent of the NCCAOM. To demonstrate successful completion of the requirements, the applicant shall submit the following:

(A) (1) Evidence that the apprenticeship preceptor either is licensed as an acupuncturist in the state in which the individual practices acupuncture or is a diplomate of acupuncture; and

(2) a copy of the notes, records, or other documentation maintained by the preceptor conducting the apprenticeship or tutorial program providing evidence of the educational materials used in the apprenticeship and documenting the number of hours taught and the subjects covered; or

(B) an official school transcript;

(2) evidence of a current clean needle technique (CNT) certificate obtained from the CCAOM, NCCAOM, or any entity determined to be the equivalent by the board; and

(3) proof that the applicant has been engaged in the practice of acupuncture and has had at least 1,500 patient visits in three of the last five years. The applicant shall provide any of the following for the board's review:

(A) Affidavits from at least two people who have practiced acupuncture with the applicant, including office partners, clinic supervisors, and any other individuals approved by the board;

(B) a copy of each continuing education certificate obtained within the last three years;

(C) a copy of the applicant's patient appointment books; or

(D) a copy of the applicant's patient charts.

(b) Each applicant shall provide any additional documentation requested by the board.

100 - 76 - 4. Exempt license; description of professional activities.

(a) Each person applying for an exempt license shall specify on the application all professional activities related to the practice of acupuncture that the person will perform if issued an exempt license.

(b) The professional activities performed by each individual holding an exempt license shall be limited to the following:

(1) Performing administrative functions, including peer review, utilization review, and expert opinions; and

(2) providing direct patient care services gratuitously or providing supervision, direction, or consultation for no compensation. Nothing in this subsection shall prohibit an exempt license holder from receiving payment for subsistence allowances or actual and necessary expenses incurred in providing these services.

(c) Each person holding an exempt license shall, at the time of license renewal, specify on the renewal application all professional activities related to the practice of acupuncture that the person will perform during the renewal period.

(d) Each person who requests modification of the professional activities on that person's application or renewal application for an exempt license shall notify the board of the modification within 30 days. The request for modification shall be submitted on a form provided by the board.

(e) Each licensed acupuncturist who has held an exempt license for less than two years and requests an active license designation shall submit evidence of satisfactory completion of at least 15 contact hours of continuing education within the preceding one-year period, as specified in K.A.R. 100 – 76 – 6.

(f) Each violation of subsection (a), (c), or (d) shall constitute prima facie evidence of unprofessional conduct pursuant to K.S.A. 2017 Supp. 65 – 7616, and amendments thereto.

100 – 76 – 5.   Professional liability insurance; active license.

(a) Each person applying for an active license in acupuncture shall submit to the board, with the application, evidence that the person has obtained the professional liability insurance coverage required by K.S.A. 2017 Supp. 65 – 7609, and amendments thereto, for which the limit of the insurer's liability is at least $200,000 per claim, subject to an annual aggregate of at least $600,000 for all claims made during the period of coverage.

(b) Each licensed acupuncturist with an active license designation shall submit to the board, with the annual application for license renewal, evidence that the licensee has continuously maintained and currently holds the professional liability insurance coverage specified in subsection (a).

(c) Each licensed acupuncturist who submits an application for change of designation to active license designation shall submit to the board, with the application, evidence that the licensee currently holds the professional liability insurance coverage specified in subsection (a).

100 – 76 – 6.   Continuing education.

(a) Each licensee shall complete at least 30 contact hours of approved continuing education within the 24 months preceding each renewal date in an even-numbered year, except as specified in subsection (b).

(b) A licensee initially licensed less than 12 months before a renewal date when continuing education is required shall not be required to submit evidence of completion of the continuing education required by subsection (a) for the first renewal period. Each licensee initially licensed more than one year but less than two years before a renewal date when continuing education is required shall complete at least 15 contact hours of approved continuing education within the licensure period.

(c) Each licensee shall maintain evidence of successful completion of all continuing education activities for five years from the date of completion of the activity. Evidence of successful completion of the continuing education activities required by subsections (a) and (b) may be requested by the board.

(d) Upon request by a licensee, an extension of up to six months may be granted by the board if the licensee cannot meet the requirements of subsection (a) or (b) due to a substantiated medical condition, natural disaster, death of a spouse or an immediate family member, or any other similar circumstance that renders the licensee incapable of meeting the requirements of subsection (a) or (b). Each request shall include a plan for completing the required continuing education activities.

(e) A contact hour shall consist of 50 minutes of approved continuing education activities. Meals and breaks shall not be included in the calculation of contact hours.

(f) All continuing education activities shall be related to the practice of acupuncture and shall pertain to any of the following:

(1) Clinical skills;

(2) clinical techniques;

(3) educational principles when providing service to patients, families, health professionals, health professional students, or the community;

(4) health care and the health care delivery system;

(5) problem solving, critical thinking, medical recordkeeping, and ethics;

(6) policy;

(7) biomedical science; or

(8) research.

(g) Continuing education activities shall consist of the following:

(1) Offerings. "Offerings" shall mean any offerings approved by the NCCAOM, by NCCAOM state affiliates, or by an entity with standards substantially equivalent to the standards of the NCCAOM as determined by the board or any other offerings approved by the board, subject to the limitation specified in paragraph (g) (9) (A).

(2) Lecture. "Lecture" shall mean a live discourse for the purpose of instruction given before an audience.

(3) Panel. "Panel" shall mean the presentation of multiple views by several professional individuals on a given subject, with none of the views considered a final solution.

(4) Workshop. "Workshop" shall mean a series of meetings designed for intensive study, work, or discussion in a specific field of interest.

(5) Seminar. "Seminar" shall mean directed advanced study or discussion in a specific field of interest.

(6) Symposium. "Symposium" shall mean a conference of more than a single session organized for the purpose of discussing a specific subject from various viewpoints and by various speakers.

(7) In-service training. "In-service training" shall mean an educational presentation given

to employees during the course of employment that pertains solely to the enhancement of acupuncture skills in the evaluation, assessment, or treatment of patients.

(8) Administrative training. "Administrative training" shall mean a presentation that enhances the knowledge of an acupuncturist on the topic of quality assurance, risk management, reimbursement, statutory requirements, or claim procedures.

(9) Self-instruction. "Self-instruction" shall mean either of the following:

(A) Reading professional literature. A maximum of four contact hours for each continuing education cycle shall be awarded. Each licensee shall maintain a log of all professional literature read as a continuing education activity; or

(B) completion of a correspondence, audio, video, or internet course approved by the NCCAOM, by NCCAOM state affiliates, or by an entity with standards substantially equivalent to the standards of the NCCAOM as determined by the board or any other continuing education offerings approved by the board, for which a printed verification of successful completion is provided by the person or organization offering the course.

(10) Continuing education activity presentation. "Continuing education activity presentation" shall mean the preparation and presentation of a continuing education activity that meets the requirements of this subsection. Three contact hours shall be awarded for each hour spent presenting.

(h) No contact hours shall be awarded for any continuing education activity that is repeated within a 48-month period.

100 – 76 – 7. Unprofessional conduct; definitions.

Each of the following terms, as used in K.S.A. 2017 Supp. 65 – 7616 and amendments thereto and this article of the board's regulations, shall have the meaning specified in this regulation:

(a) "Unprofessional conduct" shall mean any of the following:

(1) Soliciting patients through the use of fraudulent or false advertisements or profiting by the acts of those representing themselves to be agents of the licensee;

(2) representing to a patient that a manifestly incurable disease, condition, or injury can be permanently cured;

(3) assisting in the care or treatment of a patient without the consent of the patient or the patient's legal representative;

(4) using any letters, words, or terms as an affix on stationery or in advertisements or otherwise indicating that the person is entitled to practice any profession regulated by the board or any other state licensing board or agency for which the person is not licensed;

(5) willful betrayal of confidential information;

(6) advertising professional superiority or the performance of professional services in a superior manner;

（7）advertising to guarantee any professional service or to perform any professional service painlessly;

（8）engaging in conduct related to the practice of acupuncture that is likely to deceive, defraud, or harm the public;

（9）making a false or misleading statement regarding the licensee's skill or the efficacy or value of the treatment or remedy prescribed by the licensee or at the licensee's direction, in the treatment of any disease or other condition of the body or mind;

（10）commission of any act of sexual abuse, misconduct, or other improper sexual contact that exploits the licensee-patient relationship, with a patient or a person responsible for health care decisions concerning the patient;

（11）using any false, fraudulent, or deceptive statement in any document connected with the practice of acupuncture, including the intentional falsifying or fraudulent altering of a patient record;

（12）obtaining any fee by fraud, deceit, or misrepresentation;

（13）failing to transfer a patient's records to another licensee when requested to do so by the patient or by the patient's legally designated representative;

（14）performing unnecessary tests, examinations, or services that have no legitimate purpose;

（15）charging an excessive fee for services rendered;

（16）repeated failure to engage in the practice of acupuncture with that level of care, skill, and treatment that is recognized by a reasonably prudent similar practitioner as being acceptable under similar conditions and circumstances;

（17）failure to keep written medical records that accurately describe the services rendered to each patient, including patient histories, pertinent findings, examination results, and test results;

（18）delegating professional responsibilities to a person if the licensee knows or has reason to know that the person is not qualified by training, experience, or licensure to perform those professional responsibilities;

（19）failing to properly supervise, direct, or delegate acts that constitute the practice of acupuncture to persons who perform professional services pursuant to the licensee's direction, supervision, order, referral, delegation, or practice protocols;

（20）committing fraud or misrepresentation in applying for or securing an original, renewal, or reinstated license;

（21）willfully or repeatedly violating the act, any implementing regulations, or any regulations of the secretary of health and environment that govern the practice of acupuncture;

（22）unlawfully practicing any profession regulated by the board in which the licensed acupuncturist is not licensed to practice;

（23）failing to report or reveal the knowledge required to be reported or revealed pursuant to K.S.A. 2017 Supp. 65 – 7621, and amendments thereto;

(24) failing to furnish the board, or its investigators or representatives, any information legally requested by the board;

(25) incurring any sanction or disciplinary action by a peer review committee, a governmental agency or department, or a professional association or society for conduct that could constitute grounds for disciplinary action under the act or this article of the board's regulations;

(26) failing to maintain a policy of professional liability insurance as required by K.S.A. 2017 Supp. 65 – 7609, and amendments thereto, and K.A.R. 100 – 76 – 5;

(27) knowingly submitting any misleading, deceptive, untrue, or fraudulent representation on a claim form, bill, or statement;

(28) giving a worthless check or stopping payment on a debit or credit card for fees or moneys legally due to the board;

(29) knowingly or negligently abandoning medical records;

(30) engaging in conduct that violates patient trust and exploits the licensee-patient relationship for personal gain; or

(31) obstructing a board investigation, including engaging in one or more of the following acts:

(A) Falsifying or concealing a material fact;

(B) knowingly making or causing to be made any false or misleading statement or writing; or

(C) committing any other acts or engaging in conduct likely to deceive or defraud the board.

(b) "Advertisement" shall mean all representations disseminated in any manner or by any means that are for the purpose of inducing or that are likely to induce, directly or indirectly, the purchase of professional services.

(c) "False advertisement" shall mean any advertisement that is false, misleading, or deceptive in a material respect. In determining whether any advertisement is misleading, the following shall be taken into account:

(1) Representations made or suggested by statement, word, design, device, or sound, or any combination of these; and

(2) the extent to which the advertisement fails to reveal facts material in the light of the representations made.

100 – 76 – 8.   Professional incompetency; definition.

As used in K.S.A. 2017 Supp. 65 – 7616 and amendments thereto and this article of the board's regulations, professional incompetency shall mean any of the following:

(a) One or more instances involving failure to adhere to the applicable standard of care to a degree that constitutes gross negligence, as determined by the board;

(b) repeated instances involving failure to adhere to the applicable standard of care to a degree that constitutes ordinary negligence, as determined by the board; or

(c) a pattern of practice or other evidence of incapacity or incompetence to engage in the practice of acupuncture.

100 - 76 - 9. Patient records; adequacy.

(a) Each licensed censed acupuncturist shall maintain an adequate record for each patient for whom the licensee performs a professional service.

(b) Each patient record shall meet the following requirements:

(1) Be legible;

(2) contain only those terms and abbreviations that are or should be comprehensible to similar licensees;

(3) contain adequate identification of the patient;

(4) indicate the date on which each professional service was provided;

(5) contain all clinically pertinent information concerning the patient's condition;

(6) document what examinations, vital signs, and tests were obtained, performed, or ordered and the findings and results of each;

(7) specify the patient's initial reason for seeking the licensee's services and the initial diagnosis;

(8) specify the treatment performed or recommended;

(9) document the patient's progress during the course of treatment provided by the licensee; and

(10) include all patient records received from other health care providers, if those records formed the basis for a treatment decision by the licensee.

(c) Each entry shall be authenticated by the person making the entry, unless the entire patient record is maintained in the licensee's own handwriting.

(d) Each patient record shall include any writing intended to be a final record, but shall not require the maintenance of rough drafts, notes, other writings, or recordings once this information is converted to final form. The final form shall accurately reflect the care and services rendered to the patient.

(e) For purposes of the act and this regulation, an electronic patient record shall be deemed to be a written patient record if both of the following conditions are met:

(1) Each entry in the electronic record is authenticated by the licensee.

(2) No entry in the electronic record can be altered after authentication.

100 - 76 - 10. Release of records.

(a) Each licensed acupuncturist shall, upon receipt of a signed release from a patient, furnish a copy of the patient record to the patient, to another licensee designated by the patient, or to the patient's legally designated representative, unless withholding records is permitted by law or furnishing records is prohibited by law.

(b) Any licensee may charge a person or entity for the reasonable costs to retrieve or reproduce a patient record. A licensee shall not condition the furnishing of a patient record to another licensee upon prepayment of these costs.

(c) Each violation of this regulation shall constitute prima facie evidence of unprofessional conduct pursuant to K.S.A. 2017 Supp. 65 – 7616, and amendments thereto.

100 – 76 – 11. Free offers.

Each licensed acupuncturist who offers to perform a free examination, service, or procedure for a patient shall perform only the examination, service, or procedure specified in the offer. Before any additional examination, service, or procedure is performed, the licensee shall explain the nature and purpose of the examination, service, or procedure and specifically disclose to the patient, to the greatest extent possible, the cost of the additional examination, service, or procedure.

100 – 76 – 12. Business transactions with patients; unprofessional conduct.

(a) Non-health-related goods or services. A licensed acupuncturist offering to sell a non-health-related product or service to a patient from a location at which the licensee regularly engages in the practice of acupuncture shall have engaged in unprofessional conduct, unless otherwise allowed by this subsection. A licensed acupuncturist shall not have engaged in unprofessional conduct by offering to sell a non-health-related product or service if all of the following conditions are met:

(1) The sale is for the benefit of a public service organization.

(2) The sale does not directly or indirectly result in financial gain to the licensee.

(3) No patient is unduly influenced to make a purchase.

(b) Business opportunity. A licensed acupuncturist shall have engaged in unprofessional conduct if all of the following conditions are met:

(1) The licensee recruits or solicits a patient either to participate in a business opportunity involving the sale of a product or service or to recruit or solicit others to participate in a business opportunity.

(2) The sale of the product or service directly or indirectly results in financial gain to the licensee.

(3) The licensee recruits or solicits the patient at any time that the patient is present in a location at which the licensee regularly engages in the practice of acupuncture.

Missouri

Annotated Missouri Statutes

324.475. Definitions

For the purposes of sections 324.475 to 324.499, the following terms mean:

(1) "Acupuncture", the use of needles inserted into the body by piercing of the skin and related modalities for the assessment, evaluation, prevention, treatment or correction of any abnormal physiology or pain by means of controlling and regulating the flow and balance of energy in the body so as to restore the body to its proper functioning and state of health;

(2) "Acupuncturist", any person licensed as provided in sections 324.475 to 324.499 to practice acupuncture as defined in subdivision (1) of this section;

(3) "Auricular detox technician", a person trained solely in, and who performs only, auricular detox treatment. An auricular detox technician shall practice under the supervision of a licensed acupuncturist. Such treatment shall take place in a hospital, clinic or treatment facility which provides comprehensive substance abuse services, including counseling, and maintains all licenses and certifications necessary and applicable;

(4) "Auricular detox treatment", a very limited procedure consisting of acupuncture needles inserted into specified points in the outer ear of a person undergoing treatment for drug or alcohol abuse or both drug and alcohol abuse;

(5) "Board", the state board of chiropractic examiners established in chapter 331;

(6) "Committee", the Missouri acupuncture advisory committee;

(7) "Department", the department of commerce and insurance;

(8) "Director", the director of the division of professional registration;

(9) "Division", the division of professional registration;

(10) "License", the document of authorization issued by the board for a person to engage in the practice of acupuncture.

324.478.　Missouri acupuncturist advisory committee created, duties, members, terms

1. There is hereby created within the division of professional registration a committee to be known as the "Missouri Acupuncturist Advisory Committee". The committee shall consist of five members, all of whom shall be citizens of the United States and registered voters of the state of Missouri. The director of the division of professional registration shall appoint the members of the committee for terms of four years; except as provided in subsection 2 of this section. Three committee members shall be acupuncturists. Such members shall at all times be holders of licenses for the practice of acupuncture in this state; except for the members of the first committee who shall meet the requirements for licensure pursuant to sections 324.475 to 324.499. One member shall be a current board member of the Missouri state board for chiropractic examiners. The remaining member shall be a public member. All members shall be chosen from lists submitted by the director of the division of professional registration. The president of the Acupuncture Association of Missouri in office at the time shall, at least ninety days prior to the expiration of the term of a board member, other than the public member, or as soon as feasible after a vacancy on the board otherwise occurs, submit to the director of the division of professional registration a list of five acupuncturists qualified and willing to fill the vacancy in question, with the request and recommendation that the director appoint one of the five persons so listed, and with the list so submitted, the president of the Acupuncture Association of Missouri shall include in his or her letter of transmittal a description of the method by which the names were chosen by that association.

2. The initial appointments to the committee shall be one member for a term of one year, one member for a term of two years, one member for a term of three years and two members for a term of four years.

3. The public member of the committee shall not be and never has been a member of any profession regulated by the provisions of sections 324.475 to 324.499, or the spouse of any such person; and a person who does not have and never has had a material financial interest in either the providing of the professional services regulated by the provisions of sections 324.475 to 324.499 or an activity or organization directly related to the profession regulated pursuant to sections 324.475 to 324.499.

4. Any member of the committee may be removed from the committee by the director for neglect of duty required by law, for incompetency or for unethical or dishonest conduct. Upon the death, resignation, disqualification or removal of any member of the committee, the director shall appoint a successor. A vacancy in the office of any member shall only be filled for the unexpired term.

5. The acupuncturist advisory committee shall:

(1) Review all applications for licensure;

(2) Advise the board on all matters pertaining to the licensing of acupuncturists;

(3) Review all complaints and/or investigations wherein there is a possible violation of sections 324.475 to 324.499 or regulations promulgated pursuant thereto and make recommendations and referrals to the board on complaints the committee determines to warrant further action, which may include a recommendation for prosecuting violations of sections 324.475 to 324.499 to an appropriate prosecuting or circuit attorney;

(4) Follow the provisions of the board's administrative practice procedures in conducting all official duties;

(5) Assist the board, as needed and when requested by the board, in conducting any inquiry or disciplinary proceedings initiated as a result of committee recommendation and referral pursuant to subdivision (3) of this subsection.

324.481. Duties of board — rulemaking authority — acupuncturist fund created, use of

1. The board shall upon recommendation of the committee license applicants who meet the qualifications for acupuncturists, who file for licensure, and who pay all fees required for this licensure.

2. The board shall:

(1) Maintain a record of all board and committee proceedings regarding sections 324.475 to 324.499 and of all acupuncturists licensed in this state;

(2) Annually prepare a roster of the names and addresses of all acupuncturists licensed in this state, copies of which shall be made available upon request to any person paying the fee therefor;

(3) Set the fee for the roster at an amount sufficient to cover the actual cost of publishing and distributing the roster;

(4) Adopt an official seal;

(5) Prescribe the design of all forms to be furnished to all persons seeking licensure under sections 324.475 to 324.499;

(6) Prescribe the form and design of the license to be issued under sections 324.475 to 324.499;

(7) Inform licensees of any changes in policy, rules or regulations;

(8) Upon the recommendation of the committee, set all fees, by rule, necessary to administer the provisions of sections 324.475 to 324.499.

3. The board may with the approval of the advisory committee:

(1) Issue subpoenas to compel witnesses to testify or produce evidence in proceedings to deny, suspend or revoke licensure;

(2) Promulgate rules pursuant to chapter 536 in order to carry out the provisions of sections 324.475 to 324.499 including, but not limited to, regulations establishing:

(a) Standards for the practice of acupuncture;

(b) Standards for ethical conduct in the practice of acupuncture;

(c) Standards for continuing professional education;

(d) Standards for the training and practice of auricular detox technicians, including specific enumeration of points which may be used.

4. Any rule or portion of a rule, as that term is defined in section 536.010, that is promulgated to administer and enforce sections 324.475 to 324.499, shall become effective only if the agency has fully complied with all of the requirements of chapter 536, including but not limited to, section 536.028, if applicable, after August 28, 1998. If the provisions of section 536.028 apply, the provisions of this section are nonseverable and if any of the powers vested with the general assembly pursuant to section 536.028 to review, to delay the effective date, or to disapprove and annul a rule or portion of a rule are held unconstitutional or invalid, the purported grant of rulemaking authority and any rule so proposed and contained in the order of rulemaking shall be invalid and void, except that nothing in this section shall affect the validity of any rule adopted and promulgated prior to August 28, 1998.

5. All funds received by the board pursuant to the provisions of sections 324.240 to 324.275 shall be collected by the director who shall transmit the funds to the department of revenue for deposit in the state treasury to the credit of the "Acupuncturist Fund" which is hereby created.

6. Notwithstanding the provisions of section 33.080 to the contrary, money in this fund shall not be transferred and placed to the credit of general revenue until the amount in the fund at the end of the biennium exceeds three times the amount of the appropriation from the acupuncturist fund for the preceding fiscal year. The amount, if any, in the fund which shall lapse is that amount in the fund which exceeds the appropriate multiple of the appropriations from the acupuncturist fund for the preceding fiscal year.

324.484. Persons exempt from licensing requirements

1. Nothing in sections 324.475 to 324.499 shall be construed to apply to physicians and surgeons licensed pursuant to sections 334.010 to 334.265 or chiropractic physicians licensed pursuant to chapter 331; except that, if such physician or surgeon or chiropractic physician, with or without a current certification in meridian therapy, uses the title, licensed acupuncturist, then the provisions of sections 324.475 to 324.499 shall apply.

2. No license to practice acupuncture shall be required for any person who is an auricular detox technician, provided that such person performs only auricular detox treatments as defined in section 324.475, under the supervision of a licensed acupuncturist and in accordance with regulations promulgated pursuant to sections 324.475 to 324.499. An auricular detox technician may not insert acupuncture needles in any other points of the ear or body or use the title, licensed acupuncturist.

324.487. Qualifications for licensure

1. It is unlawful for any person to practice acupuncture in this state, unless such person:

(1) Possesses a valid license issued by the board pursuant to sections 324.475 to 324.499; or

（2）Is engaged in a supervised course of study that has been authorized by the committee approved by the board, and is designated and identified by a title that clearly indicates status as a trainee, and is under the supervision of a licensed acupuncturist.

2. A person may be licensed to practice acupuncture in this state if the applicant:

（1）Is twenty-one years of age or older and is actively certified as a Diplomate in Acupuncture by the National Commission for the Certification of Acupuncture and Oriental Medicine; and

（2）Submits to the committee an application on a form prescribed by the committee; and

（3）Pays the appropriate fee.

3. The board shall issue a certificate of licensure to each individual who satisfies the requirements of subsection 2 of this section, certifying that the holder is authorized to practice acupuncture in this state. The holder shall have in his or her possession at all times while practicing acupuncture, the license issued pursuant to sections 324.475 to 324.499.

324.490.　Expiration of licenses

1. Licenses issued pursuant to sections 324.475 to 324.499 shall expire every other year. Renewal applications shall be submitted to the division along with the appropriate renewal fee.

2. A license to practice acupuncture which is not renewed on or before the date of its expiration becomes invalid. Such license may be restored by complying with the provisions of section 324.493.

324.493.　Restoration of license, procedure

Any acupuncturist who fails to renew such acupuncturist's license on or before the date of its expiration may restore such license as follows:

（1）If the application for renewal is submitted to the committee not more than two years after the expiration of the applicant's last license, by payment of the appropriate fee and by providing all documentation required by the committee by rule; or

（2）If the application for renewal is submitted to the committee more than two years after the expiration of the applicant's last license, by payment of the appropriate fee, and by reapplying as provided in subdivisions（1）and（2）of subsection 2 of section 324.487.

324.496.　Authority of the board — complaints, procedure — limitation of liability

1. The board, with recommendation by the committee, may refuse to issue, renew or reinstate any license required by sections 324.475 to 324.499 for one or any combination of causes stated in subsection 2 of this section. The board shall notify the applicant in writing of the reasons for the refusal and shall advise the applicant of his or her right to file a complaint with the administrative hearing commission as provided by chapter 621.

2. The board, with recommendation by the committee, may cause a complaint to be filed with the administrative hearing commission as provided by chapter 621 against any holder of any license issued pursuant to sections 324.475 to 324.499 or any person who has failed to renew or has surrendered his or her license for any one or any combination of the following causes:

(1) The person has been finally adjudicated and found guilty, or entered a plea of guilty or nolo contendere, in a criminal prosecution pursuant to the laws of any state, of the United States, or of any country, for any offense directly related to the duties and responsibilities of the occupation, as set forth in section 324.012, regardless of whether or not sentence is imposed;

(2) Use of fraud, deception, misrepresentation or bribery in securing any license issued pursuant to sections 324.475 to 324.499 or in obtaining permission to take any examination given or required pursuant to sections 324.475 to 324.499;

(3) Obtaining or attempting to obtain any fee, charge, tuition or other compensation by fraud, deception or misrepresentation;

(4) Incompetency, misconduct, gross negligence, fraud, misrepresentation or dishonesty in the performance of the functions or duties of the profession regulated by sections 324.475 to 324.499;

(5) Violation of, or assisting or enabling any person to violate, any provision of sections 324.475 to 324.499, or of any lawful rule or regulation adopted pursuant to such sections;

(6) Impersonation of any person holding a license or allowing any person to use his or her certificate or diploma from any school or certification entity;

(7) Disciplinary action against the holder of a license or other right to practice the profession regulated by sections 324.475 to 324.499 granted by another state, territory, federal agency or country upon grounds for which revocation or suspension is authorized in this state;

(8) A person is finally adjudged insane or incompetent by a court of competent jurisdiction;

(9) Issuance of a license based upon a material mistake of fact;

(10) Use of any advertisement or solicitation which is false, misleading or deceptive to the general public or persons to whom the advertisement or solicitation is primarily directed;

(11) Use of any controlled substance, as defined in chapter 195, or alcoholic beverage to an extent that such use impairs a person's ability to perform the work of any profession licensed or regulated by sections 324.475 to 324.499.

3. Any person, organization, association or corporation who reports or provides information to the division, board or committee pursuant to the provisions of sections 324.475 to 324.499 and who does so in good faith and without negligence shall not be subject to an action for civil damages as a result thereof.

4. After the filing of a complaint pursuant to subsection 2 of this section, the proceedings shall be conducted in accordance with the provisions of chapter 621. Upon a finding by the administrative hearing commission that the grounds, provided in subsection 2 of this section, for disciplinary action are met, the board may, upon recommendation of the committee, singly or in combination, censure or place the person named in the complaint on probation, suspension or revoke the license of the person on such terms and conditions as the division deems appropriate.

324.499. Violations, penalty — right to sue

1. Any person who violates any provision of sections 324.475 to 324.499 is guilty of a class B misdemeanor.

2. All fees or other compensation received for services which are rendered in violation of sections 324.475 to 324.499 shall be refunded.

3. The board on behalf of the committee may sue in its own name in any court in this state to enforce the provisions of sections 324.475 to 324.499. The board may investigate any alleged violations of sections 324.475 to 324.499 referred to it by the committee, may institute actions for penalties provided in this section and shall enforce generally the provisions of sections 324.475 to 324.499.

4. Upon application by the board, the attorney general may, on behalf of the board, request that a court of competent jurisdiction grant an injunction, restraining order or other order as may be appropriate to enjoin a person from:

(1) Offering to engage or engaging in the performance of any acts or practices for which a certificate of registration or authority, permit or license is required upon a showing that such acts or[1] practices were performed or offered to be performed without a certificate of registration or authority, permit or license; or

(2) Engaging in any practice or business authorized by a certificate of registration or authority, permit or license, issued pursuant to sections 324.475 to 324.499 upon a showing that the holder presents a substantial probability of serious harm to the health, safety or welfare of any resident of this state or client or patient of the licensee.

5. Any action brought pursuant to this section may be in addition to, or in lieu of, any penalty provided by sections 324.475 to 324.499 and may be brought concurrently with other actions to enforce the provisions of sections 324.475 to 324.499.

Missouri Code of State Regulations

Chapter 1. General Rules

20 CSR 2015 - 1.010. Complaint Handling and Disposition

PURPOSE: This rule establishes a procedure for the receipt, handling, and disposition of requests for information and complaints.

(1) All complaints shall be made in writing addressed to the Missouri Acupuncture Advisory Committee, 3605 Missouri Boulevard, PO Box 1335, Jefferson City, MO 65102 and fully identify the complainant by name and address. Verbal or telephone communications will not be considered or processed as complaints. The person making these communications will be

asked to file a written statement. No member of the Advisory Committee for Acupuncturists may file a complaint with the advisory committee while holding that office, unless that member is excused from further advisory committee deliberation or activity concerning the matters alleged within that complaint. Any division staff member or the advisory committee may file a complaint pursuant to this rule in the same manner as any member of the public.

(2) Upon receipt of a complaint in proper form, the board or advisory committee may investigate the actions of the licensee, applicant, registrant, or unlicensed individual or entity against whom the complaint is made. Each complaint received under this rule shall be acknowledged in writing and the complainant be notified of the ultimate disposition of the complaint.

(3) The advisory committee will maintain each complaint received under this rule. The complaint file will contain a record of each complainant's name and address; subject(s) of the complaint; the date each complaint is received by the advisory committee; a brief statement of the complaint, including the name of any person injured or victimized by the alleged acts or practices; and the ultimate disposition of the complaint.

20 CSR 2015 – 1.020.   Acupuncturist Credentials, Name and Address Changes

PURPOSE: This rule specifies the title used by a licensed acupuncturist and requirements for maintaining current licensee information.

(1) Any person licensed as an acupuncturist shall use the abbreviations L. AC. or the licensure title Licensed Acupuncturist after the licensee's name and ensure that the license bears the current legal name of the licensee.

(2) A licensee whose name or address has changed shall, within thirty (30) days of such change —

(A) Notify the advisory committee via regular mail at PO Box 1335, Jefferson City, MO 65102, fax at 573/751/0735 or email at acupuncture@pr.mo.gov. A name change requires a copy of the document authorizing the name change; and

(B) Destroy the license bearing the former name.

(3) A licensed acupuncturist shall use only those educational credentials in association with the license that have been earned at an acceptable educational institution as defined in 20 CSR 2015 – 4.020 and that are related to acupuncture.

20 CSR 2015 – 1.030.   Fees

PURPOSE: This rule establishes the various fees and charges for the Acupuncturist Advisory Committee.

(1) All fees shall be paid by cashier's check, personal check, money order, or other method approved by the division and must be made payable to the Acupuncturist Advisory Committee.

(2) No fee will be refunded should any license be surrendered, suspended, or revoked

during the term for which the license is issued.

(3) The fees are established as follows:

(A) Acupuncturist Application Fee $200.00

(B) Acupuncturist Biennial Renewal Fee $100.00

(C) Fingerprinting Fee Amount to be determined by the Missouri State Highway Patrol

(D) Insufficient Funds Check Charge Fee $25.00

(E) Late Renewal Fee $50.00

(4) Fees may be returned to an applicant or licensee, at the advisory committee's discretion, with the applicant or licensee submitting a written request to the advisory committee explaining the reason the fee should be returned.

Chapter 2. Acupuncturist Licensure Requirements

20 CSR 2015 - 2.010. Application for Licensure

PURPOSE: This rule outlines the requirements for applying for licensure as an acupuncturist.

(1) Application for licensure shall be made on a form provided by the Acupuncturist Advisory Committee. Applications may be obtained by written request to the advisory committee at PO Box 672, Jefferson City, MO 65102 - 0672, or by calling the advisory committee office at (573) 751 - 1655 or contacting the advisory committee by e-mail at acupunct@ mail. state. mo.us.

(2) The application shall be printed in black ink, signed, notarized, and accompanied by all documents required by the advisory committee and the application fee as defined in 20 CSR 2015 - 1.030 (3) (A). Documentation includes, and is not limited to, the following:

(A) Two (2) sets of fingerprints. Any fees due for a fingerprint background check shall be paid by the applicant directly to the Missouri State Highway Patrol or its approved vendor(s);

(B) Proof that the applicant is at least twenty-one (21) years of age as demonstrated by one (1) of the following;

1. Driver's license or identification (ID) card issued by a state or jurisdiction of the United States provided the ID includes a photograph and date of birth;

2. ID card issued by federal, state, or local government agency or entity provided the ID includes a photograph and date of birth;

3. Certified copy of a birth certificate issued by a state, county, municipal authority or jurisdiction of the United States bearing an official seal;

4. United States citizen ID card provided that the ID includes the date of birth;

5. ID card used as a resident citizen in the United States provided the ID includes the date of birth.

(3) An applicant for licensure based upon certification by the National Commission for the Certification of Acupuncture and Oriental Medicine (NCCAOM) shall be currently certified as a

diplomate in acupuncture by NCCAOM. The applicant is responsible for authorizing NCCAOM to verify certification and notify the advisory committee.

(A) An applicant for licensure with a course of study from a school or program outside the United States may be considered in compliance with these rules if the applicant is certified as a diplomate in acupuncture by NCCAOM.

(4) A person applying for licensure based upon current licensure, certification, or registration in another state or jurisdiction of the United States shall comply with sections (1) and (2) of this rule and submit the following:

(A) Verification of licensure, certification, or registration as an acupuncturist to be provided directly to the advisory committee office from the state or jurisdiction of the United States regulatory agency that shall include:

1. Status of the applicant's license;

2. License original issue date and if there has been any lapse in the license;

3. License expiration date; and

4. Information regarding any complaints, investigations, or disciplinary action.

20 CSR 2015 − 2.020.   License Renewal, Restoration and Continuing Education

PURPOSE: This rule outlines the requirements for the renewal and restoration of licensure and the required continuing education to maintain a license.

(1) A license shall be renewed on or before the expiration date of the license by submitting the completed renewal form along with the renewal fee. Failure of a licensee to receive the notice and application to renew the license shall not excuse the licensee from the requirements of section 324.487, RSMo to renew that license.

(2) Receipt of the renewal form and fee postmarked after the expiration date of the license shall cause the license to become not current and a licensee who continues to practice without a valid license shall be deemed to be practicing in violation of sections 324.475 to 324.499, RSMo and subject to the penalties contained therein.

(3) Prior to the expiration date of the license and as a condition of the license renewal, a licensed acupuncturist shall complete thirty (30) hours of continuing education within the two (2) -year licensure period. Continuing education shall be related to the practice of acupuncture and include universal precautions/infection control and cardiopulmonary resuscitation (CPR) certification. For the first year of licensure continuing education hours shall not be required.

(4) A person may submit an application to restore a license that has been expired for not more than two (2) years after the expiration date. The application shall be submitted in compliance with 20 CSR 2015 − 2.010, accompanied by the required fee, and shall include documentation of completing continuing education pursuant to 20 CSR 2015 − 2.020 (3).

(5) Violation of any provision of this rule shall be grounds for discipline in accordance with section 324.496, RSMo.

Chapter 3. Standards of Practice, Code of Ethics, Professional Conduct

20 CSR 2015 – 3.010. Standards of Practice

PURPOSE: This rule establishes standards of practice for licensed acupuncturists.

(1) A licensed acupuncturist is strongly encouraged to maintain professional liability insurance coverage.

(2) Each acupuncturist shall —

(A) Practice within the scope of education and training as defined in section 324.475, RSMo;

(B) Disclose the acupuncturist's legal name on all documentation regarding the practice of acupuncture and advertisements;

(C) When offering gratuitous services or discounts in connection with acupuncture, the offer shall clearly and conspicuously state whether or not additional charges may be incurred by related services as well as the range of such additional charges;

(D) Post the license at the place of work or provide the patient documentation of licensure. Patient is defined as any individual for whom the practice of acupuncture, as defined in section 324.475 (1), RSMo is provided;

(E) Prior to performing initial acupuncture services, document in writing patient assessment information. Written patient assessment information shall include, but not be limited to the following:

1. Purpose of the visit;

2. Presence and location of pain and any preexisting conditions;

3. Allergies and current medication used and for what purpose;

4. If the patient is under the care of any health or mental health care professional;

5. Surgical history;

6. Signed consent for treatment and date signed;

7. Inform patient concerning fees and financial arrangements;

(F) Update patient records at each session. Such updated patient record information shall include, and not be limited to, the following:

1. Changes or additions regarding patient assessment;

2. Date and type of acupuncture service provided;

3. The signature of the acupuncturist and, when applicable, the name of the detox technician or acupuncture trainee that provided the acupuncture service;

(G) Provide current information concerning anticipated course of treatment;

(H) Safeguard the maintenance, storage, and disposal of records of patients so that unauthorized person(s) shall not have access to patient records; and

(I) Inform a patient regarding the limits of confidentiality when providing services.

(3) An acupuncturist shall not delegate acupuncture duties to a person that is not qualified or licensed to perform acupuncture.

(4) For the purpose of this rule, an acupuncturist shall maintain patient records for a minimum of five (5) years after the date of service is rendered, or not less than the time required by other applicable laws or regulations, if that time is longer than five (5) years.

(5) If a licensed acupuncturist discontinues practice in Missouri, the licensee shall notify the patient in writing at least thirty (30) days in advance of discontinuing practice that the patient records are available to either the patient or another licensed acupuncturist of the patient's choosing. The advisory committee may waive the thirty- (30-) day requirement if the licensee can make a showing of good cause for failing to comply.

(6) If services are to be provided by an acupuncturist trainee or detox technician the patient shall be advised in advance.

(7) Acupuncturists, auricular detox technicians, and acupuncturist trainees under the supervision of a licensed acupuncturist shall follow the standards for Clean Needle Technique (CNT) as published by the National Acupuncture Foundation in effect at the time the acupuncture service is performed, and follow universal precautions.

(A) For the purpose of this rule, "universal precautions" is an approach to infection control as defined by the Center for Disease Control (CDC). According to the concept of universal precautions, all human blood and certain body fluids are treated as if known to be infectious for Human Immunodeficiency Virus (HIV), Hepatitis B Virus (HBV), and other blood borne pathogens.

(8) All disposable needles shall be disposed of immediately after use and placed in a biohazard container pursuant to the U. S. Department of Labor, Occupational Safety and Health Administration (OSHA).

(9) When reusable needles are used, a basic, double sterilization procedure protocol shall be utilized. Specific procedures of the protocol are outlined in the Clean Needle Technique Manual published by the National Acupuncture Foundation.

(10) After each patient, an antibacterial product shall be used on all equipment that does not penetrate the skin, come into direct contact with needles, or is made of rubber or plastic.

20 CSR 2015 – 3.020.　Code of Ethics

PURPOSE: This rule establishes the code of ethics for applicants and acupuncturists.

(1) All applicants and licensees shall —

(A) Demonstrate behavior that reflects integrity, supports objectivity, and fosters trust in the profession of acupuncture;

(B) Conduct business and activities relating to acupuncture with honesty and integrity;

(C) Respect and protect the legal and personal rights of the patient/client, including the right to informed consent, refusal of treatment, and refrain from endangering patient health, safety, or welfare;

(D) Refuse to participate in illegal or unethical acts, or conceal illegal, unethical, or incompetent acts of others;

(E) When conducting research, comply with federal, state, and local laws or rules and applicable standards of ethical procedures regarding research with human subjects;

(F) Comply with all state and federal laws and regulations regarding the practice of acupuncture;

(G) Not allow the pursuit of financial gain or other personal benefit to interfere with the exercise of sound professional judgment and skills;

(H) Within the limits of the law, report to the advisory committee all knowledge pertaining to known or suspected violations of the laws and regulations governing the practice of acupuncture.

(2) An acupuncturist shall not —

(A) Encourage unnecessary or unjustified acupuncture services;

(B) Engage in any verbally or physically abusive behavior with a patient/client, detox technician or trainee;

(C) Exploit a patient/client, detox technician, or trainee for the purpose of financial gain. For the purpose of this rule exploitation is defined as any relationship between the acupuncturist, patient/client, technician, or trainee that may cause harm to the patient/client, technician, or trainee;

(D) Accept gifts or benefits intended to influence a referral, decision, or treatment that are primarily for personal gain;

(E) Engage in or exercise influence concerning sexual activity with a patient, trainee(s), or detox technician during an ongoing professional relationship with such person or within six (6) months after termination of such professional relationship:

Chapter 4. Supervision of Auricular Detox Technicians and Acupuncturist Trainees

20 CSR 2015 - 4.010.　Supervision of Auricular Detox Technicians

PURPOSE: This rule outlines the requirements for supervision of auricular detox technicians.

(1) An auricular detox technician (hereinafter technician) shall insert and remove acupuncture needles in the auricle of the ear only. The points where a technician shall insert needles are limited specifically to the points known as Shen Men, Lung, Liver, Kidney, and Sympathetic as described and located by the National Acupuncture Detox Association (NADA) or other national entity approved by the advisory committee.

(2) When providing supervision to a technician, a licensed acupuncturist shall have supervisory meetings with the technician a minimum of four (4) hours per month and be

available on-site, by telephone or pager, when the technician is providing services as defined in 20 CSR 2015 – 4.010 (1).

(A) A minimum of two (2) hours per month shall consist of face-to-face supervision, at no less than fifty (50) continuous minutes per supervisory meeting, and include observing the technician inserting and removing the acupuncture needles in the auricle of the ear.

(B) The remaining two (2) hours per month of supervisory meetings may be face-to-face or via electronic communication to include telephone contact, Internet such as email, video tape, or simultaneous visual and verbal interaction via the Internet.

(3) The licensed acupuncturist must exercise professional judgment when determining the number of technicians s/he can safely and effectively supervise to ensure that quality care is provided at all times.

(4) Any duties assigned to a technician must be determined and supervised by a licensed acupuncturist and not exceed the level of training, knowledge, skill, and competence of the detox technician being supervised. An acupuncturist may delegate to a technician only specific tasks that are not evaluative, assessment oriented, task selective, or recommending in nature.

(5) When providing supervision of a technician, a licensed acupuncturist is responsible for the oversight of the auricular detoxification procedures only. When referring to procedures provided by a technician, only the terms auricular detoxification or auricular detox shall be used.

(6) Duties or functions that a technician shall not perform include, and are not limited to:

(A) Interpretation of referrals or prescriptions for acupuncture services;

(B) Evaluative procedures;

(C) Development, planning, adjusting, or modification of acupuncture treatment procedures;

(D) Acting on behalf of the acupuncturist in any matter related to direct patient care that requires judgement or decision making; and

(E) Acupuncture performed independently or without supervision of a licensed acupuncturist.

20 CSR 2015 – 4.020. Supervision of Acupuncturist Trainees

PURPOSE: This rule outlines the requirements for supervision of acupuncturist trainees.

(1) An acupuncturist trainee (trainee) shall practice acupuncture on members of the public while under the direct supervision of a licensed acupuncturist. For the purpose of this rule direct supervision is the control, direction, instruction, and regulation of a student at all times.

(2) In order to qualify as a trainee, the individual shall be enrolled in a course of study authorized by the advisory committee and not receive compensation for any acupuncture provided by the trainee.

(3) Acupuncture programs certified by the Accreditation Commission for Acupuncture and Oriental Medicine (ACAOM) are considered acceptable programs for the training of acupuncture.

(4) Programs that are not certified by ACAOM shall consist of a curriculum that is at least three (3) academic years in length with a minimum of one hundred five (105) semester credits

or one thousand nine hundred five (1,905) hours of study. The curriculum shall be composed of at least:

(A) Forty-seven (47) semester credits [seven hundred five (705) clock hours] in Oriental medical theory, diagnosis and treatment techniques in acupuncture and related studies;

(B) Twenty-two (22) semester credits [six hundred sixty (660) clock hours] in clinical training; and

(C) Thirty (30) semester credits [four hundred fifty (450) clock hours] in biomedical clinical sciences; and

(D) Six (6) semester credits, [ninety (90) clock hours] in counseling, communication, ethics, and practice management.

(5) Any duties assigned to an acupuncturist trainee must be supervised by a licensed acupuncturist and not exceed the level of training, knowledge, skill, and competence of the individual being supervised. The licensed acupuncturist is responsible for the acts or actions performed by any acupuncturist trainee functioning in the acupuncture setting.

Michigan

Michigan Compiled Laws Annotated

333.16501. Definitions

(1) As used in this part:

(a) "Acupressure" means a form of manual therapy in which physical pressure is applied to various points on the body.

(b) "Acupuncture" means the insertion and manipulation of needles through the surface of the human body. Acupuncture includes, but is not limited to, laser acupuncture, electroacupuncture, pricking therapy, dry needling, and intramuscular stimulation.

(c) "Acupuncturist" means an individual who is licensed under this part to engage in the practice of acupuncture.

(d) "Cupping" means the placement of a specially designed cup on the body to create suction.

(e) "Dermal friction" means the use of repeated, closely timed, unidirectional press-stroking with a smooth-edged instrument over a lubricated area of the body.

(f) "Dietary counseling" means the process of advising a patient about healthy food choices and healthy eating habits in accordance with East Asian medical theory.

(g) "Dry needling" means a rehabilitative procedure using filiform needles to penetrate the skin or underlying tissues by targeting only myofascial trigger points and muscular and connective tissues to affect change in body structures and functions for the evaluation and management of neuromusculoskeletal pain and movement impairment. Dry needling does not include the stimulation of auricular points or other acupuncture points.

(h) "East Asian medicine techniques" includes, but is not limited to, acupuncture, manual therapy, moxibustion, heat therapy, dietary counseling, therapeutic exercise, acupressure, cupping, dermal friction, homeopathy, lifestyle coaching, and treatment with herbal medicines.

(i) "Heat therapy" means the use of heat in therapy, such as for pain relief and health.

(j) "Herbal medicine" means the internal and external use of a plant or a plant extract, a mineral, or an animal product, that is not a prescription drug as that term is defined in section 17708.[1]

(k) "Homeopathy" means the use of a highly diluted natural remedy from the plant, mineral, and animal domain.

(l) "Lifestyle coaching" means the process of advising a patient about healthy lifestyle choices and habits in accordance with East Asian medical theory.

(m) "Manual therapy" means the application of an accurately determined and specifically directed manual force to the body, excluding a high-velocity, low-amplitude thrust to the spine.

(n) "Moxibustion" means burning the dried plant *Artemisia vulgaris* on or very near the surface of the skin as a form of therapy.

(o) "Practice of acupuncture", subject to subsection (2), means the use of traditional and contemporary East Asian medical theory to assess and diagnose a patient, to develop a plan to treat the patient, and to treat the patient through East Asian medicine techniques.

(p) "Practice of chiropractic" means that term as defined in section 16401.[2]

(q) "Practice of massage therapy" means that term as defined in section 17951.[3]

(r) "Practice of medicine" means that term as defined in section 17001.[4]

(s) "Practice of osteopathic medicine and surgery" means that term as defined in section 17501.[5]

(t) "Practice of physical therapy" means that term as defined in section 17801.[6]

(u) "Registered acupuncturist" means an individual who is registered or otherwise authorized under this part before the effective date of the rules promulgated under section 16525[7] regarding licensure.

(v) "Systematic acupuncture education" means a course of education that covers the foundation of acupuncture science and theory, channel and point location, needling techniques, approaches to diagnosis and therapy, and patient management.

(w) "Therapeutic exercise" means a range of physical activities that help restore and build physical strength, endurance, flexibility, balance, and stability.

(2) For purposes of this part, practice of acupuncture does not include the practice of medicine, the practice of osteopathic medicine and surgery, the practice of physical therapy, the practice of occupational therapy, the practice of podiatric medicine and podiatric surgery, the practice of nursing, the practice of dentistry, the practice of massage therapy, or the practice of chiropractic.

(3) In addition to the definitions in this part, article 1[8] contains general definitions and principles of construction applicable to all articles in the code and part 161[9] contains definitions applicable to this part.

333.16511. Use of words, titles, and letters

(1) Except as otherwise provided in this part, beginning on the effective date of rules promulgated under section 16525[1] regarding licensure, an individual shall not use the words, titles, or letters "acupuncturist", "certified acupuncturist", "registered acupuncturist", "licensed acupuncturist", "L. Ac.", or a similar word or initial that indicates that the individual is an acupuncturist, unless he or she is authorized under this part to use the terms and in a way prescribed in this part. However, for a period not to exceed 36 months from the effective date of the rules promulgated under section 16525 regarding licensure, a registered acupuncturist may, without a license under this part, continue to use the titles "acupuncturist", "registered acupuncturist", or "certified acupuncturist" and engage in the practice of acupuncture.

(2) Until the effective date of the rules promulgated under section 16525 regarding licensure, an individual shall not use the words, titles, or letters "acupuncturist", "certified acupuncturist", or "registered acupuncturist", or a combination of the words, titles, or letters, with or without qualifying words or phrases, unless he or she is registered under this part.

(3) Until the effective date of the rules promulgated under section 16525 regarding licensure, neither of the following is subject to this part:

(a) A physician who is licensed under part 170[2] or part 175.[3]

(b) An individual who is certified by the National Acupuncture Detoxification Association.

333.16513. Licensure requirement; applicability

(1) Beginning on the effective date of rules promulgated under section 16525[1] regarding licensure, an individual shall not engage in the practice of acupuncture unless he or she is licensed under this part or is otherwise authorized under this article.

(2) In addition to the exemptions from licensure under section 16171,[2] beginning on the effective date of the rules promulgated under section 16525 regarding licensure, this part does not apply to any of the following:

(a) Except as otherwise provided in subdivision (e), an individual licensed, registered, or otherwise authorized under any other part or act who is performing activities that are considered to be within the practice of acupuncture if those activities are within the individual's scope of practice and the individual does not use the words, titles, or letters protected under section 16511.[3]

(b) A physician who is licensed under part 170[4] or part 175[5] if the physician has completed a total of not less than 300 hours of systematic acupuncture education that include not less than 100 hours of live lectures, demonstrations, and supervised clinical training specific to acupuncture.

(c) An individual who meets all of the following requirements:

(i) He or she meets the requirements for a certificate of training as an acupuncture detoxification specialist issued by the National Acupuncture Detoxification Association or an organization that the board determines is a successor organization.

(ii) He or she only uses the auricular protocol for substance use disorder prevention and treatment developed by the National Acupuncture Detoxification Association or an organization that the board determines is a successor organization.

(*iii*) When using the protocol described in subparagraph (*ii*), he or she is under the supervision of an acupuncturist or a physician licensed under part 170 or part 175.

(*iv*) He or she does not use the words, titles, or letters protected under section 16511.

(d) An individual performing acupressure, cupping, dermal friction, dietary counseling, heat therapy, herbal medicine, homeopathy, lifestyle coaching, manual therapy, or therapeutic exercise, while engaged in the practice of a profession with established standards and ethics and as long as those services are not designated as or implied to be the practice of acupuncture and the individual does not use the titles, words, or letters protected under section 16511.

(e) Dry needling by an individual licensed, registered, or otherwise authorized under any other part if dry needling is within the individual's scope of practice.

333.16515. Issuance of licenses and limited licenses; qualifications

(1) Except as otherwise provided in subsections (2) and (3), the department shall issue a license to an applicant who meets the requirements of section 16174[1] and the requirements for licensure established in rules promulgated under section 16525.[2]

(2) On or before the expiration of 36 months after the effective date of the rules promulgated under section 16525 regarding licensure, the department shall issue a license to an applicant who meets the requirements of section 16174 and 1 of the following:

(a) He or she is a registered acupuncturist.

(b) He or she has the education, training, and experience appropriate to the practice of acupuncture as established in rules promulgated under section 16525 regarding licensure. In determining whether an applicant has met the requirements for licensure under this subdivision, the department, in consultation with the board, shall promulgate rules establishing criteria for considering patient records, billing records, education records, training records, or other evidence of the applicant's education, training, and experience that is submitted to the department. An applicant shall ensure that any document that is submitted to the department under this subdivision ensures the confidentiality of a patient's identity.

(3) On or before the expiration of 36 months after the effective date of the rules promulgated under section 16525 regarding licensure, the department shall issue a limited license to an applicant who meets the requirements of section 16174, and who, at the time of the application, meets all of the following requirements:

(a) The applicant has been performing acupuncture under the supervision of a physician licensed under part 170[3] or part 175[4] for at least 2 years as of the effective date of the amendatory act that added this section. The applicant shall include the name of the physician under which he or she is engaging in the practice of acupuncture on the application for limited licensure.

(b) The applicant holds a license to engage in another health profession.

(4) An individual who is granted a limited license under subsection (3) shall comply with all of the following:

(a) He or she shall only engage in the practice of acupuncture while he or she is under the supervision of the physician named in the application for limited licensure and shall immediately notify the department if the physician named in the application is no longer willing or able to supervise the individual.

(b) He or she shall not collect payment from an insurer for performing a service that is within the practice of acupuncture. As used in this subdivision, "insurer" means that term as defined in section 106 of the insurance code of 1956, 1956 PA 218, MCL 500.106.

333.16517.   Renewal of license or limited license; promulgation of rules; continuing education requirements

(1) Notwithstanding the requirements of part 161, [1] the department, in consultation with the board, shall promulgate rules requiring a licensee seeking renewal of a license to furnish the department with satisfactory evidence that during the license cycle immediately preceding the application for renewal the licensee has attended continuing education courses or programs approved by the board in subjects related to the practice of acupuncture and designed to further educate licensees. An individual is considered to have completed the continuing education requirements described in this subsection if the department determines that the individual has met the continuing education standards of the National Certification Commission for Acupuncture and Oriental Medicine or equivalent standards as determined by the board.

(2) As required under section 16204, [2] the department, in consultation with the board, shall promulgate rules requiring each applicant for license renewal to complete as part of the educational courses or programs required under subsection (1) an appropriate number of hours or courses in pain and symptom management.

(3) In addition to the continuing education requirements of this section, the department shall require an applicant seeking renewal of a limited license granted under section 16515 (3) [3] to hold a license to engage in another health profession at the time of his or her application for renewal as a condition of renewal of his or her limited license.

333.16521.   Board of acupuncture; creation; membership

(1) The Michigan board of acupuncture is created in the department and consists of the following 13 voting members, each of whom must meet the requirements of part 161: [1]

(a) Seven acupuncturists or, until 36 months after the effective date of the rules promulgated under section 16525, [2] 7 registered acupuncturists. The members appointed under this subdivision must meet the requirements of section 16135. [3]

(b) Three physicians licensed under part 170[4] or 175, [5] at least 1 of whom has met the requirement in section 16513 (2) (b). [6]

(c) Three public members.

(2) The terms of office of individual members of the board created under this part, except those appointed to fill vacancies, expire on June 30 of the year in which the term expires pursuant to section 16122.[7]

333.16525.   Promulgation of rules; standards for licensure

(1) By March 4, 2021, the department, in consultation with the board, shall promulgate rules that establish the minimum standards for licensure as an acupuncturist and implement the licensure program for the practice of acupuncture. In promulgating rules for purposes of section 16515 (1), [1] the department, in consultation with the board, may adopt by reference the professional standards issued by a certified program that is recognized by the National Commission for Certifying Agencies. In promulgating rules for purposes of section 16515 (2) (b), the department, in consultation with the board, shall consider whether an applicant has completed systematic acupuncture education that includes live lectures, demonstrations, and supervised clinical training specific to acupuncture.

(2) The rules in effect on March 3, 2020 regarding the registration of acupuncturists remain in effect until the effective date of the rules promulgated under subsection (1).

333.16529.   Third party reimbursement or worker's compensation benefits

This part does not require new or additional third party reimbursement or mandated worker's compensation benefits for services by an individual registered or licensed as an acupuncturist under this part.

Michigan Administrative Code

Part 1. General Rules

R 338.13001.   Definitions.

Rule 1. (1) As used in these rules:

(a) "Board" means the Michigan board of acupuncture created under section 16521 of the public health code, MCL 333.16521.

(b) "Code" means the public health code 1978 PA 368, MCL 333.1101 to 333.25211.

(c) "Department" means the department of licensing and regulatory affairs.

(2) Terms defined in the code have the same meanings when used in these rules.

R 338.13002.   Training standards for identifying victims of human trafficking; requirements.

Rule 2. (1) Pursuant to section 16148 of the code, MCL 333.16148, an individual seeking licensure or registration or who is licensed or registered shall complete training in identifying victims of human trafficking that meets the following standards:

(a) Training content must cover all of the following:

(i) Understanding the types and venues of human trafficking in the United States.

(ii) Identifying victims of human trafficking in health care settings.

(iii) Identifying the warning signs of human trafficking in health care settings for adults and minors.

(iv) Resources for reporting the suspected victims of human trafficking.

(b) Acceptable providers or methods of training include any of the following:

(i) Training offered by a nationally-recognized or state-recognized health-related organization.

(ii) Training offered by, or in conjunction with, a state or federal agency.

(iii) Training obtained in an educational program that has been approved by the board for initial licensure or registration, or by a college or university.

(iv) Reading an article related to the identification of victims of human trafficking that meets the requirements of subdivision (a) of this subrule and is published in a peer review journal, health care journal, or professional or scientific journal.

(c) Acceptable modalities of training may include any of the following:

(i) Teleconference or webinar.

(ii) Online presentation.

(iii) Live presentation.

(iv) Printed or electronic media.

(2) The department may select and audit a sample of individuals and request documentation of proof of completion of training. If audited by the department, an individual shall provide an acceptable proof of completion of training, including either of the following:

(a) Proof of completion certificate issued by the training provider that includes the date, provider name, name of training, and individual's name.

(b) A self-certification statement by an individual. The certification statement must include the individual's name and either of the following:

(i) For training completed pursuant to subrule (1) (b) (i) to (iii) of this rule, the date, training provider name, and name of training.

(ii) For training completed pursuant to subrule (1) (b) (iv) of this rule, the title of article, author, publication name of peer review journal, health care journal, or professional or scientific journal, and date, volume, and issue of publication, as applicable.

(3) Pursuant to section 16148 of the code, MCL 333.16148, the requirements specified in subrule (1) of this rule apply to an applicant for license renewal beginning July 2, 2018 and to an applicant for initial licensure beginning April 22, 2021.

R 338.13003. Telehealth.

Rule 3. (1) An acupuncturist shall obtain consent before providing a telehealth service pursuant to section 16284 of the code, MCL 333.16284.

(2) An acupuncturist providing a telehealth service shall do both of the following:

(a) Act within the scope of his or her practice.

(b) Exercise the same standard of care applicable to a traditional, in-person health care service.

R 338.13004. Adoption of standards.

Rule 4. The National Certification Commission for Acupuncture and Oriental Medicine's (NCCAOM) national standards of competence in acupuncture and Oriental medicine as set forth in the document titled, "NCCAOM Certification Handbook," effective January 1, 2019, is approved by the board and adopted by reference in these rules. The document is available for inspection and distribution at the cost of 10 cents per page from the Department of Licensing and Regulatory Affairs, Bureau of Professional Licensing at 611 W. Ottawa St. P. O. Box 30670, Lansing, Michigan 48909 and at no cost from NCCAOM at www.nccaom.org or National Certification Commission for Acupuncture and Oriental Medicine, 611 W. Ottawa St. P. O. Box 30670, Lansing, Michigan 48909.

Part 2. Licensure

R 338.13005. Licensure of Michigan-registered acupuncturist; requirements.

Rule 5. Beginning on the date of promulgation of these rules, and for a period of 36 months following promulgation of these rules, the department shall issue a license to an applicant who, in addition to meeting all the requirements of the code, satisfies both of the following:

(a) Submits a completed application on a form provided by the department, together with the requisite fee.

(b) Is currently registered as an acupuncturist in this state.

R 338.13006. Licensure of non-NCCAOM certified acupuncturist; requirements.

Rule 6. (1) Beginning on the date of promulgation of these rules, and for a period of 36 months following promulgation of these rules, the department shall issue a license to an applicant who, in addition to meeting all the requirements of the code, submits a completed application on a form provided by the department, together with the requisite fee.

(2) The applicant shall demonstrate to the board that he or she has the education, training, and experience required for licensure pursuant to sections 16515 and 16525 of the code, MCL 333.16515 and 333.16525. The applicant shall satisfy all of the following:

(a) The applicant shall establish that he or she has completed a minimum of 1,245 hours of systematic acupuncture education, as that term is defined in section 16501 (1) (v) of the code, MCL 333.16501, by submitting his or her education records, training records, or other verifiable evidence of the applicant's education and training that included live lectures, demonstrations, and supervised clinical training specific to acupuncture.

(b) The applicant shall establish that he or she is certified in clean needle technique by the Council of Colleges of Acupuncture and Oriental Medicine.

(c) The applicant shall establish that he or she has provided acupuncture services to an average of 50 or more patients per year during the 4 years preceding the date of application for licensure by submitting his or her patient records, billing records, or both. The applicant shall ensure that patient confidentiality is protected on every document submitted.

(3) If documentation submitted pursuant to this rule is in a language other than English, an original, official translation must also be submitted.

R 338.13007. Licensure of NCCAOM-certified applicant; requirements.

Rule 7. Beginning on the date of promulgation of these rules, the department shall issue a license to an applicant who, in addition to meeting all the requirements of the code, satisfies both of the following:

(a) Submits a completed application on a form provided by the department, together with the requisite fee.

(b) Submits proof acceptable to the department that he or she is currently certified by NCCAOM as a Diplomate of Acupuncture or Diplomate of Oriental Medicine.

R 338.13008. Limited License; requirements; restrictions.

Rule 8. (1) Beginning on the date of promulgation of these rules, and for a period of 36 months following the promulgation of these rules, the department shall issue a limited license to an applicant who, in addition to meeting the requirements of the code, meets all of the following:

(a) The applicant provides documentation that he or she has been performing acupuncture under the supervision of a physician licensed under part 170 of the code, MCL 333.17001 to 333.17097, or part 175 of the code, MCL 333.17501 to 333.17556, for a minimum of 2 years before March 4, 2020.

(b) The applicant submits a form provided by the department that contains the name and signature of the supervising physician acknowledging assumption of the supervisory responsibilities under section 16109 (2) of the code, MCL 333.16109.

(c) The applicant holds a license to engage in another health profession as defined in section 16105 (2) of the code, MCL 333.16105, at the time of his or her application.

(2) A limited licensee shall comply with all of the following:

(a) Engage in the practice of acupuncture only under the supervision of the physician identified pursuant to subrule (1) (b) of this rule.

(b) Notify the department if the physician identified pursuant to subrule (1) (b) of this rule is no longer willing or able to supervise the limited licensee.

(*i*) If the supervising physician is no longer willing or able to supervise the limited licensee, the limited licensee shall not provide acupuncture services until a new supervising physician licensed under part 170 or part 175 of the code is secured and the requirements of subrule (1) (b) of this rule have been met by the new supervising physician and the form, provided by the department, that contains the name and signature of the supervising physician acknowledging assumption of the supervisory responsibilities under section 16109 (2) of the code, MCL 333.16109, has been submitted to the department.

(*ii*) A limited license cannot be renewed if a supervising physician licensed under part 170 or part 175 of the code is not identified.

(c) A limited licensee shall not collect payment from an insurer for performing a service that is within the practice of acupuncture.

R 338.13010.　Licensure by endorsement; requirements.

Rule 10. (1) An applicant for an acupuncturist license by endorsement, in addition to meeting all the requirements of the code, shall submit a completed application on a form provided by the department, together with the requisite fee and satisfy both of the following:

(a) Demonstrate to the satisfaction of the department that he or she holds an active license or registration in good standing from another state on the date of filing an application for licensure by endorsement.

(b) Submit proof acceptable to the department that he or she is currently certified by NCCAOM as a Diplomate of Acupuncture or Diplomate of Oriental Medicine.

(2) An applicant's license or registration in good standing shall be verified by the licensing or registering agency of each state in which the applicant holds or ever held a license or registration as an acupuncturist. If applicable, verification must include the record of any disciplinary action taken or pending against the applicant.

R 338.13015.　Applicant with nonaccredited training; requirements — Rescinded.

R 338.13020.　Renewal of acupuncturist registration; requirements — Rescinded.

R 338.13025.　Application for relicensure; requirements.

Rule 25. An applicant whose license has lapsed may be relicensed upon submission of the appropriate documentation as noted in the table below:

(1) For an acupuncturist who has let his or her Michigan license lapse and is currently licensed in another state or Canada		Lapsed 0 – 3 years	Lapsed more than 3 years
(a)	Submits a completed application on a form provided by the department, together with the required fee	√	√
(b)	Establishes that he or she is of good moral character as defined under sections 1 to 7 of 1974 PA 381, MCL 338.41 to 338.47	√	√
(c)	Submits fingerprints as required under section 16174 (3) of the code, MCL 333.16174 (3)		√
(d)	Submits proof of having completed 30 hours of continuing education in compliance with R 338.13026 and R 338.13028 within the 2-year period immediately preceding the application for relicensure	√	√

		Lapsed 0 – 3 years	Lapsed more than 3 years
(e)	An applicant's license or registration in good standing must be verified by the licensing or registering agency of each state in which the applicant holds or ever held a license or registration as an acupuncturist. If applicable, verification must include the record of any disciplinary action taken or pending against the applicant	√	√
(2)	For an acupuncturist who has let his or her Michigan license lapse and is not currently licensed in another state or Canada	Lapsed 0 – 3 years	Lapsed more than 3 years
(a)	Submits a completed application on a form provided by the department, together with the required fee	√	√
(b)	Establishes that he or she is of good moral character as defined under sections 1 to 7 of 1974 PA 381, MCL 338.41 to 338.47	√	√
(c)	Submits fingerprints as required under section 16174 (3) of the code, MCL 333.16174 (3)		√
(d)	Submits proof of having completed 30 hours of continuing education in compliance with R 338.13026 and R 338.13028 within the 2-year period immediately preceding the application for relicensure	√	√
(e)	Possesses a current and valid NCCAOM certification as a Diplomate of Acupuncture or Diplomate of Oriental Medicine		√
(f)	An applicant's license or registration in good standing must be verified by the licensing or registering agency of each state in which the applicant holds or ever held a license or registration as an acupuncturist. If applicable, verification must include the record of any disciplinary action taken or pending against the applicant	√	√

Part 3. License Renewal, Limited License Renewal, and Continuing Education

R 338.13026.　Renewal of acupuncturist license; renewal of limited license; requirements; limitations; waiver request.

Rule 26. (1) Pursuant to section 16517 of the code, MCL 333.16517, an applicant for renewal of a license or limited license, who has been licensed for the 2-year period immediately preceding the expiration date of the license, shall accumulate 30 hours of continuing education related to the practice of acupuncture and approved by the board, pursuant to these rules, during the 2 years before the expiration date of the license.

(2) An applicant for renewal of a license or a limited license shall accumulate at least 5 hours of the required hours of continuing education in pain and symptom management related to the practice of acupuncture during each license cycle pursuant to sections 16204 (2) and 16517 (2) of the code, MCL 333.16204 and 333.16517.

(3) An applicant for renewal of a limited license, in addition to meeting the requirements of subrules (1) and (2) of this rule, shall meet all of the following:

(a) Pursuant to section 16517 (3) of the code, MCL 333.16517, the applicant shall hold an active license to engage in another health profession, as defined in section 16105 of the code, MCL 333.16105, at the time of his or her application, and as a condition of renewal of his or her limited license.

(b) The applicant shall accumulate the continuing education credits required in subrules (1) and (2) of this rule in addition to any continuing education credits accumulated for the purpose of renewing his or her other health professional license.

(c) The applicant shall submit a form, provided by the department, that contains the name and signature of his or her supervising physician acknowledging that the physician provided the supervisory responsibilities required under section 16109 (2) of the code, MCL 333.16109, during the previous license cycle and agreeing to provide those supervisory responsibilities during the next license cycle.

(4) Submission of an application for renewal constitutes the applicant's certification of compliance with this rule. An applicant shall retain documentation of satisfying the requirements of this rule for a period of 4 years from the date of applying for license renewal. The board may require an applicant to submit evidence to demonstrate compliance with this rule. Failure to comply with this rule is a violation of section 16221 (h) of the code, MCL 333.16221.

(5) The department must receive a request for a waiver under section 16205 of the code, MCL 333.16205, before the expiration date of the license.

(6) The continuing education credits earned in 1 license cycle may not be carried forward to the next license cycle.

(7) The applicant may not earn continuing education credits for completing the same activity twice within the same license cycle.

R 338.13028. Acceptable continuing education, requirements.

Rule 28. (1) The board approves for continuing education a course or activity approved by the NCCAOM as a professional development activity (PDA). One PDA credit equals 1 hour of continuing education credit that can be accumulated to satisfy the requirements of R 338.13026.

(2) Pursuant to section 16517 (1) of the code, MCL 333.16517, an individual who has met the continuing education standards of the NCCAOM is considered to have met the continuing education requirements for license renewal.

(3) If an applicant does not meet the requirements of subrule (2) of this rule, he or she

shall accumulate not less than 30 continuing education credits by participating in a course or activity approved by the NCCAOM.

R 338.13030.   Educational program standards; adoption by reference — Rescinded.

R 338.13035.   Delegation; supervision.

Rule 35. An acupuncturist shall practice under the delegation of an allopathic physician or osteopathic physician and surgeon in accordance with sections 16104, 16109, and 16215 (3) of the code, MCL 333.16104, 333.16109, and 333.16215 (3).

R 338.13040.   Patient records; retention; disposition; confidentiality — Rescinded.

R 338.13045.   Prohibited conduct — Rescinded.

Minnesota

Minnesota Statutes Annotated

147B.01. Definitions

1. Applicability. The definitions in this section apply to this chapter.

2. Acupressure. "Acupressure" means the application of pressure to acupuncture points.

3. Acupuncture practice. "Acupuncture practice" means a comprehensive system of health care using Oriental medical theory and its unique methods of diagnosis and treatment. Its treatment techniques include the insertion of acupuncture needles through the skin and the use of other biophysical methods of acupuncture point stimulation, including the use of heat, Oriental massage techniques, electrical stimulation, herbal supplemental therapies, dietary guidelines, breathing techniques, and exercise based on Oriental medical principles.

4. Acupuncture needle. "Acupuncture needle" means a needle designed exclusively for acupuncture purposes. It has a solid core, with a tapered point, and is 0.12 mm to 0.45 mm in thickness. It is constructed of stainless steel, gold, silver, or other board-approved materials as long as the materials can be sterilized according to recommendations of the National Centers for Disease Control and Prevention.

5. Acupuncture points. "Acupuncture points" means specific anatomically described locations as defined by the recognized acupuncture reference texts. These texts are listed in the study guide to the examination for the NCCAOM certification exam.

6. Acupuncture practitioner. "Acupuncture practitioner" means a person licensed to practice acupuncture under this chapter.

7. Board. "Board" means the Board of Medical Practice or its designee.

8. Repealed by Laws 2002, c. 375, art. 3, § 11.

9. Breathing techniques. "Breathing techniques" means Oriental breathing exercises taught to a patient as part of a treatment plan.

10. Cupping. "Cupping" means a therapy in which a jar-shaped instrument is attached to

the skin and negative pressure is created by using suction.

11. **Dermal friction.** "Dermal friction" means rubbing on the surface of the skin, using topical ointments with a smooth-surfaced instrument without a cutting edge that can be sterilized or, if disposable, a onetime only use product.

12. **Diplomate in acupuncture.** "Diplomate in acupuncture" means a person who is certified by the NCCAOM as having met the standards of competence established by the NCCAOM, who subscribes to the NCCAOM code of ethics, and who has a current and active NCCAOM certificate. Current and active NCCAOM certification indicates successful completion of continued professional development and previous satisfaction of NCCAOM requirements.

13. **Electrical stimulation.** "Electrical stimulation" means a method of stimulating acupuncture points by an electrical current of 0.001 to 100 milliamps, or other current as approved by the board. Electrical stimulation may be used by attachment of a device to an acupuncture needle or may be used transcutaneously without penetrating the skin.

14. **Herbal therapies.** "Herbal therapies" are the use of herbs and patent herbal remedies as supplements as part of the treatment plan of the patient.

15. Repealed by Laws 2002, c. 375, art. 3, § 11.

16. **NCCAOM.** "NCCAOM" means the National Certification Commission for Acupuncture and Oriental Medicine, a not-for-profit corporation organized under section 501 (c) (4) of the Internal Revenue Code.

16a. **NCCAOM certification.** "NCCAOM certification" means a certification granted by the NCCAOM to a person who has met the standards of competence established for either NCCAOM certification in acupuncture or NCCAOM certification in Oriental medicine.

17. **Needle sickness.** "Needle sickness" is a temporary state of nausea and dizziness that is a potential side effect to needle insertion and from which full recovery occurs when the needles are removed.

18. **Oriental medicine.** "Oriental medicine" means a system of healing arts that perceives the circulation and balance of energy in the body as being fundamental to the well-being of the individual. It implements the theory through specialized methods of analyzing the energy status of the body and treating the body with acupuncture and other related modalities for the purpose of strengthening the body, improving energy balance, maintaining or restoring health, improving physiological function, and reducing pain.

147B.02. Licensure

1. **Licensure required.** Except as provided under subdivision 4, it is unlawful for any person to engage in the practice of acupuncture without a valid license after June 30, 1997. Each licensed acupuncture practitioner shall conspicuously display the license in the place of practice.

2. **Designation.** A person licensed under this chapter shall use the title of licensed acupuncturist or L. Ac. following the person's name in all forms of advertising, professional

literature, and billings. A person may not, in the conduct of an occupation or profession pertaining to the practice of acupuncture or in connection with the person's name, use the words or letters licensed acupuncturist, Minnesota licensed acupuncturist, or any other words, letters, abbreviations, or insignia indicating or implying that a person is an acupuncturist without a license issued under this section. A student attending an acupuncture training program must be identified as a student acupuncturist.

3. Penalty. A person who violates this section is guilty of a misdemeanor and subject to discipline under section 147.091.

4. Exceptions. (a) The following persons may practice acupuncture within the scope of their practice without an acupuncture license:

(1) a physician licensed under chapter 147;

(2) an osteopathic physician licensed under chapter 147;

(3) a chiropractor licensed under chapter 148;

(4) a person who is studying in a formal course of study or tutorial intern program approved by the acupuncture advisory council established in section 147B.05 so long as the person's acupuncture practice is supervised by a licensed acupuncturist or a person who is exempt under clause (5);

(5) a visiting acupuncturist practicing acupuncture within an instructional setting for the sole purpose of teaching at a school registered with the Minnesota Office of Higher Education, who may practice without a license for a period of one year, with two one-year extensions permitted; and

(6) a visiting acupuncturist who is in the state for the sole purpose of providing a tutorial or workshop not to exceed 30 days in one calendar year.

(b) This chapter does not prohibit a person who does not have an acupuncturist license from practicing specific noninvasive techniques, such as acupressure, that are within the scope of practice as set forth in section 147B.06, subdivision 4.

5. Repealed by Laws 2004, c. 279, art. 3, § 3.

6. License by reciprocity. The board shall issue an acupuncture license to a person who holds a current license or certificate as an acupuncturist from another jurisdiction if the board determines that the standards for certification or licensure in the other jurisdiction meet or exceed the requirements for licensure in Minnesota and a letter is received from that jurisdiction that the acupuncturist is in good standing in that jurisdiction.

7. Licensure requirements.

(a) After June 30, 1997, an applicant for licensure must:

(1) submit a completed application for licensure on forms provided by the board, which must include the applicant's name and address of record, which shall be public;

(2) unless licensed under subdivision 5 or 6, submit a notarized copy of a current NCCAOM

certification;

(3) sign a statement that the information in the application is true and correct to the best of the applicant's knowledge and belief;

(4) submit with the application all fees required; and

(5) sign a waiver authorizing the board to obtain access to the applicant's records in this state or any state in which the applicant has engaged in the practice of acupuncture.

(b) The board may ask the applicant to provide any additional information necessary to ensure that the applicant is able to practice with reasonable skill and safety to the public.

(c) The board may investigate information provided by an applicant to whether the information is accurate and complete. The board shall notify an applicant of action taken on the application and the reasons for denying licensure if licensure is denied.

8. Licensure expiration. Licenses issued under this section expire annually.

9. Renewal. (a) To renew a license an applicant must:

(1) annually, or as determined by the board, complete a renewal application on a form provided by the board;

(2) submit the renewal fee;

(3) provide documentation of current and active NCCAOM certification; or

(4) if licensed under subdivision 5 or 6, meet the same NCCAOM professional development activity requirements as those licensed under subdivision 7.

(b) An applicant shall submit any additional information requested by the board to clarify information presented in the renewal application. The information must be submitted within 30 days after the board's request, or the renewal request is nullified.

(c) An applicant must maintain a correct mailing address with the board for receiving board communications, notices, and license renewal documents. Placing the license renewal application in first-class United States mail, addressed to the applicant at the applicant's last known address with postage prepaid, constitutes valid service. Failure to receive the renewal documents does not relieve an applicant of the obligation to comply with this section.

(d) The name of an applicant who does not return a complete license renewal application, annual license fee, or late application fee, as applicable, within the time period required by this section shall be removed from the list of individuals authorized to practice during the current renewal period. If the applicant's license is reinstated, the applicant's name shall be placed on the list of individuals authorized to practice.

10. Licensure renewal notice. At least 30 days before the license renewal date, the board shall send out a renewal notice to the last known address of the licensee. The notice must include a renewal application and a notice of fees required for renewal. If the licensee does not receive a renewal notice, the licensee must still meet the requirements for registration renewal under this section.

11. Renewal deadline. The renewal application and fee must be postmarked on or before June 30 of the year of renewal or as determined by the board.

12. Inactive status.

（a）A license may be placed in inactive status upon application to the board and upon payment of an inactive status fee. The board may not renew or restore a license that has lapsed and has not been renewed within two annual license renewal cycles.

（b）An inactive license may be reactivated by the license holder upon application to the board. A licensee whose license is canceled for nonrenewal must obtain a new license by applying for licensure and fulfilling all the requirements then in existence for the initial license to practice acupuncture in the state of Minnesota. The application must include：

（1）evidence of current and active NCCAOM certification；

（2）evidence of the certificate holder's payment of an inactive status fee；

（3）an annual fee；and

（4）all back fees since previous renewal.

（c）A person licensed under subdivision 5 who has allowed the license to reach inactive status must become NCCAOM certified.

12a. Licensure following lapse of licensed status；transition.（a）A licensee whose license has lapsed under subdivision 4 before January 1，2020，and who seeks to regain licensed status after January 1，2020，shall be treated as a first-time licensee only for purposes of establishing a license renewal schedule，and shall not be subject to the license cycle conversion provisions in section 147B.09.

（b）This subdivision expires July 1，2022.

13. Temporary permit. The board may issue a temporary permit to practice acupuncture to an applicant eligible for licensure under this section only if the application for licensure is complete，all applicable requirements in this section have been met，and a nonrefundable fee set by the board has been paid. The permit remains valid only until the meeting of the board at which a decision is made on the acupuncturist's application for licensure.

147B.03.　NCCAOM professional development activity requirements

1. NCCAOM requirements. Unless a person is licensed under section 147B.02，subdivision 6，each licensee is required to meet the NCCAOM professional development activity requirements to maintain NCCAOM certification. These requirements may be met through a board approved continuing education program.

2. Board approval. The board shall approve a continuing education program if the program meets the following requirements：

（1）it directly relates to the practice of acupuncture；

（2）each member of the faculty shows expertise in the subject matter by holding a degree or certificate from an educational institution，has verifiable experience in traditional Oriental medicine, or has special training in the subject area;

(3) the program lasts at least one contact hour;

(4) there are specific written objectives describing the goals of the program for the participants; and

(5) the program sponsor maintains attendance records for four years.

3. Continuing education topics.

(a) Continuing education program topics may include, but are not limited to, Oriental medical theory and techniques including Oriental massage; Oriental nutrition; Oriental herbology and diet therapy; Oriental exercise; western sciences such as anatomy, physiology, biochemistry, microbiology, psychology, nutrition, history of medicine; and medical terminology or coding.

(b) Practice management courses are excluded under this section.

4. Verification. The board shall periodically select a random sample of acupuncturists and require the acupuncturist to show evidence of having completed the NCCAOM professional development activities requirements. Either the acupuncturist, the state, or the national organization that maintains continuing education records may provide the board documentation of the continuing education program.

147B.04.　Board action on applications

1. Verification of application information. The board or Acupuncture Advisory Council established under section 147B.05, with the approval of the board, may verify information provided by an application for licensure under section 147B.02 to determine if the information is accurate and complete.

2. Notification of board action. Within 120 days of receipt of the application, the board shall notify each applicant in writing of the action taken on the application.

3. Request for hearing by applicant denied. An applicant denied licensure must be notified of the determination, and the grounds for it, and may request a hearing on the determination by filing a written statement of issues with the board within 20 days after receipt of the notice from the board. After the hearing, the board shall notify the applicant in writing of its decision.

147B.05.　Acupuncture Advisory Council

1. Creation. The advisory council to the Board of Medical Practice for acupuncture consists of seven members appointed by the board to three-year terms. Four members must be licensed acupuncture practitioners, one member must be a licensed physician or osteopathic physician who also practices acupuncture, one member must be a licensed chiropractor who is NCCAOM certified, and one member must be a member of the public who has received acupuncture treatment as a primary therapy from a NCCAOM certified acupuncturist.

2. Administration; compensation; removal; quorum. The advisory council is governed by section 15.059.

3. Duties. The advisory council shall:

(1) advise the board on issuance, denial, renewal, suspension, revocation, conditioning, or restricting of licenses to practice acupuncture;

(2) advise the board on issues related to receiving, investigating, conducting hearings, and imposing disciplinary action in relation to complaints against acupuncture practitioners;

(3) maintain a register of acupuncture practitioners licensed under section 147B.02;

(4) maintain a record of all advisory council actions;

(5) prescribe registration application forms, license forms, protocol forms, and other necessary forms;

(6) review the patient visit records submitted by applicants during the transition period;

(7) advise the board regarding standards for acupuncturists;

(8) distribute information regarding acupuncture practice standards;

(9) review complaints;

(10) advise the board regarding continuing education programs;

(11) review the investigation of reports of complaints and recommend to the board whether disciplinary action should be taken; and

(12) perform other duties authorized by advisory councils under chapter 214, as directed by the board.

147B.06. Professional conduct

1. Practice standards.

(a) Before treatment of a patient, an acupuncture practitioner shall ask whether the patient has been examined by a licensed physician or other professional, as defined by section 145.61, subdivision 2, with regard to the patient's illness or injury, and shall review the diagnosis as reported.

(b) The practitioner shall obtain informed consent from the patient, after advising the patient of the following information which must be supplied to the patient in writing before or at the time of the initial visit:

(1) the practitioner's qualifications including:

(i) education;

(ii) license information; and

(iii) outline of the scope of practice of acupuncturists in Minnesota; and

(2) side effects which may include the following:

(i) some pain in the treatment area;

(ii) minor bruising;

(iii) infection;

(iv) needle sickness; or

(v) broken needles.

(c) The practitioner shall obtain acknowledgment by the patient in writing that the patient has been advised to consult with the patient's primary care physician about the acupuncture treatment if the patient circumstances warrant or the patient chooses to do so.

(d) The practitioner shall inquire whether the patient has a pacemaker or bleeding disorder.

2. Sterilized equipment. An acupuncture practitioner shall use sterilized equipment that has been sterilized under standards of the National Centers for Disease Control and Prevention.

3. State and municipal public health regulations. An acupuncture practitioner shall comply with all applicable state and municipal requirements regarding public health.

4. Scope of practice. The scope of practice of acupuncture includes, but is not limited to, the following:

(1) using Oriental medical theory to assess and diagnose a patient;

(2) using Oriental medical theory to develop a plan to treat a patient. The treatment techniques that may be chosen include:

(i) insertion of sterile acupuncture needles through the skin;

(ii) acupuncture stimulation including, but not limited to, electrical stimulation or the application of heat;

(iii) cupping;

(iv) dermal friction;

(v) acupressure;

(vi) herbal therapies;

(vii) dietary counseling based on traditional Chinese medical principles;

(viii) breathing techniques;

(ix) exercise according to Oriental medical principles; or

(x) Oriental massage.

5. Patient records. An acupuncturist shall maintain a patient record for each patient treated, including:

(1) a copy of the informed consent;

(2) evidence of a patient interview concerning the patient's medical history and current physical condition;

(3) evidence of a traditional acupuncture examination and diagnosis;

(4) record of the treatment including points treated; and

(5) evidence of evaluation and instructions given to the patient.

6. Referral to other health care practitioners. Referral to other health care practitioners is required when an acupuncturist practitioner sees patients with potentially serious disorders including, but not limited to:

(1) cardiac conditions including uncontrolled hypertension;

(2) acute, severe abdominal pain;

(3) acute, undiagnosed neurological changes;

(4) unexplained weight loss or gain in excess of 15 percent of the body weight in less than a three-month period;

(5) suspected fracture or dislocation;

(6) suspected systemic infections;

(7) any serious undiagnosed hemorrhagic disorder; and

(8) acute respiratory distress without previous history.

The acupuncturist shall request a consultation or written diagnosis from a licensed physician for patients with potentially serious disorders.

7. Data practices. Data maintained on an acupuncture patient by an acupuncture practitioner is subject to section 144.336.

147B.07.　Discipline; reporting

For purposes of this chapter, acupuncturist licensees and applicants are subject to the provisions of sections 147.091 to 147.162.

147B.08.　Fees

1 to 3. Repealed by Laws 2017, 1st Sp., c. 6, art. 11, § 56 (a), eff. July 1, 2017.

4. Acupuncturist application and license fees.

(a) The board may charge the following nonrefundable fees:

(1) acupuncturist application fee, $150;

(2) acupuncturist annual registration renewal fee, $150;

(3) acupuncturist temporary registration fee, $60;

(4) acupuncturist inactive status fee, $50;

(5) acupuncturist late fee, $50;

(6) duplicate license fee, $20;

(7) certification letter fee, $25;

(8) education or training program approval fee, $100;

(9) report creation and generation fee, $60 per hour; and

(10) verification fee, $25.

(b) The board may prorate the initial annual license fee. All licensees are required to pay the full fee upon license renewal. The revenue generated from the fees must be deposited in an account in the state government special revenue fund.

147B.09.　License renewal cycle conversion

1. Generally. The license renewal cycle for acupuncture practitioner licensees is converted to an annual cycle where renewal is due on the last day of the licensee's month of birth. Conversion pursuant to this section begins January 1, 2020. This section governs license renewal procedures for licensees who were licensed before December 31, 2019. The conversion renewal cycle is the renewal cycle following the first license renewal after January 1, 2020. The

conversion license period is the license period for the conversion renewal cycle. The conversion license period is between six and 17 months and ends the last day of the licensee's month of birth in either 2020 or 2021, as described in subdivision 2.

2. **Conversion of license renewal cycle for current licensees.** For a licensee whose license is current as of December 31, 2019, the licensee's conversion license period begins on January 1, 2020, and ends on the last day of the licensee's month of birth in 2020, except that for licensees whose month of birth is January, February, March, April, May, or June, the licensee's renewal cycle ends on the last day of the licensee's month of birth in 2021.

3. **Conversion of license renewal cycle for noncurrent licensees.** This subdivision applies to an individual who was licensed before December 31, 2019, but whose license is not current as of December 31, 2019. When the individual first renews the license after January 1, 2020, the conversion renewal cycle begins on the date the individual applies for renewal and ends on the last day of the licensee's month of birth in the same year, except that if the last day of the individual's month of birth is less than six months after the date the individual applies for renewal, then the renewal period ends on the last day of the individual's month of birth in the following year.

4. **Subsequent renewal cycles.** After the licensee's conversion renewal cycle under subdivision 2 or 3, subsequent renewal cycles are annual and begin on the last day of the month of the licensee's birth.

5. **Conversion period and fees.**

(a) A licensee who holds a license issued before January 1, 2020, and who renews that license pursuant to subdivision 2 or 3, shall pay a renewal fee as required in this subdivision.

(b) A licensee shall be charged the annual license fee listed in section 147B.08 for the conversion license period.

(c) For a licensee whose conversion license period is six to 11 months, the first annual license fee charged after the conversion license period shall be adjusted to credit the excess fee payment made during the conversion license period. The credit is calculated by: (1) subtracting the number of months of the licensee's conversion license period from 12; and (2) multiplying the result of clause (1) by 1/12 of the annual fee rounded up to the next dollar.

(d) For a licensee whose conversion license period is 12 months, the first annual license fee charged after the conversion license period shall not be adjusted.

(e) For a licensee whose conversion license period is 13 to 17 months, the first annual license fee charged after the conversion license period shall be adjusted to add the annual license fee payment for the months that were not included in the annual license fee paid for the conversion license period. The added payment is calculated by: (1) subtracting 12 from the number of months of the licensee's conversion license period; and (2) multiplying the result of clause (1) by 1/12 of the annual fee rounded up to the next dollar.

(f) For the second and all subsequent license renewals made after the conversion license period, the licensee's annual license fee is as listed in section 147B.08.

6. Expiration. This section expires July 1, 2022.

Minnesota Rules

Chapter 2500. Chiropractors' Licensing and Practice

2500.3000.   ACUPUNCTURE.

1. Sterilization; disposal. Where nondisposable needles are used for acupuncture, the needles must be sterilized by:

A. autoclave;

B. dry heat sterilization; or

C. ethylene oxide sterilization.

Needles must be individually packaged for each patient. The individually packaged needles must either be discarded following patient treatment or sterilized according to the above methods of sterilization when nondisposable needles are used.

Needles must be disposed of according to the Infectious Waste Control Act, Minnesota Statutes, sections 116.75 to 116.83. In addition, all needles to be discarded must be sterilized and placed in a rigid puncture-resistant container before disposal. Noncorrosive needles must be used. An infectious waste disposal plan must be filed with the Department of Health.

2. Qualifications and fees. Prior to engaging in acupuncture, a licensed chiropractor must be registered with the board. Prior to initial registration, the chiropractor must complete no less than 100 hours of study, in the utilization of acupuncture. Courses or seminars offered by accredited schools, the National Acupuncturists' Association, or separately approved by the board according to parts 2500.1200 to 2500.1600 shall be accepted by the board. The chiropractor must submit certification of completion of the approved course of study along with a $100 registration fee. In addition, the applicant must have successfully completed either the National Board of Chiropractic Examiners Acupuncture Examination or the National Certification Commission for Acupuncture and Oriental Medicine (NCCAOM) Examination.

Doctors of chiropractic who are applying for licensure under the provisions of part 2500.0800 and who do not have proof of compliance with the requirements in the preceding paragraph, may satisfy the requirements by providing the board with an affidavit stating the following:

A. the doctor of chiropractic has obtained no less than 100 hours of acupuncture-related education from an educational institution approved by the board prior to the submission of this application; and

B. the doctor of chiropractic has performed no less than 500 acupuncture-related patient visits per year for at least three years preceding this application for registration.

Upon applying to the board for registration, the doctor of chiropractic must submit the affidavit in addition to a $100 registration fee. An annual renewal fee of $50 is required in order to maintain registered status with the board.

3. **Continuing education.** The doctor of chiropractic is required to fulfill the continuing education requirements as set by the board in part 2500.1200 before a renewal of registration is granted.

4. **Sanitary office or clinic.** It is unprofessional conduct to maintain unsanitary or unsafe equipment as it relates to the utilization of acupuncture.

5. **Registration certificate.** Upon receiving a registration certificate from the board, a doctor of chiropractic may utilize acupuncture to prepare for or complement a chiropractic adjustment.

6. **Exemptions.** Any doctor of chiropractic who is separately registered according to Minnesota Statutes, chapter 147B, is exempt from subparts 2 and 5.

7. **Renewals.** Within 14 days after the due date of acupuncture registration renewal, the board shall mail notices to applicants who have not completed registration.

Any registrant who fails to renew registration for more than 30 days after the due date for renewal, and who wishes to renew registration, must reapply for registration prior to providing acupuncture services, pay the initial registration fee, and pay the penalty fees in part 2500.1150.

Any registrant who fails to renew registration for more than one year but less than five years, and who wishes to renew registration, must reapply for registration prior to providing acupuncture services, pay the initial registration fee, pay the penalty fees in part 2500.1150, and complete ten hours of acupuncture-related continuing education for each year the registration was not renewed.

Any registrant who fails to renew registration for a period of more than five years and who wishes to renew registration, must reapply for registration prior to providing acupuncture services, pay the initial registration fee, pay the penalty fees in part 2500.1150, and successfully complete either the National Board of Chiropractic Examiners Acupuncture Examination or the NCCAOM Examination.

Any person continuing to provide acupuncture services while not authorized to do so is in violation of Minnesota Statutes, section 148.10.

2500.3100. INACTIVE ACUPUNCTURE REGISTRATION.

A Minnesota licensed chiropractor who has converted a Minnesota license to inactive may apply to the board for an inactive acupuncture registration. An inactive acupuncture registration is intended for those chiropractors who will be in active practice elsewhere. Upon approval of an application, the board will modify the annual acupuncture registration certificate to indicate inactive registration.

2500.3200.   ANNUAL RENEWAL OF INACTIVE ACUPUNCTURE REGISTRATION.

A registrant must complete an annual renewal application and submit the annual renewal fee for an inactive acupuncture registration as authorized under Minnesota Statutes, section 148.108.

2500.3300.   REINSTATEMENT OF INACTIVE ACUPUNCTURE REGISTRATION.

1. Generally. An inactive acupuncture registration may be reinstated to an active acupuncture registration according to items A to C:

A. completion of a board-approved application of reinstatement;

B. payment of a reinstatement fee as authorized under Minnesota Statutes, section 148.108; and

C. submission of a notarized statement from the doctor stating that the registrant has completed two hours of continuing education credits in acupuncture or acupuncture-related subjects as approved by the board for each year the registration was inactive.

2. Denial. If any of the requirements of subpart 1, items A to C, are not met by the doctor, the board shall deny approval of the application for reinstatement. A person who maintains an inactive acupuncture registration will not be required to take the NBCE acupuncture examination for the purposes of reinstatement.

2500.4000.   [Repealed, L 2014 c 291 art 4 s 59]

2500.5000.   [Repealed, L 2010 c 329 art 1 s 24]

Nebraska

Revised Statutes of Nebraska Annotated

38 – 2006. Acupuncture, defined

Acupuncture means the insertion, manipulation, and removal of acupuncture needles and the application of manual, mechanical, thermal, electrical, and electromagnetic treatment to such needles at specific points or meridians on the human body in an effort to promote, maintain, and restore health and for the treatment of disease, based on acupuncture theory. Acupuncture may include the recommendation of therapeutic exercises, dietary guidelines, and nutritional support to promote the effectiveness of the acupuncture treatment. Acupuncture does not include manipulation or mobilization of or adjustment to the spine, extraspinal manipulation, or the practice of medical nutrition therapy.

38 – 2007. Acupuncturist, defined

Acupuncturist means a person engaged in the practice of acupuncture.

38 – 2057. Acupuncture; exemptions

The provisions of the Medicine and Surgery Practice Act relating to acupuncture do not apply to:

(1) Any other health care practitioner credentialed under the Uniform Credentialing Act practicing within the scope of his or her profession;

(2) A student practicing acupuncture under the supervision of a person licensed to practice acupuncture under the Uniform Credentialing Act as part of a course of study approved by the department; or

(3) The practice of acupuncture by any person licensed or certified to practice acupuncture in any other jurisdiction when practicing in an educational seminar sponsored by a state-approved acupuncture or professional organization if the practice is supervised directly by a person licensed to practice acupuncture under the Uniform Credentialing Act.

38 - 2058.　Acupuncture; license required; standard of care

It is unlawful to practice acupuncture on a person in this state unless the acupuncturist is licensed to practice acupuncture under the Uniform Credentialing Act. An acupuncturist licensed under the Uniform Credentialing Act shall provide the same standard of care to patients as that provided by a person licensed under the Uniform Credentialing Act to practice medicine and surgery, osteopathy, or osteopathic medicine and surgery. An acupuncturist licensed under the Uniform Credentialing Act shall refer a patient to an appropriate practitioner when the problem of the patient is beyond the training, experience, or competence of the acupuncturist.

38 - 2059.　Acupuncture; consent required

The practice of acupuncture shall not be performed upon any person except with the voluntary and informed consent of such person. Information provided in connection with obtaining such informed consent shall include, but not be limited to, the following:

(1) The distinctions and differences between the practice of acupuncture and the practice of medicine;

(2) The disclosure that an acupuncturist is not licensed to practice medicine or to make a medical diagnosis of the person's disease or condition and that a physician should be consulted for such medical diagnosis;

(3) The nature and the purpose of the acupuncture treatment; and

(4) Any medical or other risks associated with such treatment.

38 - 2060.　Acupuncture; license requirements

At the time of application for an initial license to practice acupuncture, the applicant shall present to the department proof that he or she:

(1) Has graduated from, after having successfully completed the acupuncture curriculum requirements of, a formal, full-time acupuncture program at a university, college, or school of acupuncture approved by the board which includes at least one thousand seven hundred twenty-five hours of entry-level acupuncture education consisting of a minimum of one thousand didactic and five hundred clinical hours;

(2) Has successfully passed an acupuncture examination approved by the board which shall include a comprehensive written examination in acupuncture theory, diagnosis and treatment technique, and point location; and

(3) Has successfully completed a clean-needle technique course approved by the board.

Nebraska Administrative Code

1. SCOPE AND AUTHORITY.

These regulations govern the licensure of acupuncturists under Nebraska Revised Statute

(Neb. Rev. Stat.) §§ 38 – 2001 to 38 – 2063 of the Medicine and Surgery Practice Act, and the Uniform Credentialing Act.

2. DEFINITIONS.

Definitions are set out in the Medicine and Surgery Practice Act, the Uniform Credentialing Act, 172 Nebraska Administrative Code (NAC) 10, and this chapter.

(1) APPROVED ACUPUNCTURE EXAMINATION. National Certification Commission for Acupuncture and Oriental Medicine (NCCAOM) Acupuncture Comprehensive Written Examination, which is a comprehensive written examination including acupuncture theory, diagnosis and treatment technique, and the National Certification Commission for Acupuncture and Oriental Medicine (NCCAOM) Point Location Examination.

(2) BOARD APPROVED SCHOOL. A formal, full-time acupuncture program at a university, college or school of acupuncture which includes at least 1,725 hours of entry-level acupuncture education consisting of a minimum of 1,000 didactic and 500 clinical hours, and is accredited or a candidate for accreditation by the Accreditation Commission for Acupuncture and Oriental Medicine, or is accredited by another accrediting body that is recognized as such by the United States Secretary of Education.

(3) APPROVED CLEAN NEEDLE TECHNIQUE COURSE. A course in clean needle technique approved by the National Certification Commission for Acupuncture and Oriental Medicine (NCCAOM), or an equivalent course approved by the Board.

3. LICENSE REQUIREMENTS.

To obtain a license, an individual must submit a complete application provided by the Department and provide documentation demonstrating that the applicant meets the licensing requirements of Neb. Rev. Stat. §§ 38 – 2060, 172 NAC 10, and the following:

(A) Have graduated from, after having successfully completed the acupuncture curriculum requirements of an approved school;

(B) Have successfully passed an approved acupuncture examination;

(C) Have successfully completed an approved clean-needle technique course;

(D) Submit to the Department:

(i) Official transcripts submitted to the Department by the issuing institution;

(ii) Official documentation of passing score obtained on the approved acupuncture examinations; and

(iii) Official documentation showing successful completion of an approved clean-needle technique course.

4. INFORMED CONSENT.

The licensee must comply with Neb. Rev. Stat. § 38 – 2059 and present to each patient treated a voluntary and informed consent form. Each patient treated must sign and date the form stating that they have read and understood the information on the form and that they agree to acupuncture treatment. The voluntary and informed consent form must be retained in the each patient's records for a period of at least 5 years after termination of the treatment.

5. RENEWAL, WAIVER OF CONTINUING EDUCATION, AND INACTIVE STATUS.

The applicant must meet the requirements set out in 172 NAC 10. All acupuncture licenses expire on May 1 of each odd-numbered year.

6. CONTINUING COMPETENCY.

On or before the expiration date, each acupuncturist who is licensed in the State of Nebraska must, as a condition for renewal of his or her license, earn one of the following in order to meet the continuing competency requirement:

(A) 50 hours of continuing education approved by the National Certification Commission for Acupuncture and Oriental Medicine (NCCAOM);

(i) Hours are to be earned within the 24 months immediately preceding the date of expiration, except that a licensee who has earned more than the 50 hours required for license renewal for a 24-month renewal period is allowed to carry over up to 25 hours to the next 24-month renewal period; or

(B) 50 hours of Category 1 continuing education approved by the Accreditation Council for Continuing Medical Education (ACCME) or the American Osteopathic Association (AOA);

(i) Hours are to be earned within the 24 months immediately preceding the date of expiration, except that a licensee who has earned more than the 50 hours required for license renewal for a 24-month renewal period is allowed to carry over up to 25 hours to the next 24-month renewal period; or

(C) Active certification or active recertification of diplomat status with the National Certification Commission for Acupuncture and Oriental Medicine (NCCAOM) earned within the 24 months immediately preceding the date of expiration.

(1) ATTESTATION. Each licensee must submit to the Department an attestation that he or she has met the continuing competency requirement for the 24 months immediately preceding the expiration date.

(2) PROOF OF CONTINUING COMPETENCY. Each licensee is responsible for maintaining records verifying his or her attendance at continuing education programs or otherwise meeting the continuing competency requirement.

7. UNPROFESSIONAL CONDUCT.

Unprofessional conduct is set out in Neb. Rev. Stat. § 38 - 179, 172 NAC 88 as applicable to the profession of acupuncture, and this chapter.

(A) Failure to obtain a voluntary and informed consent form as referenced in 172 NAC 89 - 004; and

(B) Failure to provide the same standard of care to patients as that provided by a person licensed under the Uniform Credentialing Act to practice medicine and surgery, or osteopathic medicine and surgery.

8. REINSTATEMENT.

The applicant must meet the requirements set out in 172 NAC 10.

9. FEES.

Fees are set out in 172 NAC 2.

10. [Renumbered]

11. [Renumbered]

12. [Repealed]

13. [Renumbered]

Wisconsin

Wisconsin Statutes Annotated

451.01. Definitions

In this chapter:

(1) "Acupuncture" means promoting, maintaining or restoring health or diagnosing, preventing or treating disease based on traditional Oriental medical concepts of treating specific areas of the human body, known as acupuncture points or meridians, by performing any of the following practices:

(a) Inserting acupuncture needles.

(b) Moxibustion.

(c) Applying manual, thermal or electrical stimulation or any other secondary therapeutic technique.

(2) "Acupuncturist" means a person who is engaged in the practice of acupuncture.

451.02. Applicability

Nothing in this chapter requires a certificate under this chapter for any of the following:

(1) An individual holding a license, permit or certificate under ch. 441, 446, 447, 448, or 449 or a compact privilege under subch. IX or XI of ch. 448 who engages in a practice of acupuncture that is also included within the scope of his or her license, permit, certificate, or privilege.

(2) An individual assisting an acupuncturist in practice under the direct supervision of the acupuncturist.

(3) An individual who engages in the practice of acupuncture as part of a supervised course of study or residency program in acupuncture that is approved by the department if the individual is designated by a title that clearly indicates his or her status as a student or trainee.

451.04. Certification

(1) Acupuncturist certificate required. No person may engage in the practice of acupuncture

or use the title "acupuncturist" or any similar title unless the person is certified as an acupuncturist by the department.

(2) Acupuncturist certificate. The department shall grant an acupuncturist certificate to any individual who does all of the following:

(a) Submits an application for the certificate to the department on a form provided by the department.

(b) Pays the fee specified in s. 440.05 (1).

(c) Subject to ss. 111.321, 111.322 and 111.335, submits evidence satisfactory to the department that he or she does not have an arrest or conviction record.

(d) Subject to s. 451.08, submits evidence satisfactory to the department that he or she has completed a course of study and residency program in acupuncture that meets standards established by the department by rule.

(e) Subject to s. 451.08, passes an examination approved by the department to determine fitness as an acupuncturist.

(3) Posting of certificate. The department shall issue a certificate to each individual who satisfies the requirements in sub. (2) or s. 451.08, certifying that the holder is authorized to practice acupuncture in this state. The holder shall post the certificate in a conspicuous place in his or her place of business.

(4) Expiration and renewal. Renewal applications shall be submitted to the department on a form provided by the department on or before the applicable renewal date specified under s. 440.08 (2) (a) and shall include the applicable renewal fee determined by the department under s. 440.03 (9) (a).

451.06. Examination

Examinations shall consist of written or practical tests, or both, requiring applicants to demonstrate minimum competency in services and subjects substantially related to the practice of acupuncture.

451.08. Reciprocal certificate

Upon application and payment of the fee specified in s. 440.05 (2), the department shall grant an acupuncturist certificate to any applicant who holds an acupuncturist certificate or license in another state or territory of the United States if the department determines that the applicant has actively engaged in the practice of acupuncture for at least 5 years or that the requirements for certification or licensure in the other state or territory are substantially equivalent to the requirements under s. 451.04 (2).

451.10. Repealed by 1991 Act 39, § 3386, eff. Aug. 15, 1991

451.12. Infection control

The department shall promulgate rules relating to the prevention of infection, the sterilization of needles and other equipment or materials capable of transmitting infection and the safe disposal of potentially infectious materials. The rules shall require acupuncture needles to be thoroughly cleansed with an antiseptic solution prior to sterilization by autoclave and shall permit an acupuncturist to use needles that are presterilized, prewrapped and disposable.

451.14. Disciplinary proceedings and actions

(1) Subject to the rules promulgated under s. 440.03 (1), the department may make investigations or conduct hearings to determine whether a violation of this chapter or any rule promulgated under this chapter has occurred.

(2) Subject to the rules promulgated under s. 440.03 (1), the department may reprimand a certified acupuncturist or deny, limit, suspend or revoke a certificate under this chapter if it finds that the applicant or certified acupuncturist has done any of the following:

(a) Made a material misstatement in an application for a certificate or renewal.

(b) Engaged in conduct while practicing acupuncture which evidences a lack of knowledge or ability to apply professional principles or skills.

(c) Subject to ss. 111.321, 111.322 and 111.335, been arrested or convicted of an offense committed while certified as an acupuncturist.

(d) Advertised in a manner that is false, deceptive or misleading.

(e) Impersonated another individual who holds a certificate under this chapter or allowed another individual to use his or her acupuncturist certificate.

(f) Subject to ss. 111.321, 111.322 and 111.34, practiced acupuncture while the individual's ability to practice was impaired by alcohol or other drugs.

(g) Violated this chapter or any rule promulgated under this chapter.

(3) In addition to or in lieu of a reprimand or denial, limitation, suspension or revocation of a certificate under sub. (2), the department may assess against an applicant or certified acupuncturist a forfeiture of not less than $100 nor more than $1,000 for each violation enumerated under sub. (2).

451.16. Penalties

Any person who violates this chapter or any rule promulgated under this chapter may be fined not less than $100 nor more than $1,000 or imprisoned for not more than 90 days or both.

Wisconsin Administrative Code

SPS 70.02. Definitions.

As used in ch. 451, Stats., and chs. SPS 70 to 73:

(1) (a) "Actively engaged in the certified practice of acupuncture" means using acupuncture, under the authorization of a license, certification or registration to practice acupuncture, as the

primary means of treatment of patients, not as an adjunctive therapy, and the treatment is dependent upon a thorough understanding and application of Oriental diagnostic theories and practices.

(b) The applicant provides evidence satisfactory to the department that he or she has been "actively engaged in the certified practice of acupuncture" during the 5 years immediately preceding the application in any other state or territory of the United States. Any applicant, whether or not licensed, registered or certified to practice another healing art, shall provide the department with satisfactory evidence that the applicant:

1. Uses acupuncture based on Oriental diagnostic and therapeutic theories and practices as the primary means of treating diseases and disorders in a minimum of 100 patients with a minimum of 500 patient visits during the 12 months immediately preceding the date of the application, as demonstrated by patient records or affidavits.

2. Performs general health care in at least 70% of all patient visits, and performs specialized health care such as anesthetics, cosmetic treatments, addiction therapies or weight control in no more than 30% of patient visits.

3. Practices consistent with the standards identified in a clean needle technique course acceptable to the department.

(2) "Acupressure" means the manual stimulation of acupuncture points.

(3) "Acupuncture" has the meaning given under s. 451.01 (1), Stats.

(4) "Acupuncturist" means a person who is certified under ch. 451, Stats., to practice acupuncture.

(5) "AIDS" means acquired immunodeficiency syndrome.

(6) "Department" means the department of safety and professional services.

(7) "Herbal medicine" means the use of plant, animal and mineral substances to assist in attaining or maintaining a state of health or relief from symptoms of disease.

(8) "HIV" means human immunodeficiency virus.

(9) "Laserpuncture" means the use of lasers to stimulate acupuncture points.

(10) "Moxibustion" means the application of heat produced by burning dried moxa wool to specific points of the human body other than the burning of moxa wool directly on the skin.

(11) "NCCAOM" means the national certification commission for acupuncture and Oriental medicine.

(12) "Needle sickness" includes nausea, or dizziness, or other physical discomforts resulting from acupuncture treatment.

SPS 71.01. Application for certification.

An applicant for certification as an acupuncturist who has never practiced acupuncture or who does not qualify for certification under s. SPS 71.03, shall submit to the department:

(1) An application on a form provided by the department.

Note：Application forms are available on request to the department at 1400 East Washington Avenue, P. O. Box 8935, Madison, Wisconsin 53708.

(2) The fee specified in s. 440.05 (1), Stats.

(3) Evidence that the applicant has never been the subject of any disciplinary action by any professional or licensing authority, and subject to ss. 111.321, 111.322 and 111.335, Stats., has not been convicted of any offense substantially related to the practice of acupuncture.

(4) Evidence of successful completion of the NCCAOM examination in acupuncture, with a passing score as determined by the NCCAOM.

(5) Evidence of successful completion of course of study and residency, the equivalent of at least 2 consecutive years of fulltime education and clinical work in Oriental diagnostic and therapeutic theories and practices at a school accredited by the national accreditation commission for schools and colleges of acupuncture and Oriental medicine or the NCCAOM.

(6) Evidence of successful completion of a clean needle technique course acceptable to the department.

SPS 71.04. Renewal of certification after 5 years.

An acupuncture certificate holder who fails to renew his or her credential within 5 years following the renewal date of the certificate shall take and pass the examination required under s. SPS 71.01 (5) within one year prior to the date of application for renewal, unless the applicant provides evidence satisfactory to the department that he or she has actively engaged in the certified practice of acupuncture during the 5 years immediately preceding the application in any other state or territory of the United States.

SPS 72.03. Treatment procedures.

(1) Before any treatment commences, a patient shall be given the option, at the patient's own expense, to have treatment with disposable acupuncture needles, which have been sterilized and wrapped in accordance with s. 451.12, Stats., and maintained in accordance with s. SPS 72.02 (7).

(2) An acupuncturist shall wash his or her hands by scrubbing thoroughly for at least 10 seconds with soap or anti-microbial products between treatment of patients, immediately before an acupuncture procedure and after contact with blood or body fluids or obvious environmental contaminants.

(3) A clean field shall be maintained to protect sterility of equipment used in acupuncture treatment of each patient.

(4) A topical disinfectant shall be applied to the skin surface in the area prior to needle insertion or treatment that breaks the skin.

(5) A sterile needle shall be maintained in a sterile state prior to insertion into an acupuncture point and its shaft shall not come in contact with fingers during insertion, positioning or other manipulation.

SPS 72.07. Safe practices.

(1) No acupuncturist shall engage in any treatment which violates standards of good and accepted practice of acupuncture, or which makes use of any unsanitary or non-sterile equipment.

(2) An acupuncturist shall obtain from each patient a medical history pertinent to the patient's chief complaints.

(3) When an acupuncturist encounters a patient with a potentially serious disorder including, but not limited to, cardiac conditions, uncontrolled hypertension, acute abdominal symptoms, acute undiagnosed neurological changes, unexplained weight loss or gain in excess of 15% of body weight within a 3 month period, suspected fracture or dislocation, suspected systemic infection, communicable disease, any serious undiagnosed hemorrhagic disorder or acute respiratory distress without previous history or diagnosis, the acupuncturist shall:

(a) In a non-emergency situation, request a consultation or written diagnosis from a licensed physician prior to commencing acupuncture treatment or continuing treatment if the situation is discovered in the course of treatment.

(b) In an emergency situation, provide life support and transportation to the nearest licensed medical facility.

(4) An acupuncturist shall have on file for each patient treated a written confirmation signed by the patient and the acupuncturist acknowledging that the patient has been advised to consult a physician regarding the conditions for which such patient seeks acupuncture treatment.

SPS 73.01. Grounds for denial of certification or discipline.

For purposes of s. 451.14(2) (b), Stats., engaging in conduct while practicing acupuncture that evidences a lack of knowledge or ability to apply professional principles or skills includes, but is not limited to:

(1) Practicing acupuncture while ability is impaired by a mental or emotional disorder, physical disability, alcohol or other drugs.

(2) Violating, or aiding or abetting violation of any law, the circumstances of which substantially relate to the practice of acupuncture or other healing art.

(3) Practicing acupuncture without a current and valid certificate.

(4) Having been disciplined in another jurisdiction in any way by a certifying, registering, or licensing authority for reasons substantially the same as those set forth in s. 451.14, Stats., or in chs. SPS 70 to 73.

(5) After a request by the department, failing to cooperate in a timely manner with the department's investigation of a complaint filed against an acupuncturist. The department will apply a rebuttable presumption that an acupuncturist who takes longer than 30 days to respond to a request by the department has not acted in a timely manner.

(6) Practicing acupuncture fraudulently, beyond its authorized scope, with gross incompetence or gross negligence, with incompetence on one or more occasion, with negligence on more than one occasion, or practicing acupuncture or any secondary therapeutic technique beyond or inconsistent with training, education or experience.

(7) Refusing to provide professional services to a person solely on the basis of such person's race, color, age, sex, sexual orientation, political or religious beliefs, handicap, marital status or national origin.

(8) Failing to provide duplicate patient records when requested by the patient or the department. If the original record is not in English, the acupuncturist shall provide the duplicate in English translation performed by a competent translator. Thirty days is presumed to be a reasonable period of time in which to obtain the translation.

(9) Failing to maintain complete and accurate records of each patient visit, including patient histories, summaries of examinations, diagnoses, and treatments performed or prescribed, and referrals to other practitioners of acupuncture or any other healing art, for a period of 7 years past the most recent visit of the patient to whom the record refers, or the time the patient reaches the age of majority.

(10) Providing acupuncture without the informed consent of a patient. Informed consent requires:

(a) The disclosure to the patient of the availability of all alternate, viable modes of acupuncture treatment and the benefits and risks of these treatments, including the risks and benefits associated with the use of:

1. Acupuncture needles to stimulate acupuncture points and meridians, including the specific risks of needling certain points.

2. Use of mechanical, magnetic or electrical stimulation of acupuncture points, particularly in instances where such stimulation is applied across the midline of the trunk or in patients with a history of heart trouble.

3. Moxibustion.

4. Herbal medicine.

5. Laserpuncture.

6. Acupressure.

(b) The disclosure to the patient shall involve a disclosure of the side effects including:

1. Some pain at the site of needle insertion.

2. Minor bruising.

3. Infection and the risks from needling in the vicinity of an infection.

4. Needle sickness.

5. Broken needles.

SPS 73.02.　Use of titles.

(1) Any person certified under ch. 451, Stats., to practice acupuncture shall include the title "acupuncturist," "Wisconsin certified acupuncturist," or a similar title in advertisements of

acupuncture services.

(2) Any person certified under ch. 451, Stats., to practice acupuncture who has been conferred the degree of doctor of Oriental medicine may advertise his or her services as an acupuncturist to the public using the title "doctor of Oriental medicine" or "D.O.M.," if the title "acupuncturist," "Wisconsin certified acupuncturist," or a similar title is used in the same advertisement.

SPS 73.03.   Examples of false, deceptive or misleading advertising.

For purposes of s. 451.14(2) (d), Stats., false, deceptive or misleading advertising includes:

(1) Advertising acupuncture services using a title that includes the words "medical doctor" or the initials "M.D.," unless the acupuncturist meets the requirements of s. 448.03 (3) (a), Stats.

Note: Section 448.03 (3) USE OF TITLES. (a) No person may use or assume the title "doctor of medicine" or append to the person's name the letters "M.D." unless one of the following applies:

1. The person possesses the degree of doctor of medicine.

2. The person is licensed as a physician under this subchapter because the person satisfied the degree requirement of s. 448.05 (2) by possessing a medical degree that was conferred by a medical school recognized and listed as such by the World Health Organization of the United Nations.

(2) Advertising acupuncture services using the title "Doctor" or the abbreviation "Dr.," or "Ph.D." in connection with the practice of acupuncture unless the acupuncturist possesses a license or certificate which authorizes such use or possesses an earned doctorate degree which is in acupuncture or Oriental medicine.

Illinois

Illinois Compiled Statutes Annotated

2/1. Short title

§ 1. Short title. This Act may be cited as the Acupuncture Practice Act.

2/5. Objects and purpose

§ 5. Objects and purpose. The practice of acupuncture in the State of Illinois is hereby declared to affect the public health, safety, and welfare and to be subject to regulation and control in the public interest. It is further declared to be a matter of public interest and concern that the practice of acupuncture as defined in this Act merit and receive the confidence of the public, and that only qualified persons, as set forth by this Act, be authorized to practice acupuncture in the State of Illinois. This Act shall be liberally construed to best carry out these subjects and purposes.

2/10. Definitions

§ 10. Definitions. As used in this Act:

"Acupuncture" means evaluation or treatment that is effected by stimulating certain body points by the insertion of pre-sterilized, single-use, disposable needles, unless medically contraindicated. "Acupuncture" includes, but is not limited to, stimulation that may be effected by the application of heat, including far infrared, or cold, electricity, electro or magnetic stimulation, cold laser, vibration, cupping, gua sha, manual pressure, or other methods, with or without the concurrent use of needles, to prevent or modify the perception of pain, to normalize physiological functions, or for the treatment of diseases or dysfunctions of the body and includes the determination of a care regimen or treatment protocol according to traditional East Asian principles and activities referenced in Section 15 of this Act for which a written referral is not required. In accordance with this Section, the practice known as dry needling or intramuscular manual stimulation, or similar wording intended to describe such practice, is determined to be within the definition, scope, and practice of acupuncture. Acupuncture also includes evaluation or treatment in accordance with traditional and modern practices of East Asian medical theory, including, but not limited to, moxibustion, herbal medicinals, natural or dietary supplements, manual methods, exercise, and diet to prevent or modify the perception of pain, to normalize physiological functions, or for the treatment of diseases or dysfunctions of the body and includes activities referenced in Section 15 of this Act for which a written referral is not required. Acupuncture does not include radiology, electrosurgery, chiropractic technique, physical therapy, naprapathic technique, use or prescribing of any pharmaceuticals, or vaccines, or determination of a differential diagnosis. An acupuncturist licensed under this Act who is not also licensed as a physical therapist under the Illinois Physical Therapy Act[1] shall not hold himself or herself out as being qualified to provide physical therapy or physiotherapy services.

"Acupuncturist" means a person who practices acupuncture in all its forms, including traditional and modern practices in both teachings and delivery, and who is licensed by the Department. An acupuncturist shall refer to a licensed physician or dentist any patient whose condition should, at the time of evaluation or treatment, be determined to be beyond the scope of practice of the acupuncturist.

"Address of record" means the designated address recorded by the Department in the applicant's or licensee's application file or license file as maintained by the Department's licensure maintenance unit.

"Board" means the Board of Acupuncture appointed by the Secretary.

"Dentist" means a person licensed under the Illinois Dental Practice Act.[2]

"Department" means the Department of Financial and Professional Regulation.

"Email address of record" means the designated email address recorded by the Department in the applicant's application file or the licensee's license file as maintained by the Department's licensure maintenance unit.

"Physician" means a person licensed under the Medical Practice Act of 1987.[3]

"Referral by written order" for purposes of this Act means a diagnosis, substantiated by signature of a physician or dentist, identifying a patient's condition and recommending treatment by acupuncture as defined in this Act. The diagnosis shall remain in effect until changed by the physician or dentist who may, through express direction in the referral, maintain management of the patient.

"Secretary" means the Secretary of Financial and Professional Regulation.

"State" includes:

(1) the states of the United States of America;

(2) the District of Columbia; and

(3) the Commonwealth of Puerto Rico.

2/12. Address of record; email address of record

§ 12. Address of record; email address of record. All applicants and licensees shall:

(1) provide a valid address and email address to the Department, which shall serve as the address of record and email address of record, respectively, at the time of application for licensure or renewal of a license; and

(2) inform the Department of any change of address of record or email address of record within 14 days after such change either through the Department's website or by contacting the Department's licensure maintenance unit.

2/15. Who may practice acupuncture

§ 15. Who may practice acupuncture. No person licensed under this Act may treat human ailments otherwise than by the practice of acupuncture as defined in this Act and shall only practice acupuncture consistent with the education and certifications obtained pursuant to the requirements set forth in this Act. A physician or dentist licensed in Illinois may practice acupuncture in accordance with his or her training pursuant to this Act or the Medical Practice Act of 1987. An acupuncturist shall refer to a licensed physician or dentist, any patient whose condition should, at the time of evaluation or treatment, be determined to be beyond the scope of practice of the acupuncturist.

Nothing in this Act regarding the use of dietary supplements or herbs shall be construed to prohibit a person licensed in this State under any other Act from engaging in the practice for which he or she is licensed.

2/16. Chinese herbology; practice

§ 16. Chinese herbology; practice. No person licensed under this Act may hold himself or herself out as being trained in Chinese herbology without proof of status as a Diplomate of Oriental Medicine certified by the National Certification Commission for Acupuncture and Oriental Medicine or a substantially equivalent status that is approved by the Department or proof that he or she has successfully completed the National Certification Commission for Acupuncture and Oriental Medicine Chinese Herbology Examination or a substantially equivalent examination approved by the Department. A violation of this Section is subject to the disciplinary action described in Section 110.

2/20. Exempt activities

§ 20. Exempt activities. This Act does not prohibit any person licensed in this State from engaging in the practice for which he or she is licensed.

2/20.1. Guest instructors of acupuncture; professional education

§ 20.1. Guest instructors of acupuncture; professional education. The provisions of this Act do not prohibit an acupuncturist from another state or country, who is not licensed under this Act and who is an invited guest of a professional acupuncture association or scientific acupuncture foundation or an acupuncture training program or continuing education provider approved by the Department under this Act, from engaging in professional education through lectures, clinics, or demonstrations, provided that the acupuncturist is currently licensed in another state or country and his or her license is active and has not been disciplined, or he or she is currently certified in good standing as an acupuncturist by the National Certification Commission for Acupuncture and Oriental Medicine or similar body approved by the Department.

Licensees under this Act may engage in professional education through lectures, clinics, or demonstrations as an invited guest of a professional acupuncture association or scientific acupuncture foundation or an acupuncture training program or continuing education provider approved by the Department under this Act. The Department may, but is not required to, establish rules concerning this Section.

2/20.2. Guest practitioners of acupuncture

§ 20.2. Guest practitioners of acupuncture. The provisions of this Act do not prohibit an acupuncturist from another state or country who is not licensed under the Act from practicing in Illinois during a state of emergency as declared by the Governor of Illinois, provided that the acupuncturist is currently licensed in another state or country and his or her license is active and has not been disciplined, or he or she is certified by the National Certification Commission for Acupuncture and Oriental Medicine or similar body approved by the Department. Such practice is limited to the time period during which the declared state of emergency is in effect and may not exceed 2 consecutive weeks or a total of 30 days in one calendar year.

2/25. Powers and duties of Department

§ 25. Powers and duties of Department. The Department shall exercise powers and duties under this Act as follows:

(1) Review applications to ascertain the qualifications of applicants for licensure.

(2) Adopt rules consistent with the provisions of this Act for its administration and enforcement and may prescribe forms that shall be used in connection with this Act. The rules may define standards and criteria for professional conduct and discipline. The Department shall consult with the Board in adopting rules.

(3) The Department may at any time seek the advice and the expert knowledge of the Board on any matter relating to the administration of this Act.

2/30. Illinois Administrative Procedure Act

§ 30. Illinois Administrative Procedure Act.[1] The Illinois Administrative Procedure Act is hereby expressly adopted and incorporated herein as if all of the provisions of that Act were included in this Act, except that the provision of subsection (d) of Section 10 − 65 of the Illinois Administrative Procedure Act, which provides that at hearings the licensee has the right to show compliance with all lawful requirements for retention or continuation or renewal of the license, is specifically excluded. For the purposes of this Act, the notice required under Section 10 − 25 of the Illinois Administrative Procedure Act is deemed sufficient when mailed to the address of record.

2/35. Board of Acupuncture

§ 35. Board of Acupuncture. The Secretary shall appoint a Board of Acupuncture to consist of 7 persons who shall serve in an advisory capacity to the Secretary. Four members must hold an active license to engage in the practice of acupuncture in this State, one member shall be a chiropractic physician licensed under the Medical Practice Act of 1987[1] who is actively engaged in the practice of acupuncture, one member shall be a physician licensed to practice medicine in all of its branches in Illinois, and one member must be a member of the public who is not licensed under this Act or a similar Act of another jurisdiction and who has no connection with the profession.

Members shall serve 4-year terms and until their successors are appointed and qualified. No member may be appointed to more than 2 consecutive full terms. Appointments to fill vacancies shall be made in the same manner as original appointments for the unexpired portion of the vacated term. Initial terms shall begin upon the effective date of this amendatory Act of 1997.

The Board may annually elect a chairperson and a vice-chairperson who shall preside in the absence of the chairperson. The membership of the Board should reasonably reflect representation from the geographic areas in this State. The Secretary may terminate the appointment of any member for cause. The Secretary may give due consideration to all recommendations of the Board. A majority of the Board members currently appointed shall constitute a quorum. A vacancy in the membership of the Board shall not impair the right of a quorum to exercise the right and perform all the duties of the Board. Members of the Board shall have no liability in any action based upon any disciplinary proceeding or other activity performed in good faith as a member of the Board.

2/40. Application for licensure

§ 40. Application for licensure. Applications for original licensure as an acupuncturist shall be made to the Department in writing on forms prescribed by the Department and shall be accompanied by the required fee, which shall not be refundable.

The Department may issue a license to an applicant who submits with the application proof of each of the following:

(1) (A) graduation from a school accredited by the Accreditation Commission for Acupuncture and Oriental Medicine or a similar accrediting body approved by the Department; or (B) completion of a comprehensive educational program approved by the Department; and

(2) for applications submitted on or before December 31, 2019, passing the National Certification Commission for Acupuncture and Oriental Medicine examination or a substantially equivalent examination approved by the Department; for applications submitted on or after January 1, 2020, demonstration of status as a Diplomate of Acupuncture or Diplomate of Oriental Medicine with the National Certification Commission for Acupuncture and Oriental Medicine or a substantially equivalent credential as approved by the Department.

An applicant has 3 years from the date of his or her application to complete the application process. If the process has not been completed in 3 years, the application shall be denied, the fee shall be forfeited, and the applicant must reapply and meet the requirements in effect at the time of reapplication.

2/45. § 45. Repealed by P.A. 90 – 61, § 15, eff. July 3, 1997

2/50. Practice prohibited

§ 50. Practice prohibited. Unless he or she has been issued, by the Department, a valid, existing license as an acupuncturist under this Act, no person may use the title and designation of "Acupuncturist", "Licensed Acupuncturist", "Certified Acupuncturist", "Doctor of Acupuncture and Chinese Medicine", "Doctor of Acupuncture and Oriental Medicine", "Doctor of Acupuncture", "Oriental Medicine Practitioner", "Licensed Oriental Medicine Practitioner", "Oriental Medicine Doctor", "Licensed Oriental Medicine Doctor", "C.A.", "Act.", "Lic. Act.", "Lic. Ac.", "D. Ac.", "DACM", "DAOM", or "O.M.D." either directly or indirectly, in connection with his or her profession or business. No person licensed under this Act may use the designation "medical", directly or indirectly, in connection with his or her profession or business. Nothing shall prevent a physician from using the designation "Acupuncturist".

No person may practice, offer to practice, attempt to practice, or hold himself or herself out to practice as a licensed acupuncturist without being licensed under this Act.

This Act does not prohibit a person from applying acupuncture needles, modalities, or techniques as part of his or her educational training when he or she:

(1) is engaged in a State-approved course in acupuncture, as provided in this Act;

(2) is a graduate of a school of acupuncture and participating in a postgraduate training program;

(3) is a graduate of a school of acupuncture and participating in a review course in preparation for taking the National Certification Commission for Acupuncture and Oriental Medicine examination; or

(4) is participating in a State-approved continuing education course offered through a State-approved provider.

Students attending schools of acupuncture, and professional acupuncturists who are not licensed in Illinois, may engage in the practice of acupuncture in conjunction with their education as provided in this Act, but may not open an office, appoint a place to meet private patients, consult with private patients, or otherwise engage in the practice of acupuncture beyond what is required in conjunction with their education.

2/55. Endorsement

§ 55. Endorsement. The Department may, at its discretion, license as an acupuncturist without examination, on payment of the fee, an applicant for licensure who is an acupuncturist under the laws of another state if the requirements pertaining to acupuncture in that state were at the date of his or her licensure substantially equal to the requirements in force in Illinois on that date or if an applicant possesses individual qualifications that are substantially equal to the requirements under this Act.

An applicant has 3 years from the date of his or her application to complete the application process. If the process has not been completed in 3 years, the application shall be denied, the fee shall be forfeited, and the applicant must reapply and meet the requirements in effect at the time of reapplication.

2/60.　Exhibition of license upon request; change of address

§ 60. Exhibition of license upon request; change of address. A licensee shall, whenever requested, exhibit his or her license to any representative of the Department.

2/70.　Renewal or restoration of license; continuing education; military service

§ 70. Renewal or restoration of license; continuing education; military service. The expiration date and renewal period for each license issued under this Act shall be set by rule. The holder of a license may renew that license during the month preceding its expiration date by paying the required fee.

In order to renew or restore a license, applicants shall provide proof of having met the requirements of continuing education set forth in the rules of the Department. Continuing education sponsors approved by the Department may not use an individual to engage in clinical demonstration, unless that individual is actively licensed under this Act or licensed by another state or country as set forth in Section 20.1 of this Act.

A person who has permitted his or her license to expire or who has had his or her license on inactive status may have the license restored by submitting an application to the Department, by meeting continuing education requirements, and by filing proof acceptable to the Department of fitness to have the license restored, which may include sworn evidence certifying to active practice in another jurisdiction satisfactory to the Department and by paying the required restoration fee. If the person has not maintained an active practice in another jurisdiction satisfactory to the Department, the Department shall determine his or her fitness to resume active status and may require successful completion of a practical examination.

Any acupuncturist whose license expired while he or she was (1) in federal service on active duty with the Armed Forces of the United States or the State Militia called into service or training or (2) in training or education under the supervision of the United States preliminary to induction into the military service, however, may have his or her license restored without paying any lapsed renewal fees if within 2 years after honorable termination of service, training, or education, he or she furnishes the Department with satisfactory evidence that he or she has been so engaged and that his or her service, training, or education has been terminated.

2/75.　Inactive licenses

§ 75. Inactive licenses. A licensee who notifies the Department in writing on forms prescribed by the Department may elect to place his or her license on inactive status and shall, subject to rules of the Department, be excused from payment of renewal fees until he or she notifies the Department in writing of his or her desire to resume active status. A licensee requesting restoration from inactive status shall be required to pay the current renewal fee, shall meet the continuing education requirements, and shall be required to restore his or her license as provided in Section 70 of this Act.

2/80. Fees

§ 80. Fees. The Department shall provide by rule for a schedule of fees for the administration and enforcement of this Act, including but not limited to original licensure, renewal, and restoration. The fees shall be nonrefundable.

All fees collected under this Act shall be deposited into the General Professions Dedicated Fund and shall be appropriated to the Department for the ordinary and contingent expenses of the Department in the administration of this Act.

2/90. § 90. Repealed by P.A. 100 – 375, § 15, eff. Aug. 25, 2017

2/100. Advertisement

§ 100. Advertisement. Any person licensed under this Act may advertise the availability of professional services in the public media or on the premises where such professional services are rendered. Such advertising shall be limited to the following information:

(1) publication of the person's name, title, office hours, address and telephone number;

(2) information pertaining to the person's areas of specialization or limitation of professional practice;

(3) information on usual and customary fees for routine professional services offered, which information shall include, notification that fees may be adjusted due to complications or unforeseen circumstances;

(4) announcement of the opening of, change of, absence from, or return to business;

(5) announcement of additions to or deletions from professional registered staff; and

(6) the issuance of business or appointment cards.

This Act does not authorize the advertising of professional services that the offeror of such services is not licensed to render. Nor shall the advertiser use statements that contain false, fraudulent, deceptive, or misleading material or guarantees of success, statements that play upon the vanity or fears of the public, or statements that promote or produce unfair competition.

2/105. Unlicensed practice; civil penalty

§ 105. Unlicensed practice; civil penalty.

(a) A person who practices, offers to practice, attempts to practice, or holds himself or herself out to practice as a licensed acupuncturist without being licensed under this Act shall, in addition to any other penalty provided by law, pay a civil penalty to the Department in an amount not to exceed $10,000 for each offense as determined by the Department. The civil penalty shall be assessed by the Department after a hearing is held in accordance with the provisions set forth in this Act regarding the provision of a hearing for the discipline of a licensee.

(b) The Department has the authority and power to investigate any and all unlicensed activity.

(c) The civil penalty shall be paid within 60 days after the effective date of the order imposing the civil penalty. The order shall constitute a judgment and may be filed and execution had thereon in the same manner as any judgment from any court of record.

2/110. Grounds for disciplinary action

§ 110. Grounds for disciplinary action.

(a) The Department may refuse to issue or to renew, place on probation, suspend, revoke or take other disciplinary or non-disciplinary action as deemed appropriate including the imposition of fines not to exceed $10,000 for each violation, as the Department may deem proper, with regard to a license for any one or combination of the following causes:

(1) Violations of this Act or its rules.

(2) Conviction by plea of guilty or nolo contendere, finding of guilt, jury verdict, or entry of judgment or sentencing, including, but not limited to, convictions, preceding sentences of supervision, conditional discharge, or first offender probation, under the laws of any jurisdiction of the United States that is (i) a felony or (ii) a misdemeanor, an essential element of which is dishonesty or that is directly related to the practice of the profession.

(3) Making any misrepresentation for the purpose of obtaining a license.

(4) Aiding or assisting another person in violating any provision of this Act or its rules.

(5) Failing to provide information within 60 days in response to a written request made by the Department which has been sent by certified or registered mail to the licensee's address of record or by email to the licensee's email address of record.

(6) Discipline by another U. S. jurisdiction or foreign nation, if at least one of the grounds for the discipline is the same or substantially equivalent to one set forth in this Section.

(7) Solicitation of professional services by means other than permitted under this Act.

(8) Failure to provide a patient with a copy of his or her record upon the written request of the patient.

(9) Gross negligence in the practice of acupuncture.

(10) Habitual or excessive use or addiction to alcohol, narcotics, stimulants, or any other chemical agent or drug that results in an acupuncturist's inability to practice with reasonable judgment, skill, or safety.

(11) A finding that licensure has been applied for or obtained by fraudulent means.

(12) A pattern of practice or other behavior that demonstrates incapacity or incompetence to practice under this Act.

(13) Being named as a perpetrator in an indicated report by the Department of Children and Family Services under the Abused and Neglected Child Reporting Act[1] and upon proof by

clear and convincing evidence that the licensee has caused a child to be an abused child or a neglected child as defined in the Abused and Neglected Child Reporting Act.

(14) Willfully failing to report an instance of suspected child abuse or neglect as required by the Abused and Neglected Child Reporting Act.

(15) The use of any words, abbreviations, figures or letters (such as "Acupuncturist", "Licensed Acupuncturist", "Certified Acupuncturist", "Doctor of Acupuncture and Chinese Medicine", "Doctor of Acupuncture and Oriental Medicine", "Doctor of Acupuncture", "Oriental Medicine Practitioner", "Licensed Oriental Medicine Practitioner", "Oriental Medicine Doctor", "Licensed Oriental Medicine Doctor", "C. A.", "Act.", "Lic. Act.", "Lic. Ac.", "D. Ac.", "DACM", "DAOM", or "O.M.D.") or any designation used by the Accreditation Commission for Acupuncture and Oriental Medicine with the intention of indicating practice as a licensed acupuncturist without a valid license as an acupuncturist issued under this Act.

When the name of the licensed acupuncturist is used professionally in oral, written, or printed announcements, professional cards, or publications for the information of the public, the degree title or degree abbreviation shall be added immediately following title and name. When the announcement, professional card, or publication is in writing or in print, the explanatory addition shall be in writing, type, or print not less than 1/2 the size of that used in the name and title. No person other than the holder of a valid existing license under this Act shall use the title and designation of "acupuncturist", either directly or indirectly, in connection with his or her profession or business.

(16) Using claims of superior quality of care to entice the public or advertising fee comparisons of available services with those of other persons providing acupuncture services.

(17) Advertising of professional services that the offeror of the services is not licensed to render. Advertising of professional services that contains false, fraudulent, deceptive, or misleading material or guarantees of success, statements that play upon the vanity or fears of the public, or statements that promote or produce unfair competition.

(18) Having treated ailments other than by the practice of acupuncture as defined in this Act, or having treated ailments of as a licensed acupuncturist pursuant to a referral by written order that provides for management of the patient by a physician or dentist without having notified the physician or dentist who established the diagnosis that the patient is receiving acupuncture treatments.

(19) Unethical, unauthorized, or unprofessional conduct as defined by rule.

(20) Physical illness, mental illness, or other impairment that results in the inability to practice the profession with reasonable judgment, skill, and safety, including, without limitation, deterioration through the aging process, mental illness, or disability.

(21) Violation of the Health Care Worker Self-Referral Act.[2]

（22）Failure to refer a patient whose condition should, at the time of evaluation or treatment, be determined to be beyond the scope of practice of the acupuncturist to a licensed physician or dentist.

（23）Holding himself or herself out as being trained in Chinese herbology without being able to provide the Department with proof of status as a Diplomate of Oriental Medicine certified by the National Certification Commission for Acupuncture and Oriental Medicine or a substantially equivalent status approved by the Department or proof that he or she has successfully completed the National Certification Commission for Acupuncture and Oriental Medicine Chinese Herbology Examination or a substantially equivalent examination approved by the Department.

The entry of an order by a circuit court establishing that any person holding a license under this Act is subject to involuntary admission or judicial admission as provided for in the Mental Health and Developmental Disabilities Code[3] operates as an automatic suspension of that license. That person may have his or her license restored only upon the determination by a circuit court that the patient is no longer subject to involuntary admission or judicial admission and the issuance of an order so finding and discharging the patient and upon the Board's recommendation to the Department that the license be restored. Where the circumstances so indicate, the Board may recommend to the Department that it require an examination prior to restoring a suspended license.

The Department may refuse to issue or renew the license of any person who fails to (i) file a return or to pay the tax, penalty or interest shown in a filed return or (ii) pay any final assessment of the tax, penalty, or interest as required by any tax Act administered by the Illinois Department of Revenue, until the time that the requirements of that tax Act are satisfied.

In enforcing this Section, the Department upon a showing of a possible violation may compel an individual licensed to practice under this Act, or who has applied for licensure under this Act, to submit to a mental or physical examination, or both, as required by and at the expense of the Department. The Department may order the examining physician to present testimony concerning the mental or physical examination of the licensee or applicant. No information shall be excluded by reason of any common law or statutory privilege relating to communications between the licensee or applicant and the examining physician. The examining physicians shall be specifically designated by the Department. The individual to be examined may have, at his or her own expense, another physician of his or her choice present during all aspects of this examination. Failure of an individual to submit to a mental or physical examination, when directed, shall be grounds for suspension of his or her license until the individual submits to the examination if the Department finds, after notice and hearing, that the refusal to submit to the examination was without reasonable cause.

If the Department finds an individual unable to practice because of the reasons set forth in this Section, the Department may require that individual to submit to care, counseling, or treatment by physicians approved or designated by the Department, as a condition, term, or restriction for continued, restored, or renewed licensure to practice; or, in lieu of care, counseling, or treatment, the Department may file a complaint to immediately suspend, revoke, or otherwise discipline the license of the individual. An individual whose license was granted, continued, restored, renewed, disciplined or supervised subject to such terms, conditions, or restrictions, and who fails to comply with such terms, conditions, or restrictions, shall be referred to the Secretary for a determination as to whether the individual shall have his or her license suspended immediately, pending a hearing by the Department.

In instances in which the Secretary immediately suspends a person's license under this Section, a hearing on that person's license must be convened by the Department within 30 days after the suspension and completed without appreciable delay. The Department and Board shall have the authority to review the subject individual's record of treatment and counseling regarding the impairment to the extent permitted by applicable federal statutes and regulations safeguarding the confidentiality of medical records.

An individual licensed under this Act and affected under this Section shall be afforded an opportunity to demonstrate to the Department that he or she can resume practice in compliance with acceptable and prevailing standards under the provisions of his or her license.

2/117.   Suspension of license for failure to restitution

§ 117. Suspension of license for failure to pay restitution. The Department, without further process or hearing, shall suspend the license or other authorization to practice of any person issued under this Act who has been certified by court order as not having paid restitution to a person under Section 8A − 3.5 of the Illinois Public Aid Code or under Section 17 − 10.5 or 46 − 1 of the Criminal Code of 1961 or the Criminal Code of 2012. A person whose license or other authorization to practice is suspended under this Section is prohibited from practicing until the restitution is made in full.

2/120.   Checks or orders to Department dishonored because of insufficient funds

§ 120. Checks or orders to Department dishonored because of insufficient funds. Any person who issues or delivers a check or other order to the Department that is not honored on 2 occasions by the financial institution upon which it is drawn because of insufficient funds on account, the account is closed, or a stop payment has been placed on the check or order shall pay to the Department, in addition to the amount owing upon the check or other order, a fee of $50. If the check or other order was issued or delivered in payment of a renewal or issuance fee and the person whose license has lapsed continues to practice acupuncture without paying the renewal or issuance fee and the required $50 fee under this Section, an additional fee of $100 shall be imposed. The fees imposed by this Section are in addition to any other disciplinary provision under this Act prohibiting practice on an expired or non-renewed license. If after the expiration of 30 days from the date of the notification a person whose license has lapsed seeks a current license, he or she shall thereafter apply to the Department for restoration of the license and pay all fees due to the Department. The Department may establish a fee for the processing of an application for restoration of a license that allows the Department to pay all costs and expenses incident to the processing of this application. The Secretary may waive the fees due under this Section in individual cases where he or she finds that the fees would be unreasonably or unnecessarily burdensome.

2/130.　Injunctions; criminal offenses; cease and desist order

§ 130. Injunctions; criminal offenses; cease and desist order.

(a) If any person violates the provisions of this Act, the Secretary may, in the name of the People of the State of Illinois, through the Attorney General of the State of Illinois or the State's Attorney for any county in which the action is brought, petition for an order enjoining the violation or for an order enforcing compliance with this Act. Upon the filing of a petition in court, the court may issue a temporary restraining order, without notice or condition, and may preliminarily and permanently enjoin the violation. If it is established that the person has violated or is violating the injunction, the court may punish the offender for contempt of court. Proceedings under this Section shall be in addition to, and not in lieu of, all other remedies and penalties provided by this Act.

(b) Whenever in the opinion of the Department a person violates a provision of this Act, the Department may issue a rule to show cause why an order to cease and desist should not be entered against that person. The rule shall clearly set forth the grounds relied upon by the Department and shall allow at least 7 days from the date of the rule to file an answer to the satisfaction of the Department. Failure to answer to the satisfaction of the Department shall cause an order to cease and desist to be issued immediately.

(c) Other than as provided in Section 20 of this Act, if any person practices as an acupuncturist or holds himself or herself out as a licensed acupuncturist under this Act without being issued a valid existing license by the Department, then any licensed acupuncturist, any interested party, or any person injured thereby may, in addition to the Secretary, petition for relief as provided in subsection (a) of this Section.

2/135.　Criminal violations

§ 135. Criminal violations. Whoever knowingly practices or offers to practice acupuncture in this State without being licensed for that purpose shall be guilty of a Class A misdemeanor and for each subsequent conviction shall be guilty of a Class 4 felony. Notwithstanding any other provision of this Act, all criminal fines, moneys, or other property collected or received by the Department under this Section or any other State or federal statute, including but not limited to property forfeited to the Department under Section 505 of the Illinois Controlled Substances Act[1] or Section 85 of the Methamphetamine Control and Community Protection Act, [2] shall be deposited into the Professional Regulation Evidence Fund.

2/140.   Investigation; notice; hearing

§ 140. Investigation; notice; hearing. Licenses may be refused, revoked, suspended, or otherwise disciplined in the manner provided by this Act and not otherwise. The Department may upon its own motion or upon the complaint of any person setting forth facts that if proven would constitute grounds for refusal to issue or renew or for suspension, revocation, or other disciplinary action under this Act, investigate the actions of a person applying for, holding, or claiming to hold a license. The Department shall, before refusing to issue or renew, suspending, revoking, or taking other disciplinary action regarding a license or taking other discipline pursuant to Section 110 of this Act, and at least 30 days prior to the date set for the hearing, notify in writing the applicant or licensee of any charges made, shall afford the applicant or licensee an opportunity to be heard in person or by counsel in reference to the charges, and direct the applicant or licensee to file a written answer to the Department under oath within 20 days after the service of the notice and inform the applicant or licensee that failure to file an answer will result in default being taken against the applicant or licensee and that the license may be suspended, revoked, placed on probationary status, or other disciplinary action may be taken, including limiting the scope, nature, or extent of practice, as the Secretary may deem proper. Written notice may be served by: (1) personal delivery to the applicant or licensee; (2) mailing the notice by registered or certified mail to his or her address of record or to the place of business last specified by the applicant or licensee in his or her last notification to the Department; or (3) sending notice via email to the applicant's or licensee's email address of record. If the person fails to file an answer after receiving notice, his or her license may, in the discretion of the Department, be suspended, revoked, or placed on probationary status or the Department may take whatever disciplinary action deemed proper, including limiting the scope, nature, or extent of the person's practice or the imposition of a fine, without a hearing, if the act or acts charged constitute sufficient grounds for such action under this Act. At the time and place fixed in the notice, the Department shall proceed to hearing of the charges and both the applicant or licensee and the complainant shall be afforded ample opportunity to present, in person or by counsel, any statements, testimony, evidence, and arguments that may be pertinent to the charges or to their defense. The Department may continue a hearing from time to time. If the Board is not sitting at the time and place fixed in the notice or at the time and place to which the hearing shall have been continued, the Department may continue the hearing for a period not to exceed 30 days.

2/142.   Confidentiality

§ 142. Confidentiality. All information collected by the Department in the course of an examination or investigation of a licensee or applicant, including, but not limited to, any complaint against a licensee filed with the Department and information collected to investigate any such complaint, shall be maintained for the confidential use of the Department and may not be disclosed. The Department may not disclose the information to anyone other than law enforcement officials, other regulatory agencies that have an appropriate regulatory interest as determined by the Secretary of the Department, or a party presenting a lawful subpoena to the Department. Information and documents disclosed to a federal, State, county, or local law enforcement agency may not be disclosed by the agency for any purpose to any other agency or person. A formal complaint filed by the Department against a licensee or applicant is a public record, except as otherwise prohibited by law.

2/145. Formal hearing; preservation of record

§ 145. Formal hearing; preservation of record. The Department, at its expense, shall preserve a record of all proceedings at the formal hearing of any case involving the refusal to issue or renew a license or discipline of a licensee. The notice of hearing, complaint, and all other documents in the nature of pleadings and written motions filed in the proceedings, the transcript of testimony, the report of the hearing officer, and order of the Department shall be the record of the proceeding.

2/150. Witnesses; production of documents; contempt

§ 150. Witnesses; production of documents; contempt. Any circuit court may, upon application of the Department or its designee or of the applicant or licensee against whom proceedings under Section 140 of this Act are pending, enter an order requiring the attendance of witnesses and their testimony and the production of documents, papers, files, books, and records in connection with any hearing or investigation. The court may compel obedience to its order by proceedings for contempt.

2/152. Certification of record

§ 152. Certification of record. The Department shall not be required to certify any record to the court, file any answer in court, or otherwise appear in any court in a judicial review proceeding, unless and until the Department has received from the plaintiff payment of the costs of furnishing and certifying the record, which costs shall be determined by the Department. Exhibits shall be certified without cost. Failure on the part of the plaintiff to file a receipt in court shall be grounds for dismissal of the action.

2/154. Compelling testimony

§ 154. Compelling testimony. Any circuit court may, upon application of the Department or its designee or of the applicant or licensee against whom proceedings pursuant to Section 140 of this Act are pending, enter an order requiring the attendance of witnesses and their testimony, and the production of documents, papers, files, books, and records in connection with any hearing or investigation. The court may compel obedience to its order through proceedings for contempt.

2/155. Subpoena; oaths

§ 155. Subpoena; oaths. The Department shall have power to subpoena and bring before it any person in this State and to take testimony either orally or by deposition or both with the same fees and mileage and in the same manner as prescribed by law in judicial proceedings in civil cases in circuit courts of this State. The Department shall also have the power to subpoena the production of documents, papers, files, books, and records in connection with a hearing or investigation.

The Secretary and the hearing officer designated by the Secretary shall each have power to administer oaths to witnesses at any hearing that the Department is authorized to conduct under this Act and any other oaths required or authorized to be administered by the Department under this Act.

2/160. Findings of facts, conclusions of law, and recommendations

§ 160. Findings of facts, conclusions of law, and recommendations. At the conclusion of the hearing, the Board shall present to the Secretary a written report of its findings of fact, conclusions of law, and recommendations. The report shall contain a finding whether or not the accused person violated this Act or failed to comply with the conditions required in this Act. The Board shall specify the nature of the violation or failure to comply and shall make its recommendations to the Secretary.

The report of findings of fact, conclusions of law, and recommendations of the Board may be the basis of the order of the Department. If the Secretary disagrees in any regard with the report of the Board, the Secretary may issue an order in contravention of the report. The finding is not admissible in evidence against the person in a criminal prosecution brought for the violation of this Act, but the hearing and findings are not a bar to a criminal prosecution brought for the violation of this Act.

2/165. Hearing officer

§ 165. Hearing officer. The Secretary shall have the authority to appoint any attorney duly licensed to practice law in the State of Illinois to serve as the hearing officer in any action for discipline of a license. The hearing officer shall have full authority to conduct the hearing. The hearing officer shall report his or her findings of fact, conclusions of law, and recommendations to the Board and the Secretary. The Board shall review the report of the hearing officer and to present its findings of fact, conclusions of law, and recommendations to the Secretary.

2/170. Service of report; rehearing; order

§ 170. Service of report; rehearing; order. In any case involving the refusal to issue or renew a license or the discipline of a license, a copy of the Board's report shall be served upon the respondent by the Department, as provided in this Act for the service of the notice of hearing. Within 20 days after the service, the respondent may present to the Department a motion in writing for a rehearing that shall specify the particular grounds for rehearing. If no motion for rehearing is filed, then upon the expiration of the time specified for filing such a motion, or if a motion for rehearing is denied, then upon the denial the Secretary may enter an order in accordance with recommendations of the Board, except as provided in Section 175 of this Act. If the respondent orders from the reporting service and pays for a transcript of the record within the time for filing a motion for rehearing, the 20-day period within which the motion may be filed shall commence upon the delivery of the transcript to the respondent.

2/175. Substantial justice to be done; rehearing

§ 175. Substantial justice to be done; rehearing. Whenever the Secretary is satisfied that substantial justice has not been done in the revocation, suspension, or refusal to issue, restore, or renew a license, or other discipline of an applicant or licensee, the Secretary may order a rehearing by the same or other examiners.

2/180. Order or certified copy as prima facie proof

§ 180. Order or certified copy as prima facie proof. An order or a certified copy thereof, over the seal of the Department and purporting to be signed by the Secretary, shall be prima facie proof:

(1) that the signature is the genuine signature of the Secretary;

(2) that such Secretary is duly appointed and qualified; and

(3) that the Board and its members are qualified to act.

2/185. Restoration of license

§ 185. Restoration of license. At any time after the suspension or revocation of any license the Department may restore it to the accused person, unless after an investigation and a hearing the Department determines that restoration is not in the public interest. Where circumstances of suspension or revocation so indicate, the Department may require an examination of the accused person prior to restoring his or her license.

2/190. Surrender of license

§ 190. Surrender of license. Upon the revocation or suspension of any license, the licensee shall immediately surrender the license certificate to the Department. If the licensee fails to do so, the Department shall have the right to seize the license certificate.

2/195. Imminent danger to public; temporary suspension

§ 195. Imminent danger to public; temporary suspension. The Secretary may temporarily suspend the license of an acupuncturist without a hearing, simultaneously with the institution of proceedings for a hearing provided for in Section 140 of this Act, if the Secretary finds that evidence in his or her possession indicates that continuation in practice would constitute an imminent danger to the public. In the event that the Secretary temporarily suspends a license without a hearing, a hearing by the Department must be held within 30 days after the suspension has occurred and be concluded without appreciable delay.

2/200. Review under Administrative Review Law

§ 200. Review under Administrative Review Law.[1] All final administrative decisions of the Department are subject to judicial review under the Administrative Review Law and all rules adopted under the Administrative Review Law. The term "administrative decision" is defined as in Section 3 – 101 of the Code of Civil Procedure.[2]

Proceedings for judicial review shall be commenced in the circuit court of the county in which the party applying for review resides; however, if the party is not a resident of this State, the venue shall be Sangamon County.

2/205.   § 205. Repealed by P.A. 90 – 61, § 15, eff. July 3, 1997

2/210.   Violations; penalties

§ 210. Violations; penalties. Any person who is found to have violated any provision of this Act is guilty of a Class A misdemeanor. On conviction of a second or subsequent offense the violator shall be guilty of a Class 4 felony.

2/999.   Effective date

§ 999. Effective date. This Act takes effect upon becoming law.

Illinois Administrative Code

1140.10   Definitions

"Act" means the Acupuncture Practice Act [225 ILCS 2].

"ACAOM" means the Accreditation Commission for Acupuncture and Oriental Medicine, which is a U. S. Department of Education recognized body that accredits educational programs in the fields of acupuncture and oriental medicine.

"Acupuncturist" means a person licensed under the Acupuncture Practice Act to practice acupuncture as defined in that Act.

"Board" means the Board of Acupuncture.

"CCAOM" means the Council of Colleges of Acupuncture and Oriental Medicine.

"CE" means continuing education.

"CNT Course" means a clean needle technique course as administered by CCAOM.

"Department" means the Department of Financial and Professional Regulation.

"Director" means the Director of the Department of Financial and Professional Regulation-Division of Professional Regulation.

"Division" means the Department of Financial and Professional Regulation-Division of Professional Regulation.

"NCCAOM" means the National Certification Commission for Acupuncture and Oriental Medicine, which certifies Diplomates of Acupuncture and Diplomates of Oriental Medicine.

1140.20   Fees

The following fees shall be paid to the Division and are not refundable:

(a) Application Fees

(1) The fee for application for a license as an acupuncturist is $500.

(2) The fee for application as a continuing education sponsor is $250.

(b) Renewal Fees

(1) The fee for the renewal of an acupuncturist license shall be calculated at the rate of $250 per year.

(2) The fee for the renewal of continuing education sponsor approval is $250 for a 2-year license.

(c) General Fees

(1) The fee for the restoration of a license other than from inactive status is $20 plus payment of all lapsed renewal fees, not to exceed $1,000.

(2) The fee for the certification of a license for any purpose is $20.

(3) The fee for a roster of persons licensed as acupuncturists in this State shall be the actual cost of producing such a roster.

1140.30 Application for Licensure

(a) An applicant for licensure as an acupuncturist shall file an application with the Division that includes the following:

(1) Acupuncture Program

(A) An official transcript certifying that the applicant has graduated from a school accredited by ACAOM or a similar accrediting body approved by Division; or

(B) An official transcript certifying that the applicant has graduated from a comprehensive educational program approved by the Division in accordance with Section 1140.40;

(2) For applications submitted on or before December 31, 2019, proof of passage of the NCCAOM examinations for Acupuncture with Point Location, Biomedicine, and Foundations of Oriental Medicine or a substantially equivalent examination approved by the Division;

(3) For applications submitted on or after January 1, 2020, proof of status as a Diplomate of Acupuncture (3-year program) or Diplomate of Oriental Medicine (4-year program) with NCCAOM, or a substantial equivalent approved by the Division;

(4) Proof of successful completion of the CNT course administered by CCAOM; and

(5) The required fee specified in Section 1140.20.

(b) All documents shall be submitted to the Division in English.

(c) If the applicant has ever been licensed as an acupuncturist in another state, he/she shall also submit a certification from the state in which the applicant was originally licensed and in which the applicant is currently licensed, stating:

(1) The time during which the applicant was licensed as an acupuncturist in that jurisdiction, including the date of the original issuance of the license;

(2) A description of the examination in that jurisdiction; and

(3) Whether the file on the applicant contains any record of disciplinary actions taken or pending.

(d) When the accuracy of any submitted documentation or experience is questioned by the Division or the Board because of lack of information, discrepancies or conflicts in information given or a need for clarification, the applicant seeking licensure shall be requested to:

(1) Provide such information as may be necessary; and/or

(2) Appear for an interview before the Board to explain such relevance or sufficiency, clarify information, or clear up any discrepancies or conflicts in information.

1140.35　Guest Instructor

(a) Any person not licensed in this State to practice acupuncture who is an invited guest of a professional acupuncture association, scientific acupuncture foundation, acupuncture training program or Division approved continuing education provider may provide professional education through lectures, clinics or demonstrations as set forth in Section 20.1 of the Act.

(b) Any individual providing services pursuant to this Section shall, upon written request of the Division, provide the following:

(1) One of the following:

(A) Current certification as an active Diplomate of Acupuncture or an active Diplomate of Oriental Medicine from NCCAOM or similar body approved by the Department; or

(B) Current certification of active licensure as an acupuncturist in another state or country.

(2) Certification from an acupuncture association, scientific acupuncture foundation, acupuncture training program or approved continuing education sponsor indicating:

(A) That the person has received an invitation or appointment to teach acupuncture technique in conjunction with lecture, clinics or demonstrations;

(B) The nature of the educational services to be provided by the applicant; and

(C) The term of the invitation or contract;

(3) A copy of the applicant's current curriculum vitae.

(c) A guest instructor may engage in the application of acupuncture techniques in conjunction with the lecture, clinics or demonstration, but may not open an office, appoint a place to meet private patients, consult with private patients, or otherwise engage in the practice of acupuncture beyond what is required in conjunction with these lectures, clinics or demonstrations.

(d) If an individual providing services under the provisions of this Section desires to remain in the State and practice or teach his/her profession, he/she must apply for and receive a license to practice acupuncture. Nothing shall prohibit individuals providing services pursuant to this Section from applying for and receiving a license to practice acupuncture in this State while providing services as allowed by this Section.

1140.40　Acupuncture Programs

The Division shall approve an applicant's acupuncture program if it meets the minimum criteria of subsection (a) and of either subsection (b) or (c).

(a) The school from which the applicant has graduated:

（1）Is legally recognized and authorized by the jurisdiction in which it is located to confer an acupuncture degree;

（2）Has a faculty that comprises a sufficient number of full-time instructors to make certain that the educational obligations to the student are fulfilled. The faculty must have demonstrated competence as evidenced by appropriate degrees in their areas of teaching from professional colleges or institutions; and

（3）Maintains permanent student records that summarize the credentials for admission, attendance and grades and other records of performance.

（b）For a 3-year program, the core curriculum includes a minimum of 1905 hours or its equivalent, within no less than 27 calendar months. This must be composed of at least:

（1）795 hours（or its equivalent）in theory and treatment techniques in acupuncture and related studies.

（A）Topics shall include, but not be limited to, the following:

（i）History of Acupuncture;

（ii）Basic Theory. Topics shall include, but not be limited to, basic Yin-Yang theory, 8 principles and 5 elements; Zang（viscera）organs and Fu（bowels）organs and extraordinary organs; theory and function of channels（meridians）and collaterals; Qi, blood and body fluids; Qi tonification（supplementation）and sedation（reducing）; etiology（the causes of diseases）such as 6 exogenous, 7 emotional factors and non-internal or non-external reasons; pathology;

（iii）Point Location and Channel（Meridian）Theory. Topics shall include, but not be limited to, nomenclature and distribution of the 14 channels on the body surface — 12 regular channels, Ren（conception）channel and Du（governing）channel; classification of points; points study should include the method of locating the points, anatomic structures, classification of points, functions and indications, and contraindications; knowledge of the specific point categories, such as the Five Shu points, Yuan（source）points, Luo（connecting）points, Xi（cleft）points, Back-Shu points, Front-Mu points, Crossing points; knowledge of the 8 extraordinary channels and their corresponding points;

（iv）Acupuncture Treatment. Topics shall include, but not be limited to, the various evaluation methods utilized in acupuncture practice, differentiation of syndromes according to 8 principles, Qi and blood, Zang-Fu organs and theory of meridians and collaterals; case review, based on history of the patient and charting; the four-examination methods; measuring and recording vital signs and symptoms, to make treatment plans and future prognosis; contraindications of treatment; indications of potential risk to the patient; the need to modify standard therapeutic approach（e.g., infants and children, pregnancy）and apparently benign presentations that may have a more serious cause（hypertension, headaches）;

（v）Treatment Techniques. Topics shall include, but not be limited to, needle insertion depth, duration, manipulation and withdrawal; the appearance of Qi; Moxa application, direct and indirect, etc.; other techniques (e.g., bleeding, moxibustion, cupping, Gua Sha, 7 star); tonification and sedation techniques; knowledge relating to the treatment of acute and chronic conditions, first aid, analgesia, anesthesia, and electrical stimulation; safety issues; Oriental bodywork therapy (e.g., Tui Na, Shiatsu, Amma, acupressure, etc.); contraindication for certain conditions; and

(vi) Ethics and Practice Management. Topics shall include, but not be limited to, confidentiality; informed consent; HIPAA guidelines; understanding the scope of practice; recordkeeping; legal requirements, release of data; ethical and legal aspects of referring patients to another practitioner; professional conduct and appropriate interpersonal behavior; laws and regulations governing the practice of acupuncture; recognition and clarification of patient expectations; general liability insurance; legal requirements; professional liability insurance; risk management and quality assurance; building and managing a practice, including ethical and legal aspects of third party reimbursement; professional development.

(B) No more than 90 hours may count towards history and ethics and practice management.

(2) 660 hours (or its equivalent) in clinical training.

(A) The program must assure that each student participates in a minimum of 510 hours in the supervised care of patients using acupuncture. This portion of the clinical training, conducted under the supervision of program-approved supervisors, must consist of at least 250 student-performed treatments where students conduct patient interviews, perform diagnosis and treatment planning, perform appropriate acupuncture treatments, and follow-up on patients' responses to treatment.

(B) The supervised clinical practice must be an internship that provides the student training in all phases of patient care and must be conducted in a teaching clinic operated by the institution or in a clinical facility with a formal affiliation with the institution where the institution exercises academic oversight substantially equivalent to the academic oversight exercised for teaching clinics operated by the institution, where:

(i) Clinical instructors' qualifications meet school requirements for clinical instruction;

(ii) Regular, systematic evaluation of the clinical experience takes place; and

(iii) Clinical training supervision procedures are substantially equivalent to those within the teaching clinic operated by the institution. Student interns must receive training from a variety of clinical faculty in order to ensure that interns are exposed to different practice styles and instructional methods.

(C) The program must assure that each student acquires a minimum of 150 hours in observation.

(3) 450 hours (or its equivalent) in biomedical clinical sciences.

(A) Biomedical Clinical Sciences. Topics shall include, but not be limited to, basic science courses; biomedical and clinical concepts and terms; human anatomy and physiology; pathology and the biomedical disease model; pharmacology; the nature of the biomedical clinical process, including history taking, diagnosis, treatment and follow-up; the clinical relevance of laboratory and diagnostic tests and procedures, as well as biomedical physical examination findings; the basis and need for referral and/or consultation; the range of biomedical referral resources and the modalities they employ; and

(B) Clean Needle Technique. Topics shall include infectious diseases, sterilization procedures, needle handling and disposal, and other issues relevant to bloodborne and surface pathogens.

(c) For a 4-year program, the core curriculum includes a minimum of 2625 hours, or its equivalent, within no less than 36 calendar months. This must be composed of at least:

(1) 795 hours (or its equivalent) in theory and treatment techniques in acupuncture and related studies.

(A) Topics shall include, but not be limited to, the following:

(i) History of Acupuncture;

(ii) Basic Theory. Topics shall include, but not be limited to, basic Yin-Yang theory, 8 principles and 5 elements; Zang (viscera) organs and Fu (bowels) organs and extraordinary organs; theory and function of channels (meridians) and collaterals; Qi, blood and body fluids; Qi tonification (supplementation) and sedation (reducing), etiology (the causes of diseases) such as 6 exogenous, 7 emotional factors and non-internal or non-external reasons; pathology;

(iii) Point Location and Channel (Meridian) Theory. Topics shall include, but not be limited to, nomenclature and distribution of the 14 channels on the body surface — 12 regular channels, Ren (conception) channel and Du (governing) channel; classification of points; points study should include the method of locating the points, anatomic structures, classification of points, functions and indications, and contraindications; knowledge of the specific point categories, such as the Five Shu points, Yuan (source) points, Luo (connecting) points, Xi (cleft) points, Back-Shu points, Front-Mu points, Crossing points; knowledge of the 8 extraordinary channels and their corresponding points;

(iv) Acupuncture Treatment. Topics shall include, but not be limited to, the various evaluation methods utilized in acupuncture practice, differentiation of syndromes according to 8 principles, Qi and blood, Zang-Fu organs and theory of meridians and collaterals; case review, based on history of the patient and charting; the four-examination methods; measuring and recording vital signs and symptoms, to make treatment plans and future prognosis; contraindications of treatment; indications of potential risk to the patient; the need to modify standard therapeutic approach (e.g., infants and children, pregnancy) and apparently benign presentations that may have a more serious cause (hypertension, headaches);

(v) Treatment Techniques. Topics shall include, but not be limited to, needle insertion depth, duration, manipulation and withdrawal; the appearance of Qi; Moxa application, direct and indirect, etc.; other techniques (e.g., bleeding, moxibustion, cupping, Gua Sha, 7 star); tonification and sedation techniques; knowledge relating to the treatment of acute and chronic conditions, first aid, analgesia, anesthesia, and electrical stimulation; safety issues; Oriental bodywork therapy (e.g., Tui Na, Shiatsu, Amma, acupressure, etc.); contraindication for certain conditions; and

(ⅵ) Ethics and Practice Management. Topics shall include, but not be limited to, confidentiality; informed consent; HIPAA guidelines; understanding the scope of practice; recordkeeping: legal requirements, release of data; ethical and legal aspects of referring patients to another practitioner; professional conduct and appropriate interpersonal behavior; laws and regulations governing the practice of acupuncture; recognition and clarification of patient expectations; general liability insurance; legal requirements; professional liability insurance: risk management and quality assurance; building and managing a practice, including ethical and legal aspects of third party reimbursement; professional development.

(B) No more than 90 hours may count towards history and ethics and practice management.

(2) 450 hours (or its equivalent) in didactic Oriental herbal studies.

(A) Topics shall include, but not be limited to:

(ⅰ) Introduction to Oriental herbal medicine, development of herbal medical systems throughout the Orient, history of the development of Oriental herbal medicine in the USA, and legal and ethical considerations of herbal medicine;

(ⅱ) Basic Herbal Medicine Theory. Topics shall include, but not be limited to, plant-part terminology and significance to usage; herbal properties (e.g., concepts of herbal categories, taste, temperature, entering meridians); methods of preparation (i.e., dried, honey baked); methods of delivery (e.g., decoction, topical, timing); laws of combining, including common contraindications, prohibitions, precautions; methods of treatment (i.e., induce sweat, clearing, harmonize);

(ⅲ) Oriental Diagnostic and Treatment Paradigms. Topics shall include, but not be limited to, herbal medicine within the context of Shan Han/6 stages; Wen Bing/4 levels; Zang Fu; Chinese Internal and External Medicine;

(ⅳ) Herbal Strategies. Topics shall include, but are not limited to, methods and systems for planning, carrying out and evaluating a treatment; differentiation and modifications of herbal formula for various patterns of disharmony according to Chinese medical principles; Chinese herbal medicine protocols applied to patients with a biomedical diagnosis;

(ⅴ) Materia Medica. Includes instruction in a minimum of 300 different herbs with topics including, but not limited to, functions and meaning; visual identification, including differing methods of cutting; temperature, taste and entering meridians; taxonomy and nomenclature; introduction to Chinese names of herbs; functions and actions with a focus on classical and new developments; specific contraindications for each herb; applications of herbal dosages; current developments in individual herb research; endangered species and substitutions for them;

(ⅵ) Herbal Formulas. Includes instruction in a minimum of 150 formulas with topics including, but not limited to, traditional formula categories, functions and meanings; meanings of the traditional Chinese formula names; functions and actions with a focus on classical and new developments; specific contraindications for each formula; current development in formula research; composition and proportion of individual herbs in each formula; major modifications of formulations; patient education regarding administration, potential side effects, preparation and storage of formulas; prepared herbal formulations focusing on modifications and format of delivery;

(ⅶ) Clinical Internship and Herbal Dispensary. Topics include, but are not limited to, clinical internship in which students interview, diagnose, and write appropriate herbal formulae moving from complete supervision to independent formula development; standards of cleanliness in herbal dispensary; storage of herbs (both raw and prepared formulas), covering issues of spoilage and bugs; practice in the filling of herbal formulas in an herbal dispensary setting; Western science for herbal medicine; botany, non-botanical and horticulture (e.g., changes in the characteristics of herbs due to environmental factors) as they pertain to herbal medicine; general principles of pharmacognosy; biochemical components of herbs and natural substances; considerations of pharmaceutical interactions with reference to current texts.

(3) 870 hours (or its equivalent) in an integrated acupuncture and herbal clinical training.

(A) The program must assure that each student participates in a minimum of 700 hours in the supervised care of patients using acupuncture. This portion of the clinical training, conducted under the supervision of program-approved supervisors, must consist of at least 350 student-performed treatments in which students conduct patient interviews, perform diagnosis and treatment planning, perform appropriate acupuncture treatments, and follow up on patients' responses to treatment.

(B) The supervised clinical practice must be an internship that provides the student training in all phases of patient care and must be conducted in a teaching clinic operated by the institution or in a clinical facility with a formal affiliation with the institution under which the institution exercises academic oversight substantially equivalent to the academic oversight exercised for teaching clinics operated by the institution when:

(ⅰ) Clinical instructors' qualifications meet school requirements for clinical instruction;

(ⅱ) Regular, systematic evaluation of the clinical experience takes place; and

(ⅲ) Clinical training supervision procedures are substantially equivalent to those within the teaching clinic operated by the institution. Student interns must receive training from a variety of clinical faculty in order to ensure that interns are exposed to different practice styles and instructional methods.

(C) The program must assure that each student acquires a minimum of 150 hours in observation.

(4) 510 hours (or its equivalent) in biomedical clinical sciences.

(A) Biomedical Clinical Sciences. Topics shall include, but not be limited to, basic science courses; biomedical and clinical concepts and terms; human anatomy and physiology; pathology and the biomedical disease model; pharmacology; the nature of the biomedical clinical process, including history taking, diagnosis, treatment and follow-up; the clinical relevance of laboratory and diagnostic tests and procedures, as well as biomedical physical examination findings; the basis and need for referral and/or consultation; the range of biomedical referral resources and the modalities they employ; and

(B) Clean Needle Technique. Topics shall include infectious diseases, sterilization procedures, needle handling and disposal, and other issues relevant to bloodborne and surface pathogens.

(d) An individual who is deficient in course work may complete the required courses at a regionally accredited college or university or a school of acupuncture accredited by ACAOM. The individual will be required to submit a transcript from the program indicating successful completion of the course and a course description.

1140.50 Endorsement

(a) An applicant who is currently licensed as an acupuncturist under the laws of another state or territory of the United States who wishes to be licensed in Illinois as an acupuncturist shall file an application with the Division, together with:

(1) One of the following:

(A) For applicants licensed in another state on or before December 31, 2001, proof of one of the following:

(i) Successful completion of the NCCAOM comprehensive acupuncture examination or a substantially equivalent examination approved by the Division; or

(ii) Current certification as an active Diplomate of Acupuncture or an active Diplomate of Oriental Medicine from NCCAOM;

(B) For applicants licensed in another state after December 31, 2001, proof of:

(i) Either:

• An official transcript certifying that the applicant has graduated from a school accredited by the ACAOM or a similar accrediting body approved by the Division; or

• An official transcript certifying that the applicant has graduated from a comprehensive educational program approved by the Division in accordance with Section 1140.40; and

(ii) Proof of successful completion of the NCCAOM comprehensive acupuncture examination or a substantially equivalent examination approved by the Division; or

(C) For applicants licensed on or after January 1, 2020 in another state, current certification as an active Diplomate of Acupuncture or Diplomate of Oriental Medicine with NCCAOM or substantially equivalent credential as approved by the Division;

(2) Proof of successful completion of the CNT course as administered by CCAOM;

(3) Certification from the state of original licensure and the state in which the applicant is currently licensed and practicing as an acupuncturist, if other than original, stating the applicant's license number, the time during which the applicant was licensed in that state, a description of the licensure examination in that jurisdiction, and whether the file on the applicant contains any disciplinary actions taken or pending; and

(4) The required fee specified in Section 1140.20.

(b) The Division shall examine each endorsement application to determine whether the requirements and examination in the jurisdiction at the date of licensing were substantially equivalent to the requirements and examination of the Act or whether the applicant possesses individual qualifications that were substantially equivalent to the requirements of the Act.

(c) The Division shall either issue a license by endorsement to the applicant or notify the applicant in writing of the reasons for the denial of the application.

1140.60.　Renewals

(a) Every license issued under the Act shall expire on June 30 of odd numbered years. The holder of a license may renew such license during the month preceding the expiration date by paying the required fee. A renewal applicant will be required to complete 30 hours of continuing education in accordance with Section 1140.90.

(b) It is the responsibility of each licensee to notify the Division of any change of address. Failure to receive a renewal form from the Division shall not constitute an excuse for failure to pay the renewal fee or to renew one's license.

(c) Practicing or offering to practice on a license that has expired shall be considered unlicensed activity and shall be grounds for discipline pursuant to Section 110 of the Act.

1140.70　Inactive Status

(a) A licensed acupuncturist who notifies the Division in writing, may place his or her license on inactive status and shall be excused from paying renewal fees until he or she notifies the Division in writing of the intention to resume active status.

(b) A person seeking restoration of an acupuncturist license that has been placed on inactive status shall do so in accordance with Section 1140.80.

(c) A person whose acupuncturist license is on inactive status shall not use the title "acupuncturist" or any of the other designations listed in Section 50 of the Act in the State of Illinois. Any person violating this subsection shall be considered to be practicing without a license and shall be subject to discipline pursuant to Section 110 of the Act.

1140.80　Restoration

(a) A person seeking restoration of an acupuncturist license after it has been expired or placed on inactive status for 5 years or less shall file an application with the Division, together with the fee specified in Section 1140.20 and proof of having completed 30 continuing education

(CE) hours not more than 2 years prior to submitting the restoration application. The CE hours must have been completed and documented in accordance with Section 1140.90.

(b) A person seeking restoration of an acupuncturist license after it has been expired or placed on inactive status for more than 5 years shall file an application with the Division, on forms supplied by the Division, together with the fee specified in Section 1140.20 and proof of having completed 30 CE hours not more than 2 years prior to submitting the restoration application. The CE hours must have been completed and documented in accordance with Section 1140.90. In addition, the applicant shall submit:

(1) One of the following:

(A) Sworn evidence of active practice as a licensed acupuncturist in another state or territory of the United States within 2 years prior to submitting the restoration application. The evidence shall include a statement from the appropriate licensing board or licensing authority in the other jurisdiction that the licensee was authorized to practice during the term of active practice; or

(B) An affidavit attesting to military service as provided in Section 70 of the Act; or

(C) Proof of having successfully completed the Acupuncture with Point Location examination, Biomedicine examination, and Foundations of Oriental Medicine examination of NCCAOM or a substantially equivalent examination approved by the Division not more than 2 years prior to submitting the restoration application; or

(D) Proof of having completed educational programs or post-graduate courses related to the clinical aspects of acupuncture, including courses at a school of acupuncture accredited by ACAOM or a similar accrediting body approved by the Division, professionally oriented continuing education classes, special seminars, or any other similar program approved by the Board. The programs or courses shall not be completed more than 2 years prior to submitting the restoration application.

(i) An applicant whose license has been expired or placed on inactive status for 5 to 10 years shall submit proof of 90 hours of educational programs or courses relating to the clinical aspects of acupuncture; or

(ii) An applicant whose license has been expired or placed on inactive status for more than 10 years shall submit proof of 120 hours of educational programs or courses relating to the clinical aspects of acupuncture.

(2) Proof of having successfully completed the CNT course administered by CCAOM not more than 5 years prior to submitting the restoration application.

(c) When the accuracy of any submitted documentation or the relevance or sufficiency of the course work or experience is questioned by the Division because of lack of information, discrepancies or conflicts in information given, or a need for clarification, the licensee seeking restoration shall be requested to:

(1) Provide such information as may be necessary; and/or

(2) Appear for an interview before the Board to explain the relevance or sufficiency, clarify information or clear up any discrepancies or conflicts in information.

1140.90   Continuing Education

(a) Continuing Education Hours Requirements

(1) Every licensee who applies for renewal or restoration of an acupuncturist license shall complete 30 hours of CE relevant to the professional skills and scientific knowledge of the licensee in the practice of acupuncture.

(2) A pre-renewal period is the 24 months preceding June 30 of each odd-numbered year.

(3) One CE hour shall equal one 60-minute clock hour with not less than 50 minutes of instructional content within the hour 30 to 49 minutes of instructional content would be reported be as 0.5 CE hour and 50 to 60 minutes of instructional content would be reported as 1.0 CE hour.

(4) A renewal applicant shall not be required to comply with CE requirements for the first renewal of an Illinois acupuncturist license.

(5) Acupuncturists licensed in Illinois but residing and practicing in other states shall comply with the CE requirements set forth in this Section.

(6) CE credit hours used to satisfy the CE requirements of another state may be applied to fulfill the CE requirements of the State of Illinois if they meet the requirements for CE in Illinois.

(b) Approved Continuing Education

(1) Except for those activities listed in subsections (b) (3), (4), (5) and (6), all CE hours must be earned through sponsors approved under subsection (c) and must comply with program requirements set forth in subsection (c).

(2) A maximum of 23 hours of CE credit may be earned in a pre-renewal period for completion of self-study (including online, correspondence, audio or video) courses that are provided by a sponsor approved by the Division pursuant to subsection (c). Each self-study course shall include an examination that the licensee must pass to obtain credit.

(3) A maximum of 30 hours of CE credit may be earned in a pre-renewal period for successful completion of post-graduate courses related to the clinical aspects of acupuncture at a school of acupuncture accredited by ACAOM or a similar accrediting body approved by the Division. CE credit will be allotted at the rate of 15 CE hours for each semester hour or 10 CE hours for each quarter hour of school credit awarded.

(4) A maximum of 15 hours of CE credit may be earned in a pre-renewal period for verified teaching of coursework that is part of the curriculum of an acupuncture program accredited by ACAOM or a similar accrediting body approved by the Division and/or as an instructor of CE programs provided by a sponsor approved by the Division pursuant to subsection (c). Credit will be applied at the rate of 1.5 hours for each hour of teaching or presenting the course or

program material and only for the first presentation of the course or program (i.e., credit shall not be allowed for repetitious presentations of the same program).

(5) A maximum of 5 hours of CE credit may be earned in a pre-renewal period for completion of coursework that is part of the curriculum of an accredited college or university and/or for completion of CE programs in Illinois approved by the Division but not approved under this Part. The course or program material must be relevant to the professional skills and scientific knowledge of the licensee in the practice of acupuncture.

(6) A maximum of 5 hours of CE credit may be earned in a pre-renewal period for authoring papers published in refereed professional journals or books.

(c) Approved CE Sponsors and Programs

(1) Approved sponsor, as used in this Section, shall mean:

(A) American Association of Acupuncture and Oriental Medicine or its affiliates;

(B) Asian American Acupuncture Association, or its affiliates;

(C) Illinois Association of Acupuncture and Oriental Medicine, or its affiliates;

(D) Korean American Acupuncture Association of Illinois, or its affiliates;

(E) Chicago Korean American Acupuncture Association, or its affiliates;

(F) The National Certification Commission for Acupuncture and Oriental Medicine and individuals and organizations approved by NCCAOM to provide acupuncture CE programs; or

(G) American Society of Acupuncturists, or its affiliates;

(H) American Academy of Medical Acupuncture; or

(I) Any other person, firm, association, corporation or group that has been approved and authorized by the Division pursuant to subsection (c) (2) upon the recommendation of the Board to coordinate and present CE programs.

(2) Entities seeking registration as a CE sponsor pursuant to subsection (c) (1) (I) shall file a CE sponsor application, a sample CE program in accordance with subsection (c) (3), a sample evaluation in accordance with subsection (c) (4), and a sample certificate of attendance in accordance with subsection (c) (5) along with the fee specified in Section 1140.20. (State agencies, State colleges and State universities in Illinois shall be exempt from paying this fee.) The applicant shall also certify to the following:

(A) That all programs offered by the sponsor for CE credit will comply with the criteria in subsection (c) (3) and all other criteria in this Section;

(B) That the sponsor will be responsible for verifying attendance at each program and provide a certificate of attendance as set forth in subsection (c) (5);

(C) That, upon request by the Division, the sponsor will submit evidence necessary to establish compliance with this Section. Evidence shall be required when the Division has reason to believe that there is not full compliance with the statute and this Part and that this information is necessary to ensure compliance.

(3) All programs shall：

(A) Contribute to the advancement, extension and enhancement of the professional skills and scientific knowledge of the licensee in the practice of acupuncture that includes direct and indirect patient care, acupuncture treatment, treatment techniques, point location and theory, herbal therapy or preparation, and ethics;

(B) Foster the enhancement of general or specialized acupuncture practice and values;

(C) Be developed and presented by persons with education and/or experience in the subject matter of the program;

(D) Specify the course objectives, course content and teaching methods to be used; and

(E) Specify the number of CE hours that may be applied to fulfilling the Illinois CE requirements for acupuncturist license renewal.

(4) Each CE program shall provide a mechanism for participants to evaluate the program and the instructor.

(5) It shall be the responsibility of the sponsor to provide each participant in a program with a certificate of attendance to verify completion of the program. The sponsor's certificate of attendance shall contain：

(A) The sponsor's name, address and Illinois CE sponsor registration number;

(B) The participant's name and Illinois acupuncturist license number;

(C) The title of the program and a brief description of the subject matter;

(D) The number of hours attended by the participant;

(E) The date and location of the program; and

(F) The signature of the sponsor.

(6) The sponsor shall be responsible for assuring that each participant receives CE credit only for time spent attending the program.

(7) The sponsor shall maintain attendance records for not less than 5 years.

(8) All programs given by approved sponsors shall be open to all licensed acupuncturists and not be limited to members of a single organization or group.

(9) An approved sponsor may subcontract with individuals and organizations to provide programs in accordance with the criteria set forth in this Section.

(10) To maintain approval as a registered CE sponsor, each sponsor shall submit a renewal application in accordance with Section 1140.60, along with the renewal fee specified in Section 1140.20. Upon the Division's request, the sponsor shall provide a list of each program provided by the sponsor in the pre-renewal period, including the name of the program, a brief description of the subject matter, the number of credit hours available, the program date, and the location of the program.

(11) Upon the failure of a sponsor to comply with any of the foregoing requirements, the Division, after notice to the sponsor and hearing before and recommendation by the Board (see

68 Ill. Adm. Code 1110), shall thereafter refuse to accept for CE credit attendance at or participation in any of that sponsor's CE programs until such time as the Division receives assurances of compliance with this Section.

(12) Notwithstanding any other provision of this Section, the Division or Board may evaluate any sponsor of any approved CE program at any time to ensure compliance with the requirements of this Section.

(d) Certification of Compliance with CE Requirements

(1) Each renewal applicant shall certify, on the renewal application, full compliance with the CE requirements set forth in subsections (a) and (b).

(2) The Division may require additional evidence demonstrating compliance with the CE requirements (e.g., certificate of attendance). This additional evidence may be required in the context of the Division's random audit. It is the responsibility of each renewal applicant to retain or otherwise produce evidence of compliance.

(3) When there appears to be a lack of compliance with CE requirements, a renewal applicant shall be notified in writing, which shall include electronic communication. At that time, the Board may recommend that steps be taken to begin formal disciplinary proceedings as required by Section 10 – 65 of the Illinois Administrative Procedure Act[5 ILCS 100/10 – 65].

(e) Continuing Education Earned in Other Jurisdictions

(1) If a licensee will be earning or has earned CE hours in another state or territory for which the licensee will be claiming credit toward full compliance in Illinois and the sponsor is not approved by the Division pursuant to subsection (c), the applicant shall submit an out-of-state CE approval form, a description and schedule of the CE program, a description of the instructor's qualifications, proof of registration or attendance, and a $25 processing fee, prior to participation in the program or 90 days prior to the expiration of his or her acupuncturist license. The Board or division shall review and recommend approval or disapproval of the program using the criteria set forth in this Section.

(2) If a licensee fails to submit an out of state CE approval form within the time frame specified in subsection (e) (1), late approval may be obtained by submitting an out-of-state CE approval form, a description and schedule of the CE program, a description of the instructor's qualifications, and proof of attendance, along with the required fee. The required fee shall be a $25 processing fee plus a late fee of $10 for each CE hour for which late approval is requested. The late fee shall not exceed $150. The Board or Division shall review and recommend approval or disapproval of the program using the criteria set forth in this Section.

(f) Waiver of CE Requirements

(1) Any renewal applicant seeking renewal of a license without having fully complied with these CE requirements shall file with the Division a renewal application along with the required fee set forth in Section 1140.20, a statement setting forth the facts concerning non-compliance,

and a request for waiver of all or part of the CE requirements on the basis of these facts. A request for waiver shall be made prior to the expiration date of the license. If the Division, upon the written recommendation of the Board, finds from such affidavit or any other evidence submitted that extreme hardship has been shown for granting a waiver, the Division shall waive enforcement of the CE requirements for the license renewal for which the applicant has applied.

(2) Extreme hardship shall be determined on an individual basis by the Board and be defined as an inability to devote sufficient hours to fulfilling the CE requirements during the applicable pre-renewal period because of:

(A) Full-time service in the armed forces of the United States of America during a substantial part of the pre-renewal period;

(B) An incapacitating illness during a substantial part of the pre-renewal period, documented by a statement from a currently licensed physician;

(C) A physical inability to travel to the sites of approved programs during a substantial part of the pre-renewal period, documented by a currently licensed physician; or

(D) Any other similar extenuating circumstances.

(3) Any renewal applicant who, prior to the expiration date of the license, submits a request for a waiver, in whole or in part, pursuant to the provisions of this Section shall be deemed to be in good standing until the final decision on the application is made by the Division.

1140.100 Unprofessional Conduct

(a) Pursuant to Section 110 of the Act, unethical, unauthorized or unprofessional conduct in the practice of acupuncture shall include, but not be limited to:

(1) Procuring, attempting to procure or renewing a license by bribery or by fraudulent misrepresentation;

(2) Willfully making or filing a false report or record, willfully failing to file a report or record required by State or federal law, or willfully impeding or obstructing such filing or inducing another person to do so;

(3) Circulating untruthful, fraudulent, deceptive or misleading advertising;

(4) Willfully failing to report any violation of the Act or this Part;

(5) Willfully or repeatedly violating a lawful order of the Board or the Division previously entered in a disciplinary hearing;

(6) Accepting and performing professional responsibilities that the licensee knows, or has reason to know, he/she is not competent to perform;

(7) Delegating professional responsibilities to a person when the licensee delegating such responsibilities knows, or has reason to know, that such person is not qualified by training, experience or licensure to perform them;

(8) Gross or repeated malpractice or the failure to deliver acupuncture services with that level of care, skill and treatment that is recognized by a reasonably prudent acupuncturist with

similar professional training as being acceptable under similar conditions and circumstances;

(9) Dividing with anyone, other than physicians with whom the licensee receives referrals or another acupuncturist with whom the licensee works, any fee, commission, rebate or other form of compensation for any professional services not actually and personally rendered. Nothing contained in this subsection prohibits persons holding valid and current licenses under this Act from practicing in a partnership, limited liability partnership, limited liability company or a corporation under the Professional Corporation Act or from pooling, sharing, dividing or apportioning the fees and monies received by them or by the partnership or corporation;

(10) Engaging in immoral conduct in the commission of any act related to the licensee's practice;

(11) Engaging in sexual abuse, sexual misconduct, or sexual exploitation.

(b) The Division hereby incorporates by reference the "Code of Ethics" of the National Certification Commission for Acupuncture and Oriental Medicine, 2025 M Street NW, Suite 800, Washington DC 20036 (January 2016), with no later amendments or editions.

1140.110 Granting Variances

The Director may grant variances from this Part in individual cases when he or she finds that:

(a) The provision from which the variance is granted is not statutorily mandated;

(b) No party will be injured by the granting of the variance; and

(c) The rule from which the variance is granted would, in that particular case, be unreasonable or unnecessarily burdensome.

Indiana

Annotated Indiana Code

Chapter 1. Definitions

IC 25 − 2.5 − 1 − 1   Applicability of definitions

The definitions in this chapter apply throughout this article.

IC 25 − 2.5 − 1 − 2   "Acupuncture"

"Acupuncture" means a form of health care employing traditional and modern Oriental medical concepts, Oriental medical diagnosis and treatment, and adjunctive therapies and diagnostic techniques for the promotion, maintenance, and restoration of health and the prevention of disease.

IC 25 − 2.5 − 1 − 2.1   "Acupuncturist"

"Acupuncturist" means an individual to whom a license to practice acupuncture in Indiana has been issued under IC 25 − 2.5 − 2.

IC 25 − 2.5 − 1 − 2.5   "Agency"

"Agency" refers to the Indiana professional licensing agency established by IC 25 − 1 − 5 − 3.

IC 25 − 2.5 − 1 − 3   "Board"

"Board" refers to the medical licensing board.

IC 25 − 2.5 − 1 − 4   Repealed by P.L.1 − 2006, SEC.588, eff. Mar.24, 2006

IC 25 − 2.5 − 1 − 5   "Practice of acupuncture"

"Practice of acupuncture" means the insertion of acupuncture needles, the application of moxibustion to specific areas of the human body based upon Oriental medical diagnosis as a primary mode of therapy, and other means of applying acupuncture under this chapter.

Chapter 2. License and Qualifications

IC 25 − 2.5 − 2 − 1   Requirements for license

Except as provided in section 3 of this chapter, to qualify for a license under this article, an individual must satisfy the following requirements:

(1) Complete an application for licensure in accordance with the rules adopted by the board.

(2) Pay the fees established by the board.

(3) Not have been convicted of a crime that has a direct bearing on the applicant's ability to practice competently as determined by the board.

(4) Not have had disciplinary action taken against the applicant or the applicant's license by the board or by the licensing agency of another state or jurisdiction by reason of the applicant's inability to safely practice acupuncture with the reasons for discipline still being valid as determined by the board or by a national certification agency.

(5) Show to the satisfaction of the board that the applicant has:

(A) current active status as a diplomate in acupuncture of the National Certification Commission for Acupuncture and Oriental Medicine;

(B) successfully completed a three (3) year postsecondary training program or acupuncture college program that:

(i) is accredited by;

(ii) is a candidate for accreditation by; or

(iii) meets the standards of;

the National Accreditation Commission for Schools and Colleges of Acupuncture and Oriental Medicine; and

(C) successfully completed a clean needle technique course approved by the National Certification Commission for Acupuncture and Oriental Medicine.

IC 25 – 2.5 – 2 – 2 Issuance of license

Except as provided in section 4 of this chapter, the board shall issue a license to an individual who:

(1) meets the conditions of section 1 of this chapter; and

(2) is otherwise qualified for licensure under this article.

IC 25 – 2.5 – 2 – 3 Applicants licensed in other state or licensed in related field

(a) An applicant may, upon the payment of a fee established by the board, be granted a license if the applicant:

(1) submits satisfactory evidence to the board that the applicant has been licensed to practice acupuncture in another state or authorized in another country to practice acupuncture;

(2) meets the requirements of section 1 (1) through 1 (4) of this chapter; and

(3) shows to the satisfaction of the board that the applicant has:

(A) successfully completed a clean needle technique course substantially equivalent to a clean needle technique course approved by a national acupuncture association approved by the board;

(B) successfully completed a three (3) year postsecondary training program or acupuncture college program that meets the standards substantially equivalent to the standards for a three (3) year postsecondary training program or acupuncture college program approved by a national acupuncture association approved by the board; and

(C) passed an examination substantially equivalent to the examination required by a national acupuncture association approved by the board.

(b) An applicant may, upon the payment of a fee established by the board, be granted a professional's license to practice acupuncture if the applicant submits satisfactory evidence to the board that the applicant is a:

(1) chiropractor licensed under IC 25 – 10;

(2) dentist licensed under IC 25 – 14; or

(3) podiatrist licensed under IC 25 – 29;

with at least two hundred (200) hours of acupuncture training.

(c) The board shall:

(1) compile, at least once every two (2) years, a list of courses and institutions that provide training approved for the purpose of qualifying an individual for a professional's license under subsection (b); and

(2) adopt rules that set forth procedures for the case by case approval of training under subsection (b).

(d) If an individual's license described in subsection (b) (1), (b) (2), or (b) (3) is subject to any restrictions as the result of disciplinary action taken against the individual by the board that regulates the individual's profession, the same restrictions shall be applied to the individual's professional's license to practice acupuncture.

(e) An individual's professional's license issued under subsection (b) shall be suspended if the individual's license described under subsection (b) (1), (b) (2), or (b) (3) is suspended.

(f) An individual's professional's license issued under subsection (b) shall be revoked if the individual's license described under subsection (b) (1), (b) (2), or (b) (3) is revoked.

(g) The practice of acupuncture by an individual issued a professional's license under subsection (b) is limited to the scope of practice of the individual's license described in subsection (b) (1), (b) (2), or (b) (3).

IC 25 – 2.5 – 2 – 4　Refusal to issue license

The board may refuse to issue a license to an applicant for licensure if:

(1) the board determines during the application process that the applicant committed an act that would have subjected the applicant to disciplinary sanction under section 1 (4) of this chapter if the applicant had been licensed in Indiana when the act occurred; or

(2) the applicant has had a license revoked under IC 25 – 1 – 1.1.

IC 25 – 2.5 – 2 – 5　Expiration and renewal of license; reinstatement of invalid license

Effective: July 1, 2018

(a) Subject to IC 25 − 1 − 2 − 6(e), a license issued by the board expires on the date established by the agency under IC 25 − 1 − 5 − 4 in each even-numbered year.

(b) To renew a license, an acupuncturist must:

(1) pay a renewal fee not later than the expiration date of the license; and

(2) submit proof of a current active certificate in acupuncture by the National Certification Commission for Acupuncture and Oriental Medicine.

(c) If an individual fails to pay a renewal fee on or before the expiration date of a license, the license becomes invalid without further action by the board.

(d) If an individual holds a license that has been invalid for not more than three (3) years, the board shall reinstate the license if the individual meets the requirements of IC 25 − 1 − 8 − 6(c).

(e) If more than three (3) years have elapsed since the date a license expired, the individual who holds the license may seek reinstatement of the license by satisfying the requirements for reinstatement under IC 25 − 1 − 8 − 6(d).

IC 25 − 2.5 − 2 − 6 Denial, suspension, or revocation of license

The board may deny, suspend, or revoke a license, require remedial education, or issue a letter of reprimand, if an applicant or licensed acupuncturist does any of the following:

(1) Engages in false or fraudulent conduct that demonstrates an unfitness to practice acupuncture, including:

(A) making a misrepresentation in connection with an application for a license or an investigation by the board;

(B) attempting to collect fees for services that were not performed;

(C) false advertising, including guaranteeing that a cure will result from an acupuncture treatment; or

(D) dividing, or agreeing to divide, a fee for acupuncture services with another person for referring the patient.

(2) Fails to exercise proper control over the acupuncturist's practice by:

(A) aiding an unlicensed person in practicing acupuncture;

(B) delegating professional responsibilities to a person the acupuncturist knows or should know is not qualified to perform; or

(C) insufficiently supervising unlicensed personnel working with the acupuncturist in the practice.

(3) Fails to maintain records in a proper manner by:

(A) failing to keep written records describing the course of treatment for each patient;

(B) refusing to provide upon request patient records that have been prepared for or paid for by the patient; or

(C) revealing personally identifiable information about a patient, without the patient's consent, unless otherwise allowed by law.

(4) Fails to exercise proper care of a patient, including:

(A) abandoning or neglecting a patient without making reasonable arrangements for the continuation of care; or

(B) exercising or attempting to exercise undue influence within the relationship between the acupuncturist and the patient by making sexual advances or requests for sexual activity or by making submission to sexual conduct a condition of treatment.

(5) Displays substance abuse or mental impairment to the degree that it interferes with the ability to provide safe and effective treatment.

(6) Is convicted, pleads guilty, or pleads no contest to a crime that demonstrates an unfitness to practice acupuncture.

(7) Fails, in a negligent manner, to practice acupuncture with the level of skill recognized within the profession as acceptable under the circumstances.

(8) Violates willfully any provision of this article or rule of the board.

(9) Has had a license denied, suspended, or revoked in another jurisdiction for a reason that would be grounds for denial, suspension, or revocation of a license under this article. IC 25 - 2.5 - 2 - 7 Auricular acupuncture.

(a) This section may not be construed to prohibit licensed acupuncturists from practicing auricular acupuncture.

(b) An individual who is not an acupuncturist licensed under this article may practice auricular acupuncture for the purpose of treating alcoholism, substance abuse, or chemical dependency if the individual:

(1) provides the board with documentation of successful completion of a board approved training program in acupuncture for the treatment of alcoholism, substance abuse, or chemical dependency that meets or exceeds the standards of training set by the National Acupuncture Detoxification Association;

(2) provides the board with documentation of successful completion of a clean needle technique course;

(3) provides auricular acupuncture services within the context of a state, federal, or board approved alcohol, substance abuse, or chemical dependency program under the supervision of a licensed acupuncturist; and

(4) maintains the ethical standards under this article and under rules adopted by the board.

Chapter 3. Unlawful Practice

IC 25 - 2.5 - 3 - 1 Applicability of chapter

This chapter does not apply to the following:

(1) A health care professional acting within the scope of the health care professional's

license, certification, or registration.

(2) A student practicing acupuncture under the direct supervision of a licensed acupuncturist as part of a course of study approved by the board.

IC 25 – 2.5 – 3 – 2 Use of acupuncturist title

An individual may not use the title "licensed acupuncturist" or "acupuncturist" unless the acupuncturist is licensed under this article.

IC 25 – 2.5 – 3 – 3 Unlicensed practice of acupuncture

(a) Subject to section 1 of this chapter, it is unlawful to practice acupuncture without a license issued under this article.

(b) If a licensed acupuncturist practices acupuncture on a patient after having obtained a written letter of referral or written diagnosis of the patient from a physician licensed under IC 25 – 22.5, the physician is immune from civil liability relating to the patient's or acupuncturist's use of that diagnosis or referral except for acts or omissions of the physician that amount to gross negligence or willful or wanton misconduct.

IC 25 – 2.5 – 3 – 4 Violations

A person who knowingly or intentionally violates this article commits a Class B misdemeanor.

Indiana Administrative Code

Rule 1. Definitions

844 IAC 13 – 1 – 1 Applicability

The definitions in this rule apply throughout this article.

844 IAC 13 – 1 – 2 "Acupuncture" defined

(a) "Acupuncture" means the evaluation and treatment of persons affected through a method of stimulation of a certain point or points on or immediately below the surface of the body by the insertion of presterilized, single-use, disposable needles, unless medically contraindicated, with or without the application of heat, electronic stimulation, or manual pressure to prevent or modify the perception of pain to normalize physiological functions, or for the treatment of certain diseases or dysfunctions of the body.

(b) The term does not include:

(1) radiology, electrosurgery, chiropractic technique, physical therapy, use or prescribing of any drugs, medications, serums, or vaccines; or

(2) determination of an allopathic differential diagnosis.

844 IAC 13 – 1 – 3 "Acupuncturist" defined

"Acupuncturist" means an individual to whom a license has been issued to practice acupuncture in Indiana and includes both a licensed acupuncturist and licensed professional acupuncturist.

844 IAC 13 - 1 - 4 "ADS" defined

(a) "ADS" means acupuncture detoxification specialist.

(b) ADS is:

(1) limited to the use of five (5) points in accordance with NADA protocol; and

(2) for the purpose of treating alcoholism, substance abuse, or chemical dependency as defined by IC 25 - 2.5 - 2 - 7.

(c) An ADS is a person who:

(1) has met the minimum requirements as stated in 844 IAC 13 - 3 - 1;

(2) is functioning in a dependent relationship with a physician licensed by the board or an acupuncturist licensed by the board; and

(3) is performing under his or her supervision a task or combination of tasks traditionally performed in a chemical dependency treatment program under the law for the purpose of treating alcoholism, substance abuse, or chemical dependency.

844 IAC 13 - 1 - 5 "Board" defined

"Board" refers to the medical licensing board of Indiana.

844 IAC 13 - 1 - 6 "Licensed professional acupuncturist" defined

(a) "Licensed professional acupuncturist" refers to the holder of a professional's license under IC 25 - 2.5 - 2 - 3 (b).

(b) An licensed professional acupuncturist is a:

(1) chiropractor licensed under IC 25 - 10;

(2) dentist licensed under IC 25 - 14; or

(3) podiatrist licensed under IC 25 - 29;

with at least two hundred (200) hours of acupuncture approved by the board.

844 IAC 13 - 1 - 7 "Licensed acupuncturist" defined

"Licensed acupuncturist" refers to the holder of a license under IC 25 - 2.5 - 2 - 1 or IC 25 - 2.5 - 2 - 3 (a).

844 IAC 13 - 1 - 8 "NADA" defined

"NADA" refers to the National Acupuncture Detoxification Association.

844 IAC 13 - 1 - 9 "Supervising acupuncturist" defined

"Supervising acupuncturist" means a medical doctor, osteopathic physician, licensed professional acupuncturist, or licensed acupuncturist approved by the board to supervise and be responsible for a particular ADS. The supervisor is not to supervise more than a total of twenty (20) ADS at any one (1) time.

844 IAC 13 - 1 - 10 "Under the direction and supervision of the licensed acupuncturist" defined

"Under the direction and supervision of the licensed acupuncturist", as referred to in this rule with reference to ADS, means that the supervising physician or affiliate licensed acupuncturist shall be reasonably available and responsible at all times for the direction and the actions of the practitioner being supervised when services are being performed by the practitioner. The patient's care shall always be the responsibility of the supervising physician or affiliate licensed acupuncturist.

Rule 2. Licensure

844 IAC 13 – 2 – 1　Application

An applicant for acupuncture licensure shall submit the following information:

(1) An application in a form and manner prescribed by the board.

(2) Two (2) recent passport-quality photographs of the applicant, approximately two (2) inches by two (2) inches in size, signed in black ink along the bottom.

(3) The fee specified in section 6 of this rule.

(4) Original or verification of proof of current active status as a diplomate in acupuncture of the National Certification Commission for Acupuncture.

(5) Transcript from the training program or acupuncture college program of completion of three (3) years of postsecondary training program or acupuncture college that is approved by the National Accreditation Commission for Schools and Colleges of Acupuncture and Oriental Medicine.

(6) A notarized copy of proof of completion of a clean needle technique course approved by the National Certification Commission for Acupuncture and Oriental Medicine.

(7) Verification from all states in which the applicant has been or is currently licensed, which statement shall include whether the applicant has ever been disciplined in any manner.

(8) Otherwise meets the requirements of IC 25 – 2.5 – 2 – 1.

844 IAC 13 – 2 – 2　Licensure in another state or authorized in another country

An applicant who is licensed in another state or authorized in another country to practice acupuncture shall submit the following information:

(1) An application in a form and manner prescribed by the board.

(2) Two (2) recent passport-quality photographs of the applicant, approximately two (2) inches by two (2) inches in size, signed in black ink along the bottom.

(3) The fee specified in section 6 of this rule.

(4) Evidence from the state or country that the applicant holds or has held a license or is authorized to practice acupuncture in another country to the board that the qualifications are substantially equivalent as those specified in section 1 of this rule.

(5) A notarized copy or original verification of proof of current active status as a diplomate in acupuncture of the National Certification Commission for Acupuncture.

(6) A transcript in the original language of issuance and a translation from the training program or acupuncture college program of completion of three (3) years of postsecondary training program or acupuncture college that is approved or substantially equivalent to the National

Accreditation Commission for Schools and Colleges of Acupuncture and Oriental Medicine.

(7) A notarized copy of proof of completion of a clean needle technique course approved by the National Certification Commission for Acupuncture and Oriental Medicine.

(8) Verification from all states in which the applicant has been or is currently licensed, which statement shall include whether the applicant has ever been disciplined in any manner.

(9) Otherwise meets the requirements of IC 25 − 2.5 − 2 − 1.

844 IAC 13 − 2 − 3　Licensure by tutorial program (Expired)

844 IAC 13 − 2 − 4　Affiliated professional's license to practice acupuncture

An applicant who is licensed as a chiropractor licensed under IC 25 − 10, a dentist licensed under IC 25 − 14, and a podiatrist licensed under IC 25 − 29 may be granted a professional's license upon submission of the following information:

(1) An application in a form and manner prescribed by the board.

(2) Two (2) recent passport-quality photographs of the applicant, approximately two (2) inches by two (2) inches in size, signed in black ink along the bottom.

(3) The fee specified in section 6 of this rule.

(4) An official certificate from the school or program which is an approved college or university of learning accredited by an accrediting agency that has been approved by the United States Department of Education where the applicant obtained two hundred (200) hours of acupuncture training.

(5) Verification from all states in which the applicant has been or is currently licensed, which statement shall include whether the applicant has ever been disciplined in any manner.

(6) Otherwise submits proof of current licensure in Indiana as a chiropractor, a podiatrist, or a dentist.

844 IAC 13 − 2 − 5　List of courses and institutions that provide training for a professional's license

(a) A list of courses and institutions that provide training approved for the purpose of qualifying an individual for an affiliated professional's license shall be available from the board through the health professions bureau.

(b) If a program or course is not listed, the board shall review each program on a case-by-case basis.

(c) The aforementioned information shall be submitted for the board's review.

844 IAC 13 − 2 − 6　Fees

The board shall charge and collect the following fees:

Application for licensure	$150
Affiliated professional's license	$150

Application for certification as an ADS	$10
Renewal fee for acupuncturist (does not apply for professional's license)	$100 per biennium
Renewal fee for professional's license (as an additional fee to be paid upon renewal of the primary license)	$100
Renewal fee for acupuncture detoxification specialist	$20 per biennium
Penalty fee for failure to renew	$150
Duplicate wall license	$10
Verification for licensure	$10

Rule 3. Supervision

844 IAC 13 - 3 - 1　Acupuncture detoxification specialist; certification

(a) An applicant may practice acupuncture detoxification protocol under the supervising acupuncturist within the context of a state, federal, or board approved alcohol, substance abuse, or chemical dependency program upon approval of the board.

(b) The ADS shall provide the board with the following documentation:

(1) An application in a form and manner prescribed by the board.

(2) Must be eighteen (18) years or older.

(3) Two (2) recent passport-quality photographs of the applicant.

(4) The fee specified in 844 IAC 13 - 2 - 6.

(5) A notarized copy of a high school diploma or general educational development diploma.

(6) A notarized copy of documentation of successful completion of a board approved training program in acupuncture for the treatment of alcoholism, substance abuse, or chemical dependency that meets or exceeds the standards of training by the National Acupuncture Detoxification Association.

(7) A notarized copy of proof of completion of a clean needle technique course approved by the National Certification Commission for Acupuncture and Oriental Medicine or National Acupuncture Detoxification Association.

(8) A list of all supervisors.

(9) Otherwise meets the requirements of IC 25 - 2.5 - 2 - 7.

844 IAC 13 - 3 - 2　Acupuncture detoxification specialist; supervision

(a) The supervising acupuncturist shall be physically present or readily available at all times that treatment is being administered by the ADS.

(b) A licensed acupuncturist who intends to supervise an ADS shall register his or her intent to do so with the board on a form approved by the board prior to commencing supervision of a ADS. The supervising acupuncturist shall include the following information on the form supplied by the board:

(1) The name, business address, and telephone number of the supervising acupuncturist or physician.

(2) The current license number of the acupuncturist or physician.

(3) A description of the setting in which the ADS will practice under the supervising acupuncturist or physician, including the specialty, if any, of the supervising acupuncturist or physician.

(4) A statement that the supervising acupuncturist or physician will do the following:

(A) Exercise continuous supervision over the ADS in accordance with IC 25 − 27.5 − 6 and this article.

(B) Review all functions performed by the ADS one (1) time per month and maintain adequate documentation at all times. The supervisor must sign-off on and date the patient chart.

(C) At all times, retain professional and legal responsibility for the care rendered by the ADS.

(5) Detailed description of the process maintained by the acupuncturist, licensed professional acupuncturist, or physician for evaluation of the ADS's performance.

(c) The supervising acupuncturist, licensed professional acupuncturist, or physician shall, within fifteen (15) days, notify the board when the supervising relationship with the ADS is terminated, and the reason for such termination.

(d) If for any reason an ADS discontinues working at the direction and/or under the supervision of the physician, licensed professional acupuncturist, or licensed acupuncturist under which the ADS was registered, such ADS and physician, licensed professional acupuncturist, or licensed acupuncturist shall inform the board, in writing, within fifteen (15) days of such event and his or her approval shall terminate effective the date of the discontinuation of employment under the supervising physician, licensed professional acupuncturist, or licensed acupuncturist, which termination of approval shall remain in effect until such time as a new application is submitted by the same or another physician, licensed professional acupuncturist, or licensed acupuncturist approved by the board. The physician, licensed professional acupuncturist, or licensed acupuncturist and ADS, in such written report, shall inform the board of the specific reason for the discontinuation of employment of the ADS, and/or of the discontinuation of supervision by the physician or licensed to whom the ADS was registered.

Rule 4. License Renewal

844 IAC 13 − 4 − 1　Licensure renewal

(a) A renewal application shall be submitted to the bureau on or before September 30 of each even-numbered year on a form provided by the bureau.

(b) The application shall be accompanied by the renewal fee required by 844 IAC 13 − 2 − 6.

(c) A licensee must sign the renewal application provided by the bureau that verifies that the applicant holds a current active certification by the National Certification Commission for Acupuncture and Oriental Medicine.

(d) A person who holds a license as an acupuncturist must renew biennially as required by IC 25 − 2.5 − 2 − 5.

(e) A person who fails to renew his or her license within three (3) years after its expiration may not renew it, and it may not be restored, reissued, or reinstated thereafter, but that person may apply for and obtain a new license if he or she meets all of the requirements.

844 IAC 13 − 4 − 2   Licensure renewal for licensed professional acupuncturist

(a) A renewal application for chiropractors, dentists, and podiatrists shall be submitted to the bureau on or before the date of the renewal of the primary license. Therefore the renewal of a:

(1) chiropractor's acupuncture license shall be submitted to the bureau on or before July 1 of each even-numbered year simultaneously with the renewal of the chiropractor license;

(2) dentist's acupuncture license shall be submitted to the bureau on or before March 1 of each even-numbered year simultaneously with the renewal of the dental license; and

(3) podiatrist's acupuncture license shall be submitted to the bureau on or before June 30 of the fourth odd-numbered year simultaneously with the renewal of the podiatrist license.

(b) The renewal fee shall be in addition to the renewal fee of the primary license.

(c) A renewal application must be signed, indicating that the practitioner is currently licensed as a chiropractor, dentist, or podiatrist in Indiana.

844 IAC 13 − 4 − 3   Certification renewal for acupuncture detoxification specialist

(a) A renewal application shall be submitted to the bureau on or before September 30 of each even-numbered year on a form provided by the bureau. The application shall be accompanied by the renewal fee required by 844 IAC 13 − 2 − 6.

(b) A person who holds a certification as an ADS must renew biennially as required by IC 25 − 2.5 − 2 − 5.

844 IAC 13 − 4 − 4   Address; change of name

(a) Each licensed acupuncturist, licensed professional acupuncturist, or certified ADS shall inform the board, in writing, of all changes of address or name within fifteen (15) days of the change.

(b) A licensed acupuncturist, licensed professional acupuncturist, or certified ADS failure to receive notification of renewal due to failure to notify the board of a change of address or name shall not constitute an error on the part of the board or bureau, nor shall it exonerate or otherwise excuse the licensed acupuncturist, licensed professional acupuncturist, or certified

ADS from renewing such license.

Rule 5. Standards of Professional Conduct

844 IAC 13 - 5 - 1   Duties of acupuncturist

(a) An acupuncturist in the conduct of his or her practice of acupuncture shall abide by, and comply with, the standards of professional conduct in this rule.

(b) An acupuncturist shall maintain the confidentiality of all knowledge and information regarding a patient, including, but not limited to, the patient's diagnosis, treatment and prognosis, and all records relating thereto, about which the acupuncturist may learn or otherwise be informed during the course of, or as a result of, the patient-acupuncturist relationship. Information about a patient shall be disclosed by an acupuncturist when required by law or when authorized by the patient or those responsible for the patient's care.

(c) An acupuncturist shall give a truthful, candid, and reasonably complete account of the patient's condition to the patient or to those responsible for the patient's care, except where an acupuncturist reasonably determines that the information is or would be detrimental to the physical or mental health of the patient or, in the case of a minor or incompetent person, except where an acupuncturist reasonably determines that the information would be detrimental to the physical or mental health of those responsible for the patient's care.

(d) The acupuncturist shall give reasonable written notice to an active patient or those responsible for the patient's care when the acupuncturist withdraws from a case so that another acupuncturist may be employed by the patient or by those responsible for the patient's care. An acupuncturist shall not abandon a patient. As used in this section, "active patient" means a person whom the acupuncturist has examined, cared for, or otherwise consulted with, during the two (2) year period prior to retirement, discontinuation of practice of acupuncture, or leaving or moving from the community.

(e) An acupuncturist who withdraws from a case, except in emergency circumstances, shall, upon written request, make available to his or her patient all records, test results, histories, diagnoses, files, and information relating to the patient that are in the acupuncturist's custody, possession, or control, or copies of such documents herein before described.

(f) An acupuncturist shall exercise reasonable care and diligence in the diagnosis and treatment of patients based upon approved scientific principles, methods, treatments, professional theory, and practice.

(g) An acupuncturist shall not represent, advertise, state, or indicate the possession of any degree recognized as the basis for licensure to practice acupuncture unless the acupuncturist is actually licensed on the basis of such degree in the state or states in which he or she practices.

(h) An acupuncturist shall obtain consultation whenever requested to do so by a patient or by those responsible for a patient's care.

(i) An acupuncturist who has personal knowledge based upon a reasonable belief that another acupuncturist has engaged in illegal, unlawful, incompetent, or fraudulent conduct in the practice of acupuncture shall promptly report such conduct to the board. Further, an acupuncturist who has personal knowledge of any person engaged in, or attempting to engage in, the unauthorized practice of acupuncture shall promptly report such conduct to the board.

844 IAC 13 − 5 − 2   Fees for services

(a) Fees charged by an acupuncturist for his or her professional services shall compensate the acupuncturist only for the services actually rendered.

(b) An acupuncturist shall not divide a fee for professional services with another practitioner who is not a partner, employee, or shareholder in a professional corporation unless the:

(1) patient consents to the employment of the other practitioner after a full disclosure that a division of fees will be made; and

(2) division of fees is made in proportion to actual services performed and responsibility assumed by each practitioner.

(c) An acupuncturist shall not pay or accept compensation from a practitioner for referral of a patient.

844 IAC 13 − 5 − 3   Responsibility for employees

An acupuncturist shall be responsible for the conduct of each and every person employed by the acupuncturist for every action or failure to act by the employee or employees in the course of the employee's relationship with the acupuncturist, provided, however, that an acupuncturist shall not be responsible for the action of persons he or she may employ whose employment by the acupuncturist does not relate directly to the acupuncturist's practice of acupuncture.

844 IAC 13 − 5 − 4   Referral

(a) A licensed acupuncturist may only provide services upon the referral of a licensed medical doctor or doctor of osteopathic medicine. This subsection does not apply to licensed professional acupuncturist.

(b) An acupuncturist may, whenever the acupuncturist believes it to be beneficial to the patient, send or refer a patient to a qualified specific health care provider. Prior to any such referral, however, the acupuncturist shall examine and/or consult with the patient to reasonably determine that a condition exists in the patient that would be within the scope of practice of the specific health care provider to whom the patient is referred.

844 IAC 13 − 5 − 5   Discontinuation of practice

(a) An acupuncturist, upon his or her retirement, upon discontinuation of the practice of acupuncture, or upon leaving or moving from a community shall notify all of his or her active patients, in writing, or by publication once a week for three (3) consecutive weeks in a newspaper of general circulation in the community, that he or she intends to discontinue his or her practice of acupuncture in the community and shall encourage his or her patients to seek the services of another licensed practitioner. The acupuncturist discontinuing his or her practice shall make reasonable arrangements with his or her active patients for the transfer of his or her records, or copies thereof, to the succeeding practitioner or an acupuncture association approved by the board.

(b) Nothing provided in this section shall preclude, prohibit, or prevent an acupuncturist from selling, conveying, or transferring for valuable consideration, the acupuncturist's patient records to another licensed practitioner who is assuming his practice, provided that written notice is given to patients as provided in this section.

844 IAC 13 - 5 - 6 Advertising

(a) An acupuncturist shall not, on behalf of himself or herself, a partner, an associate, or any other practitioner or specific health care provider affiliated with the acupuncturist, use, or participate in the use of, any form of public communication containing a false, fraudulent, materially misleading, or deceptive statement or claim.

(b) In order to facilitate the process of informed selection of an acupuncturist by the public, an acupuncturist may advertise services through the public media, including, but not limited to, a telephone directory, acupuncturists' directory, newspaper or other periodical, radio or television, or through a written communication not involving personal contact.

(c) If the advertisement is communicated to the public by radio, cable, or television, it shall be prerecorded, approved for broadcast by the acupuncturist, and a recording and transcript of the actual transmission shall be retained by the acupuncturist for a period of three (3) years from the last date of broadcast.

(d) If the acupuncturist advertises a fee for acupuncture material, service, treatment, consultation, examination, or other procedure, the acupuncturist must provide that material, service, or procedure for no more than the fee advertised.

(e) Unless otherwise conspicuously specified in the advertisement, an acupuncturist who publishes or communicates fee information in a publication that is published more than one (1) time per month shall be bound by any representation made therein for a period of thirty (30) days after the publication date. An acupuncturist who publishes or communicates fee information in a publication that is published once a month or less frequently shall be bound by any representation made therein until the publication of the succeeding issue unless a shorter time is conspicuously specified in the advertisement. An acupuncturist who publishes or communicates fee information in a publication that has no fixed date for publication for a succeeding issue shall be bound by any representation made therein for one (1) year, unless a shorter period of time is conspicuously specified in the advertisement.

(f) Unless otherwise specified in the advertisement, an acupuncturist who broadcasts fee information by radio, cable, or television shall be bound by any representation made therein for a period of ninety (90) days after such broadcast.

(g) An acupuncturist who places an advertisement using a corporation name or trade name is required to identify the location or locations at which the acupuncture service will be provided. The name of the acupuncturist who will provide the acupuncture services must be identified at that location.

844 IAC 13 – 5 – 7   Failure to comply

Failure to comply with the standards of professional conduct and competent practice of acupuncture may result in disciplinary proceedings against the offending acupuncturist. All acupuncturists licensed in Indiana shall be responsible for having knowledge of the standards of conduct and competent practice established by IC 25 – 2.5.

Rule 6. Revocation or Suspension of License

844 IAC 13 – 6 – 1   License revocation; duties of licensees

In any case where a practitioner's license has been revoked, the person shall do the following:

(1) Promptly notify, or cause to be notified, in the manner and method specified by the board, all patients then in the care of the practitioner, or those persons responsible for the patient's care, of the revocation and of the practitioner's consequent inability to act for or on their behalf in the practitioner's professional capacity. Such notice shall advise all patients to seek the services of another practitioner in good standing of their own choice.

(2) Promptly notify, or cause to be notified, all health care facilities where such practitioner has privileges of the revocation accompanied by a list of all patients then in the care of such practitioner.

(3) Notify, in writing, by first class mail, the following organizations and governmental agencies of the revocation of licensure:

(A) The Indiana department of public welfare.

(B) Social Security Administration.

(C) The board or equivalent agency of each state in which the person is licensed to practice acupuncture.

(D) The National Certification Commission for Acupuncture and Oriental Medicine.

(4) Make reasonable arrangements with the licensee's active patients for the transfer of all patient records, studies, and test results, or copies thereof, to a succeeding practitioner employed by the patient or by those responsible for the patient's care.

(5) Within thirty (30) days after the date of license revocation, the practitioner shall file an affidavit with the board showing compliance with the provisions of the revocation order and with 844 IAC 7, which time may be extended by the board. Such affidavit shall also state all other jurisdictions in which the practitioner is still licensed.

(6) Proof of compliance with this section shall be a condition precedent to any petition for reinstatement.

844 IAC 13 - 6 - 2　License suspension; duties of licensees

(a) In any case where a person's license has been suspended, the person shall, within thirty (30) days from the date of the order of suspension, file with the board an affidavit that states the following:

(1) All active patients then under the practitioner's care have been notified in the manner and method specified by the board of the practitioner's suspension and consequent inability to act for or on their behalf in a professional capacity. Such notice shall advise all such patients to seek the services of another practitioner of good standing of their own choice.

(2) All health care facilities where such practitioner has privileges have been informed of the suspension order.

(3) Reasonable arrangements were made for the transfer of patient records, studies, and test results, or copies thereof, to a succeeding practitioner employed by the patient or those responsible for the patient's care.

(b) Proof of compliance with this section shall be a condition precedent to reinstatement.

844 IAC 13 - 6 - 3　Reinstatement (Expired)

844 IAC 13 - 6 - 4　Petitions for reinstatement; filing fee (Expired)

Rule 7. Notification of Practice Location

844 IAC 13 - 7 - 1　Professional sign; notification of public; facility requirements

(a) A practitioner has a duty and responsibility in the establishment of an office for the practice of acupuncture to maintain a sign clearly visible to the public indicating the name or names of all practitioners practicing at that location. The minimum requirements on the sign are the practitioner's name and title.

(b) The practitioner's title may be written as follows:

(1) If a practitioner is licensed under this article, the practitioner may refer to themselves as either an acupuncturist or a licensed acupuncturist.

(2) If the practitioner is a professional, the practitioner may use:

(A) the doctorate initials, such as D.C., D.D.S., or D.P.M.; or

(B) acupuncturist.

(c) A sign may not be misleading to the public.

(d) A practitioner has a duty and responsibility in the establishment of an office for the practice of acupuncture to maintain a safe and hygienic facility adequately equipped to provide acupuncture services.